By the Editors of Consumer Guide®

with the

PPAG

Pediatric Pharmacy Advocacy Group, Inc.

Children's Prescription Drugs

A Parent's Guide to the Most

Commonly Recommended

Drugs for Children

Publications International, Ltd.

This publication was written and reviewed by the **Pediatric Pharmacy Advocacy Group, Inc. (PPAG)**. The PPAG is a non-profit voluntary organization of pharmacists and health care providers who strive to improve the lives of children. The sole purpose of the organization is to promote safe and effective medication use in children through communication, education, patient care, and research.

Principal reviewer: **Kellie McQueen, Pharm.D.,** Executive Director, PPAG

Contributing writers (drug profiles) from the Pediatric Pharmacy Advocacy Group, Inc.:

Varsha Bhatt-Mehta, Pharm.D., Clinical Assistant Professor of Pharmacy, College of Pharmacy, University of Michigan and Clinical Pharmacist, C.S. Mott Children's Hospital, Ann Arbor, MI

Helen Beckman Fiechtner, Pharm.D., Associate Professor, College of Pharmacy, South Dakota State University and Clinical Pharmacist, South Dakota Children's Hospital, Sioux Falls, SD

James H. Krull, Pharm.D., Clinical Pharmacist, Pediatric Intensive Care Center, Riley Hospital for Children, Indianapolis, IN

Anne Lesko, Pharm.D., Clinical Coordinator, Bone Marrow Transplant, Hematology/Oncology Clinical Specialist, Children's Hospital Medical Center, Cincinnati, OH

Christopher Lomax, Pharm.D., Director, Pharmacy Services, Children's Hospital of Los Angeles, CA

Merrell Magelli, Pharm.D., BCPP, Clinical Coordinator, Children's Hospital, Omaha, NE

Editorial assistance: **Emily Engelbrecht, Pharm.D.; Maryann Travaglini, Pharm.D.**

Contributing writer (chapter text): **Rebecca Dougherty Williams** is a freelance writer specializing in health and medical topics. She holds a master's degree in journalism from the University of Maryland, College Park, and writes regularly for *FDA Consumer,* the magazine of the U.S. Food & Drug Administration.

Illustrations: **Yoshi Miyake**

Cover photo: **Rob Goldman/FPG International**

CONTENTS

Introduction

Childhood is healthier today than ever before, thanks in part to modern prescription medicines. A century ago there were no antibiotics to fight infections, no bronchodilators to manage asthma, and no vaccines to prevent diseases such as smallpox or polio. Many children died from these diseases; those who survived often did so with lifelong disabilities.

Prescription drugs have eliminated much of the fear parents had of childhood illnesses. Parents no longer watch helplessly as their children suffer; instead they rely on medications to ease their children's pain and symptoms, minimize or cure the illness, and prevent the damage untreated illnesses can cause. Medications are so much a part of contemporary life that children receive an average of eight to nine prescription drugs by their fifth birthdays. That number certainly increases if nonprescription medications are also included.

Even though drugs are used frequently, they involve some degree of risk. Parents must be cautious and knowledgeable about giving any medication. A drug is only safe and effective when used correctly. Given incorrectly it can be ineffective and even dangerous.

To give medication appropriately, parents need to understand that children are not simply small adults. They often have different symptoms of a disease and their bodies do not absorb and distribute medicine the same way adult bodies do. Also, medications may not cause the same side effects in children. While barbiturates make adults feel sluggish, for example, they make children hyperactive. Amphetamines, which stimulate adults, can calm children.

Parents of young children need to be particularly careful. Specific information on dosage and side effects in children is minimal or lacking for many medications. This is because only 25 to 35 percent of all drugs on the market are approved by the Food and Drug Administration (FDA) for use in children. As a consequence, child dosage forms often are not available. Pharmacists must compound suspensions or liquids to achieve the desired concentration or dosage form of the product, thus increasing the risk of errors. Parents need to be well informed about the indication, dose, concentration, and potential side effects of any medication prescribed for their child.

Children's Prescription Drugs provides the information parents need to administer medications safely to their children up to 18 years of age. (Information for adult usage is not necessarily included. Refer to adult references.) You'll find detailed information, compiled by pediatric pharmacists, about hundreds of drugs in a concise, easy-to-read format. The drug profiles include information about administration, storage, dosage form and strength, how long it takes for the drug to be effective, side effects, possible drug interactions, symptoms of overdose, how the drug works, and much more. The preceding chapters provide essential information about storing and administering medications, coping with side effects, and immunizations.

Although we've tried to anticipate all the questions you might have and the information you will need about your children's medications, this book is not a substitute for your child's doctor and pharmacist. They should be your first source for information about giving a drug to your child. This book was designed to help you ask educated questions and make informed decisions about your child's medications. It is an accurate and quick reference guide for your home that will allow you to give medication to your child safely and effectively.

Chapter 1

What to Keep in Your Medicine Cabinet

When you become a parent, it's time to dust off that old scouting motto "be prepared." For as surely as the sun rises every morning, you will be called upon to minister to a wide array of injuries, bites, sniffles, rashes, splinters, and illnesses. Laying in supplies will help you deal confidently and efficiently with the inevitable minor emergencies. Make sure your medicine cabinet includes the following:

Adhesive bandages. Keep a good supply of these at home and in the car. Also stock sterile bandages, gauze pads, and elastic bandages to cover larger cuts and scrapes.

Antibacterial cream. For more serious cuts or scrapes when soap and water is not available.

Antihistamine. To relieve allergic reactions from pollens and insect bites. Available in tablet, capsule, and liquid forms.

Bulb syringe. These are usually sent home with newborns and are very useful for aspirating a baby's nose. Children older than two or three years of age can blow their own noses.

Calamine lotion or hydrocortisone cream (½ percent). To relieve itching from rashes and insect bites.

Cotton swabs and balls. For applying lotions and cleaning wounds and eyes.

Decongestant. Helpful for older children with hives, hay fever, or allergies. However, check with your child's doctor before giving a decongestant to any child younger than two years of age.

Diaper rash ointment. Rashes develop from exposure to the diaper and to wetness, bacteria from bowel or urine, or harsh cleansing agents. Light and air will kill those germs and clear up most rashes. Ointments are helpful for dry or cracked skin. If you suspect a yeast infection, or if the rash is persistent or consists of large blisters or open sores, call your child's doctor.

Heating pad or hot water bottle. Useful for easing the pain of ear infections or muscle injuries in adolescents. Be careful to avoid burns, and never let a child sleep with a heating pad.

Hydrogen peroxide or soap. Useful for cleaning small cuts.

Ice packs. For reducing swelling after an injury. Not all ice packs need to be stored in the freezer. For convenience at home or while traveling you can purchase a pack that is stored at room temperature and turns cold when squeezed forcefully.

Measuring devices for medicine. Never use a regular tableware teaspoon to measure liquid medicine. A one-teaspoon dose of medicine should measure five milliliters. However, a tableware teaspoon can vary from two to seven milliliters, making it impossible to measure an accurate dose of medicine. If the teaspoon is too small, your child won't get a sufficient dose; if it's too large, your child will get too much. If the medicine you are using came with a measuring device, always use that device to measure that medication. Otherwise, use one of the following:

Syringe. These are convenient for giving medication to infants who can't drink from a cup. You can squirt the medicine toward the back of the child's mouth where it's less likely to spill out. Syringes are also convenient for storing a dose. Many come with a plastic cylinder sheath for travel.

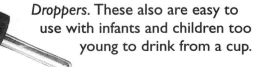

Droppers. These also are easy to use with infants and children too young to drink from a cup.

Be sure to hold the dropper at eye level when measuring and give the dose quickly because droppers drip.

Cylindrical dosing spoons. These are especially convenient to use with children who can drink from a cup but are likely to spill. The spoon looks like a test tube with a spoon formed at the top end. Small children can hold the long tube easily and the small spoon fits well in their mouths. You can also use these devices to direct medicine into a baby's mouth.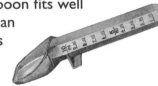

 Dosage cups. Use these for children who can drink from a cup. Be sure to check the numbers carefully on the side, and hold the cup straight at eye level when measuring.

Oral rehydration therapy. Prevents dehydration from diarrhea and vomiting. These therapies, such as Pedialyte, are fluids made of salts, sugars, and water. They are available over the counter and often can be found near the infant formula.

Pain and fever relievers. Choose acetaminophen or ibuprofen products in tablet, liquid, or suppository forms such as Children's Tylenol, Tempra, Liquiprin, Children's Panadol, Pediaprofen, and Children's Motrin or their store-brand equivalents. Aspirin is no longer routinely given to children or teenagers to reduce fever or pain because it increases the risk of Reye syndrome, a rare but potentially fatal condition, if given following viral illnesses such as the flu or chicken pox.

Petroleum jelly. Useful for lubricating rectal thermometers.

Rubbing alcohol (70 percent isopropyl alcohol). Useful for cleaning thermometers, tweezers, and the skin. Do not use alcohol for rubdowns to reduce fever as it can be harmful if inhaled.

Saline nose drops. Check first with your pediatrician, but many will recommend saline nose drops to help loosen nasal mucus when your baby has a cold.

Scissors. For cutting gauze pads, sterile bandages, and adhesive tape.

Sunscreen. Choose a sunscreen with an SPF (sun protection factor) of at least 15. Protecting your child's skin during outside play is essential as most skin cancers begin in childhood. That's because an estimated 50 to 80 percent of one's lifetime sun exposure occurs before 18 years of age. Repeated painful or blistering sunburns during childhood can double the chances of developing skin cancer in adulthood. Babies younger than six months should be totally protected from sun exposure. All sunscreen brands, including generics, are effective and safe. Oil-free sunscreens marked "non-comedogenic" or "won't clog pores" are good for acne-prone teens. Some children may be allergic to certain sunscreen ingredients, such as oxybenzone, so test the product on a small patch of skin before using it on larger areas.

Syrup of ipecac. Treats some accidental poisoning by inducing vomiting. Use it carefully *only* after receiving instructions from a poison control center or your child's doctor. Some types of poisonings should *not* be treated by inducing vomiting. Syrup of ipecac is available over the counter.

Thermometer. For determining a child's temperature. There are several varieties to choose from:

Glass thermometer. These come in both rectal and oral forms. The rectal thermometer has a stubbier tip and is used primarily with infants and small children who are not able to hold the oral thermometer under their tongue for three minutes. (Don't worry if the thermometer breaks and your child accidentally swallows the mercury. Thermometers contain elemental mercury, which is a nonpoisonous and harmless form of the metal.) Glass thermometers can also be used in your child's armpit (called an axillary reading). When speaking to the doctor, be sure to mention which method you have used to take your child's temperature. Remember that axillary readings are one degree lower than oral readings, which are one degree lower than rectal readings. A reading of 97.6°F is a normal axillary reading, while 98.6°F is normal for an oral reading, and 99.6°F is normal for a rectal reading.

Digital. For oral, rectal, or axillary use, this type of thermometer takes a much faster reading and displays the temperature on a small screen. These are more expensive than standard glass thermometers, but the speed is often worth the price.

Tympanic membrane thermometer. Formerly available only in hospitals and doctors' offices, these devices are now for sale to the public. They are fast (readings take only one or two seconds), easy to use (just insert the tip in your child's ear), and painless, but they are also the most expensive.

Forehead strip. These are not very accurate.

Tweezers, small nail clippers. For removing splinters and clipping hangnails.

Chapter 2

Answers to Questions Parents Frequently Ask

Parents usually have many questions about their children's medications and illnesses, questions that often go unasked during a quick sick visit or a hurried phone call to the pediatrician. The following are answers to questions parents frequently ask—or wish they had asked.

1. What's the difference between nonprescription and prescription drugs?

Drugs that are habit-forming or unsafe to use without the supervision of a licensed medical practitioner are required to be made available only by prescription. Of course, nonprescription medications still may be harmful and should be given appropriately and only when necessary. Talk to the doctor about what to do if your child gets sick. Some illnesses can be treated at home, some require a call to the pediatrician's office, and some will necessitate an office visit. Ask the doctor what situations constitute an emergency. If you're unsure if it's safe or appropriate to use a particular nonprescription medication, be sure to talk to the doctor first.

2. What's the difference between generic and brand-name drugs? How do I choose?

When drugs are made by pharmaceutical companies to be sold, the drug has a generic name and a brand name. Generic and brand-name products will include the same active drug but may include different types or amounts of inactive ingredients. These differences may change the way the drug is handled by the body or alter the taste or odor of the medication. Generic and brand-name drugs are interchangeable when the safety and therapeutic outcomes are identical. Ask your child's doctor or the pharmacist if you have any questions about the efficacy of one over the other. In general, generic drugs cost less than brand-name drugs. Prescription and non-prescription products may be marketed in generic or brand-name form.

3. How high should my child's temperature be before I treat it? And which medication should I choose?

Although parents tend to be concerned about fever, it is not usually dangerous. Research suggests that only fevers of 107 or 108 degrees Fahrenheit do permanent damage. The extra heat from mild fevers may, in fact, protect your child's body against viruses, bacteria, and fungi causing illness. The immune system appears to be boosted by a higher body temperature, and some microorganisms are unable to survive during fever.

Low-grade fevers don't need to be treated unless your child cannot eat or sleep well. If the fever rises above 101 or 102 degrees Fahrenheit (38.3 degrees Celsius) and is preventing your child from eating or sleeping well, you can treat it with products such as acetaminophen or ibuprofen to bring it down. Never give aspirin to treat fever in a child. Do not give any nonprescription medication to a baby younger than three months of age without first speaking with the doctor.

These are standard definitions for fever:

Rectal:	over 100.4°F
Oral:	over 99.5°F
Axillary:	over 98.6°F

4. If one of my children is taking an antibiotic and the other one gets sick, can I give some of the same medication to another child?

No! Sharing prescription medications simply is not safe for several reasons. The medication may not be the right one for another child; treating an infection with the wrong drug may make it worse instead of better. In addition, children respond to the same drug differently and may require different dosages. The child who became ill first needs the drug in the amount and for the time prescribed or it may not be effective. If another child needs medication, consult the doctor.

5. Can I keep leftover medication in case my child gets sick again?

No, unless your child has a long-term medical problem and you've been instructed by the doctor to do so. Otherwise, use prescription medications only for the length of time printed on the label, and destroy any remaining medication. Do not use a drug after the expiration date printed on the container. Cough syrups, suppositories, and liquid antibiotics have shorter shelf lives than other products.

6. What does it mean when the prescription says to give the medication "3 times a day" or "4 times a day"? Do I need to wake my child up during the night?

It depends on the medication. It can be confusing, but "four times a day" and "every six hours" do not necessarily mean the same thing. If the label on the medication tells you to give the medicine four times a day, it means the child should have four doses within the waking hours at equally spaced intervals. On the other hand, "every six hours" means each dose must be given six hours after the last one, and the child must be awakened at the appropriate time if necessary. This instruction may also appear on the prescription as "every six hours around the clock."

Check with your child's doctor or the pharmacist to make sure you understand the dosing intervals and amounts. If you don't, your child may not get the full benefit of the drug or the side effects may be worse. Some antibiotics, for example, can cause an upset stomach if the

doses are taken too close together. To avoid middle-of-the-night doses, ask the doctor if the drug can be spread out during the day, or whether there's an alternative drug that can be taken.

7. Can I cut an adult tablet, capsule, or suppository and give part of it to my child?

This is not advisable. It is impossible to get a precise dose for a child from an adult dosage form. Cutting tablets, suppositories, or capsules made for adults should be done by a pharmacist with experience in compounding children's dosages. Anyone younger than 12 years of age should only take medications labeled for children unless otherwise instructed by the doctor. Some adult medications are dangerous for children and some contain aspirin, which should not be given to a child.

8. Are there ever times when I shouldn't be giving my child medication prescribed or recommended by the doctor?

Americans love to medicate—some would say too much. And two of the favorites, cold medications and antibiotics, are often overused. Cold medicines such as decongestants and antihistamines will not make a cold go away faster, although they may make a child more comfortable. Antibiotics will not kill cold-causing viruses either. Overuse of antibiotics encourages resistance from the infecting organism and may increase the development of allergies to the drug.

Watch your child for any unexpected or undesired reaction to medication. If your child seems worse after taking a medication, develops a rash, or has trouble breathing, discontinue the medication and call the doctor immediately.

You should also call the doctor immediately if you suspect there's been a mistake concerning the prescription. Check the prescription when you pick it up. Does the label give the correct dose and frequency? Don't hesitate to ask the pharmacist or your child's doctor about what the drug should look like and how much of it you should have.

9. How do I know if my child is having an adverse reaction to the medication?

Most reactions to medications are mild and can be treated at home after consulting the pharmacist or your child's doctor. If your child experiences wheezing; swelling of the face, lips or throat; vomiting; diarrhea; dizziness; or fainting, contact the doctor immediately and seek care as necessary. Take along the medicine in its original container if you go to the emergency room.

10. What do I do if my child vomits after a dose of medicine?

It depends on whether the medication has been in the stomach long enough to be absorbed into the body. Most medication is out of the stomach and on its way through the bloodstream within 30 minutes after taking it. So if your child vomits long after taking a dose of medicine, it's probably not a problem. However, if your child vomits immediately after taking the medication, give another dose. If you are unsure of the amount vomited, or if your child is vomiting repeatedly, call the doctor or pharmacist for advice.

11. How can I tell if my baby is doing better since he isn't talking yet?

Babies are effective communicators—they just don't use words yet. Instead, they use body language. You can tell a lot about how a baby is feeling by watching his or her behavior. Is your baby eating well? Alert after a sound night's sleep? Having normal bowel movements? Registering a normal temperature? Smiling and cooing? Then the baby is probably on the road to recovery. If your baby is fussy, feverish, won't eat well, has diarrhea or is vomiting, is listless, or just doesn't seem "right," call the doctor. It takes time for any recovery. But for mild illnesses such as ear infections, a baby should be feeling better within 48 hours after taking antibiotics.

12. If my child's infection is improving, can I stop giving the antibiotic before the prescription indicates?

No. Always give the medication according to the doctor's prescription instructions. Stopping a child's medication too soon can cause a relapse or other complications. Some infections require long periods of therapy even though the symptoms may disappear in a day or two. A full course of therapy is necessary to ensure complete recovery.

13. How do I know if a product contains aspirin?

Check the list of active ingredients on the label. If it says aspirin, salicylate, subsalicylate, or salicylamide, don't use it for children younger than 16 years of age. Aspirin is hidden in many nonprescription medications, such as Pepto-Bismol, so read the label carefully. Doctors rarely recommend aspirin for children as it can increase the risk of Reye syndrome, a serious and sometimes fatal condition.

Chapter 3

What You Should Know About Your Child's Medication

The label can't tell you everything you need to know about your child's medication. Pharmacies sometimes provide written information sheets with prescription medications, but you can't rely solely on them. Although it takes some extra time, be sure you know the answers to the following questions about any prescription or nonprescription medication you are giving to your child. The answers will ensure that your child receives the medication's full benefit.

1. Why is this drug being prescribed? What is it designed to do?

2. Should this medication be given on an empty stomach or after eating? Would any particular food (such as milk) interfere with this drug?

3. Can this medication be mixed with food? (Mixing can help disguise the taste of medicine.)

4. What side effects might I expect? Is there anything I can do to lessen them?

5. Is this drug likely to cause an allergic reaction? What would those symptoms be?

6. How will this medication react with other drugs my child may take (including nonprescription medicines)?

7. How should this medication be stored?

8. Does this medication come in another form? (Chewable tablets, for instance, are more easily transported than liquids and are preferable when your child can't swallow pills whole.)

9. Is there a less expensive, equally safe and effective generic or nonprescription equivalent?

10. When should we begin to see improvement? How will we know the medication is working?

11. What should I do if I forget to give my child a dose?

12. What if my child spits up the dose I just gave?

13. If there is any medication left, should I keep it in case my child has the same illness again?

Chapter 4

How to Store Medications

Prescription and nonprescription medications need to be stored safely. That means keeping them out of the hands of children and in the proper environment. The first requires a sturdy lock and vigilance; the second requires attention to the particular requirements of each drug.

Safety first. All medications, whether prescription or nonprescription, should be stored in a locked cabinet well out of your child's reach. Even nonprescription medications, which people generally consider very safe, can be toxic and dangerous if misused. Plastic child safety locks or latches will usually suffice, but if your child is adept at opening them, use a combination or key lock. Never leave medications unattended in the presence of a child, even for a few seconds.

Location, location, location. Keeping medications in the right location and at the right temperature will ensure they remain potent. The best location for most medications is in a locked medicine cabinet on a high shelf in a hall closet with a door that locks. Your child won't be able to get to the medications, and they will be kept properly at room temperature, away from direct sunlight. Don't keep medicines in the bathroom, where heat and humidity can affect their stability. Temperature fluctuations in the kitchen (especially in cabinets near the stove) also make it a poor location for storing medications.

Medications that must be refrigerated should be kept on the refrigerator's top shelf. Instruct your child that the refrigerator is off limits. Use a refrigerator lock if necessary to keep your child from opening the door.

Always be sure you know at what temperature your medications should be kept. Ask the pharmacist and check the label for specific directions. The following are common temperature instructions and what they mean:

Keep away from excessive cold: Don't expose to temperatures lower than 36°F (2°C)

Refrigerate: Keep between 36° and 46°F (2° to 8°C)

Keep cool: Keep between 46° and 59°F (8° to 15°C)

Store at room temperature: Keep between 59° and 86°F (15° to 30°C)

Do not expose to excessive heat: Keep away from temperatures higher than 104°F (40°C)

Containers for medication. Keep all medications in their original containers, which are designed to protect them from moisture and light. If removed, the drug may lose strength and effectiveness. And don't combine medications; this can lead to confusion, errors, and even chemical interactions.

Pharmacists are required to put drugs in bottles with child-resistant caps. Don't switch to a bottle that's easier for you to open—children also may find it easier to open. Remember that child-resistant doesn't mean childproof. Children older than five years of age may be able to open most medicine bottles, so teach them that drugs can be harmful if not taken correctly and that they need supervision before taking anything.

Medication disposal. Do not keep medication past the expiration date, even if it appears normal. Expired medication may be ineffective and even can be dangerous. If your medication does not display an expiration date, throw it out after one year.

On the road. For travel, keep medications with first-aid equipment in a locked box. Make sure you keep the medication at the recommended temperature and avoid extreme heat or cold. Remember, a car can become very hot or cold. If necessary, take the storage box with you to the motel room or into the restaurant when you stop to eat.

Chapter 5

Giving Medications

Even if you were an eight-armed octopus, you might still wish you had an extra set of arms when giving medication to your baby or child. Whether children squirm and flail or simply clamp their mouths shut, they can be decidedly uncooperative when it comes to taking medicine. You'll need good technique, sophisticated strategy, tact, humor, flexibility, and negotiating skill to conquer your child's fears and resistance to taking medication.

TECHNIQUE

If you don't give the medication correctly, it may be ineffective or cause side effects. An estimated 10 to 30 percent of medications aren't effective because they have been given incorrectly. To do it right, you have to give the exact amount of medicine prescribed at the scheduled time, for the specified duration, and in the appropriate manner. Always read the label, follow the directions carefully, and use the right equipment for measuring and administering the medication. Remember to wash your hands first.

Liquids. Many pediatric drugs come in liquid form because that's what children swallow most easily. Liquid medications are often suspensions, a mixture of the powdered drug dissolved in a liquid. These drugs must be shaken before each use because the drug settles to the bottom of the bottle. If you don't shake it well, your child could get a dose that's too weak or too strong. Liquid medicines should be measured with one of the standard dosing instruments, such as plastic dosing cups, oral syringes, droppers, and cylindrical dosing spoons. (See Chapter 1, pages 5–6, for more information about measuring devices.) Never use a common teaspoon from your tableware since it does not provide an exact dose. A teaspoon of medication is always 5 milliliters; a tablespoon of medication is 15 milliliters.

Giving liquids to a baby can seem challenging and intimidating. If the medicine can be taken on an empty stomach, give it before a feeding when the baby is hungriest and most eager to accept something new in the mouth. To prevent choking, prop the baby in a stable infant seat (angled if he can't yet sit up) or hold the baby in the normal feeding position, wedging one of the arms against your body and leaving both of your hands free for control. If another adult is available, one of you can hold the baby while the other gives the medication. Gently squeeze the baby's cheeks on either side with your thumb and index finger to open the mouth. You can also try making a "cheek pocket" by using your finger to pull out a corner of the baby's mouth. Then, using a dropper, syringe, or cylindrical dosing spoon, release the liquid medicine against the side of the mouth, or into the "cheek pocket," toward the back of the tongue. For large doses, release a little at a time so the baby won't gag. Stroke the baby under the chin to encourage swallowing while still holding the cheeks together so the medicine won't spill out. Don't squirt the medicine directly down the throat or the baby may choke or gag and spit it out.

If you're not successful using these methods, pour the medication into a small cup and dip your little finger into it. Then let your baby suck it off your finger. Older babies and toddlers may cooperate better if you let them guide the dropper or cylindrical spoon into their mouths.

Since the medication may taste bad, let your child suck on a popsicle first to partially numb the mouth. Follow up with more popsicle after the dose is taken. Refrigerating the liquid can also improve its taste, but check first with the pharmacist or your child's doctor to be sure the medication can be refrigerated. You can also try diluting the medication with another liquid such as apple juice to help disguise the taste. Again, check first with the pharmacist or doctor.

Eyedrops and Eye Ointments. Wash your hands. Tilt your child's head back and slightly to one side so the affected eye is lowest; that way any excess will run off toward your child's ear, not toward the other eye. Do not touch the applicator to the affected eye area. Contaminating the applicator can cause reinfection or spread the infection to other areas of the body. With one hand, gently pull down the lower lid to form a pouch below the eye. If you're using drops, drop the prescribed amount of medication into the pouch. Wait about one minute between drops if more than one drop is prescribed. The eye only can absorb one drop at a time; any excess will drip out. If you're using an ointment, squeeze a small amount (approximately 1/8 to 1/4 inch) in a line along the pouch. After giving the drops or ointment, have your child close the eyes. Apply slight pressure with your finger at the corner of the eye next to the nose for a minute or two. This will prevent loss of medication through the duct that drains fluid from the surface of the eye into the nose and throat. Do not let your child rub the eyes. Wipe off excess medication with a clean tissue.

Eardrops. Warm eardrops by rolling the bottle between your hands for several minutes. Tilt your child's head to one side, with the affected ear pointing up toward the ceiling. For children younger than three years of age, use one hand to pull the side of the outer ear outward and downward. For children older than three years of age, pull the outer ear outward and upward. The angle of the ear canal changes as your child grows, necessitating the position change. When instilling the drops, avoid touching the sides or edge of the ear with the dropper to prevent contamination from the ear canal. Direct the drops against the wall of the ear canal, not directly into the ear. Your child should lie still for a few minutes so the medicine will stay in the ear and be absorbed. Then administer drops in the other ear if necessary.

Nose Drops. Try to clear some of the mucus out of your child's nose before administering nose drops. If old enough, the child should blow his or her nose. Otherwise, use a bulb syringe to suck out the mucus or gently twirl a moist cotton swab inside each nostril; just be careful not to insert the swab too far. Tilt your child's head back slightly so the nostrils are pointing toward the ceiling. Placing a pillow under the shoulders may help to position your child correctly. Insert the dropper into the nostril, but not too far. Gently

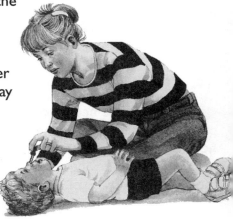

squeeze the dropper to instill the prescribed number of drops. Have your child remain in this position for a couple minutes to make sure the drops have entered the nasal passages.

Rectal Suppositories. Ask your pharmacist if the suppositories can be stored in the refrigerator to make them easier to handle. Suppositories stored at room temperature may become too soft to insert. If so, chill the suppository in the refrigerator for 30 minutes before inserting it (ask your pharmacist first) or run it under cold water with the foil wrapper still on. Babies should be positioned facedown across your knees. An older child should lie on one side with knees drawn up to the chest. Remove any foil wrapper. Then moisten with water or coat it with petroleum jelly. Gently insert it high into the rectum, about ½ to 1 inch beyond the sphincter. Hold the cheeks of the buttocks closed for several minutes to prevent your child from expelling the suppository. If you have long fingernails, use rubber gloves.

Topical Creams and Lotions. The most common mistake parents make when applying topical medications is giving too much. Only apply the exact amount prescribed. Often a thin, even layer is sufficient. Wash your hands first and do not stick a cotton swab or other applicator into the bottle or tube. Pour or squeeze out the amount of medicine you need onto a gauze pad, cotton swab, or cotton ball, and then apply it to the skin. Keep your child's hands busy with a toy. If your child gets some of the medication on the hands, wash it off immediately before the hands find their way to the child's mouth.

STRATEGIES

Sometimes you need more than just the proper technique to get the medicine down; you need strategies that work with children of different ages. The following are some parent-tested tactics that can win your child's cooperation.

Use stories, songs, or rhymes. Ask your librarian for books about children taking medicine. Or make them up yourself—a good story can help children overcome their fears.

Offer choices. This works best with children older than three years of age. "Do you want the orange medicine first or the red?" "Do you want to sit on the bed or in your chair?"

Put work before pleasure. "We cannot go outside to play until you take your medicine. Tell me when you're ready."

Work as a team. Enlist your child's help. "What can we do to make it taste better?" will prompt more cooperation than "Take your medicine or else!" Then suggest some ideas such as, "Try holding your nose while you swallow" or "We could mix this with juice if you drink it all." Let the child hold the spoon for control if necessary.

Get help. A small toddler can often out-wiggle one adult. It's easier if one adult holds the child while the other gives the medicine. Or use an infant seat or car seat to hold the baby still.

Explain the consequences. In a nonthreatening voice, talk about the consequences of not taking the medication. "Do you remember how much your ear hurt last night? It may be worse tonight unless you take this medicine."

Try a different drug form. Children older than five years of age may accept a pill or chewable tablet better than a bitter-tasting liquid. Some medications come in forms that can be sprinkled on food. For children who have trouble swallowing pills, you can buy a special glass that delivers the pill into the mouth automatically with the first gulp of liquid.

Give information. When appropriate, teach your child about the illness and how the medicine works.

Chapter 6

Coping with Side Effects

Along with their therapeutic benefits, drugs may have undesirable side effects. Some side effects are simply inconvenient or uncomfortable while others are life threatening. Some side effects last for a short time while others have more long-term effects. Fortunately, severe and long-term side effects occur relatively infrequently.

Know What to Expect. It's crucial that you know what side effects to expect from any drug you give your child so you can ease the symptoms and seek medical attention when necessary. If you have concerns about any side effects, even if they are minor, be sure to call your child's doctor. The doctor may be able to minimize or eliminate the side effects by prescribing a different medication or changing your child's dose, dosing schedule, or the way the drug is given. At the very least, the doctor can assure you that the medication's benefits far outweigh its side effects.

Managing Side Effects. Each drug profile in this book contains a section on side effects. The section tells you which side effects are more common, less common, and which require a call to the doctor. Use the following table to help make your child more comfortable when experiencing side effects.

Common Minor Side Effects

Side Effect	Management
Constipation	Increase the amount of fiber in your child's diet, give plenty of fluids,* increase your child's physical activity.*
Decreased sweating	Keep your child out of the sun and heat.
Diarrhea	Give lots of water to replace lost fluids; call the doctor if diarrhea lasts longer than three days.
Dizziness	Have your child avoid activities that require balance, such as riding a bicycle; have your child get up slowly after lying down or sitting.
Drowsiness	Have your child avoid activities that require alertness, such as playing on swings or other playground equipment.
Dry mouth	Give your child hard candy or ice chips to suck on or sugarless gum to chew.
Dry nose and throat	Use a humidifier or vaporizer.
Fluid retention (mild)	Minimize your child's salt intake; have your child keep his or her legs elevated if possible.
Headache	Give acetaminophen;* have your child lie down in a quiet place.
Insomnia	If possible, give the last dose of the drug earlier in the day;* ask your doctor about an exercise program.
Itching	Have your child take frequent cool baths or showers; ask your child's doctor about a topical or systemic medication to control itching.
Nasal congestion	Consult your pharmacist or your child's doctor.
Palpitations (mild)	Have your child rest often and avoid tension; limit your child's intake of caffeine-containing products such as coffee, tea, cola, and chocolate; your child should avoid nicotine use.
Upset stomach	Give the drug with milk or food.*

*Consult your child's doctor or pharmacist first.

Chapter 7

Overdose and Poisoning

You may have a difficult time cajoling your child to take the medication prescribed for an infection. But at another time, in another place, your child may find medication irresistible. Attractive packages, bright colors, and interesting flavors make medications very tempting to children, especially when they see their parents and their grandparents taking them.

Medication's visual appeal and children's natural curiosity can be a lethal combination. Any drug, whether prescription or nonprescription, can be poisonous if your child swallows a sufficient quantity. Even a small amount can be harmful to children because of differences in metabolism and body size. Iron supplements, nonprescription diet pills, sleep-preventing or enhancing drugs, decongestants, antihistamines, and antidepressants are especially dangerous.

Children younger than six years of age are most at risk of accidental poisoning, but older children and teenagers can become victims, too. Iron supplements are the most common cause of drug poisoning in children younger than six years of age; they taste sweet and can be mistaken for candy. As little as 600 milligrams of iron (four high-dose pills) can be fatal to a young child.

SYMPTOMS OF POISONING

Most drugs work fairly quickly in a child's system. Sudden vomiting, dizziness, or lethargy can signal poisoning. An overdose of iron causes abdominal pain and severe vomiting, followed by collapse. An overdose of aspirin triggers rapid breathing, ringing in the ears, nausea, over-excitement, and, eventually, loss of consciousness. Be suspicious if you smell medicine on your child's breath, see traces of it around the mouth, or find an open medicine bottle nearby.

IN CASE OF POISONING

If you suspect your child has swallowed medication, call the nearest poison control center or your child's doctor immediately. Do not use syrup of ipecac before you have spoken with the poison control center or the doctor. Some poisons should be expelled from your child's stomach by vomiting as soon as possible. Others are better left in the stomach temporarily because they will do additional damage as they come back up through the esophagus and throat.

The poison control center or the doctor will need accurate information about your child's age, weight, the name of the drug ingested, and whether your child has vomited or eaten recently. If you go to the emergency room, take the bottle of medicine with you.

HOW TO PREVENT POISONING

The following safety precautions will help you minimize the risk of an accidental poisoning:

- Keep pills in their original containers and secure the cap carefully after every use.

- Keep medication in a hard-to-reach cabinet with a childproof lock. Do not keep it on the countertop, kitchen table, or nightstand.

- Do not store medications in the kitchen near snacks or sweets. This can confuse children.

- Do not rely on a child-resistant cap to deter your child. Child-resistant does not mean childproof. Legally, a cap can be called child-resistant if 80 percent of five-year-olds require more than five minutes to open it. That means the other 20 percent can open it faster.

- If your child spends time at the home of a grandparent or another adult, take along a childproof lock for the medicine cabinet.

Chapter 8

Immunizations

Immunizations are the best medical insurance available. They help keep your children healthy by providing lifelong protection against certain virulent diseases. Polio, whooping cough, diphtheria, and mumps killed or permanently disabled thousands of children before vaccines for them became available. Today, thanks to immunizations, those diseases and others are rare or, such as smallpox, completely eradicated.

WHAT'S THE RISK?

In recent years parents have become concerned about the risks of immunizations. In some ways, this concern is itself a luxury parents owe to the success of immunizations in preventing disease. Freed from the specter of terrible, life-threatening childhood illnesses, some parents wonder if immunizations are harmful or even necessary.

The benefits of immunizations, however, far outweigh any risk. In fact, the risks are extremely low. For example, the risk of permanent brain damage from the pertussis (whooping cough) vaccine is 1 in 500,000 to 1 million. However, whooping cough kills 8 out of every 1,000 children younger than three years of age who contract the disease. Fifty percent of those who contract tetanus will die; polio paralyzes 50 percent of its victims.

Just because you haven't seen a case of measles doesn't mean your unvaccinated child cannot contract it. Unvaccinated children can catch even the most uncommon infectious diseases. As vaccination rates sagged in the 1980s, the number of measles cases surged from 1,500 in 1983 to 55,000 between 1989 and 1991, according to the National Centers for Disease Prevention and Control (CDC). Of those cases, 132 died. If you have any concerns about vaccinating your children, discuss them with your child's doctor.

HOW THEY WORK

Vaccinations work by stimulating the body to protect itself against disease. Doctors use two types of immunization, active or passive. Active immunization is achieved by injecting a weakened or killed virus or bacterium into the body, stimulating the body's natural defense system. The body produces substances known as antibodies which fight invading organisms. The antibodies, carried in the bloodstream, remain in the body for years, sometimes a lifetime, to protect it against that particular disease. Passive immunization involves injecting ready-made antibodies that usually have been extracted from the blood of animals in which immunity has been induced for the sole purpose of producing a vaccine. Passive immunization is only temporary but will protect someone who is already infected until the body can produce its own antibodies.

REQUIRED IMMUNIZATIONS

School-age children and those attending a licensed day-care center or home are required to be immunized. There are required immunizations against nine diseases—diphtheria, tetanus, pertussis, *Haemophilus influenzae* type b, hepatitis B virus, measles, mumps, rubella, and polio—as of June, 1996.

HIB

The Hib vaccine protects against *Haemophilus influenzae* type b, a potentially deadly bacterial infection. Before the vaccine was approved, this bacteria affected 1 in 200 children younger than five years of age. Hib often caused meningitis, an infection that can lead to death or cause brain or hearing damage. Hib can also infect blood, joints, bones, soft tissues, the throat, and the membrane surrounding the heart.

Approved in 1990, the Hib vaccine has nearly eradicated Hib infections among vaccinated children in the United States. There are a number of brand-name products available, including one that combines Hib and DTP vaccines. Side effects for the Hib vaccine are minor, consisting mostly of low-grade fever and soreness at the site of the injection.

DTP

DTP inoculates against diphtheria, tetanus, and pertussis (whooping cough). It is given at 2, 4, 6, and 15 months of age, with a booster between 4 and 6 years and again at 11 to 12 years. (Children older than 7 years of age should receive only diphtheria and tetanus, not pertussis.) Diphtheria is a highly infectious bacterial disease of the mouth, nose, and throat causing a sore throat and cough. The windpipe and tonsils can be covered with a fine web of gray membrane, causing fever, weakness, and suffocation. If untreated, pneumonia, heart failure, and paralysis can develop. This disease is rare since the vaccine was approved.

Tetanus is a serious infection that invades a cut in the skin. Rusty metal, gravel, and dirt all carry the tetanus bacterium. Once in the body, it produces a toxin that causes muscle spasms. Tetanus first attacks jaw muscles, causing lockjaw. In more severe cases it attacks the breathing muscles. Tetanus is fatal in 30 percent of cases. After the first round of tetanus shots given during infancy, your child will need a tetanus booster every 10 years throughout life.

Pertussis, or whooping cough, is a very dangerous infection in children younger than one year of age. Bacteria clog the airways with mucus, causing a severe cough that sounds like a "whoop." The cough lasts about two months and gives rise to other infections such as pneumonia

or bronchitis. The pertussis vaccine prevents most cases of this infection, but it does have a number of side effects. Many children will have fever, soreness at the site of the injection, and irritability. In rare cases, the vaccine causes very high fever and convulsions. An acellular vaccine (made from portions of the cells instead of whole cells) is available for children who have had bad reactions to the regular vaccine. It is approved for the fourth dose, given between 15 and 18 months of age, and the last dose, given before your child enters school.

HEPATITIS B

Hepatitis B is a viral disease that attacks the liver, causing nausea, fever, weakness, loss of appetite, and jaundice. It eventually can cause liver failure and death. It is transmitted through contaminated blood and body fluids. Children are not at high risk for getting hepatitis B unless they are born to mothers with the infection. However, attempts to vaccinate high-risk groups (IV drug users, homosexual men, and health care workers), have had limited success. It's easier to require children to get vaccinated before they attend school.

The hepatitis B vaccine requires two or three doses depending on the brand used, and conveys lifelong protection. There are no serious reactions to the vaccine.

POLIO

At the height of the polio epidemic in 1952, more than 20,000 people—mostly children—caught this serious disease. The first symptoms are fever, sore throat, headache, and a stiff neck. The disease can lead to death, but more commonly it causes paralysis of the lower limbs and chest, making walking and breathing difficult or impossible. There is no cure for the disease.

Two polio vaccines have eradicated this disease from the western hemisphere and almost entirely from the world. The oral polio vaccine

(OPV), taken as drops in the mouth, is used most frequently. It is given at 2, 4, and 15 months of age and again between 4 and 6 years. Unfortunately, the oral vaccine can cause polio itself. The risk is very low—no more than 1 in 1.5 million. It is greatest for people who have immune deficiencies such as AIDS and cancer.

Children with immune deficiencies, or children who live with adults who have immune deficiencies, should be given the inactivated polio vaccine (IPV). This vaccine is given by injection. Adults not vaccinated for polio might want to get the IPV before any child in their homes receives the oral dose.

MMR

The MMR vaccine protects against measles, mumps, and rubella (German measles). Measles is highly contagious and causes a spotty rash, fever, cough, and sometimes ear infections and pneumonia. Measles is much more debilitating for babies younger than two years of age and for adults than it is for elementary school children. In severe cases it can infect the brain, causing convulsions, hearing loss, mental retardation, and even death.

Given at 15 months and again between 4 and 6 years of age, the vaccine has few side effects. Some children will develop mild pain in the joints, fever, a spotty rash, and swelling of the lymph glands.

Mumps is a viral infection causing painful, swollen salivary glands under the jaw, fever, and headache. Mumps usually strikes children between 5 and 15 years of age. In adults, it can be a very serious disease, causing meningitis or hearing loss. Male teenagers and adults may have painful swelling of the testicles for several days. The disease is much more difficult for them.

Rubella, also called German measles, is not a great risk for children but is very serious when caught by a pregnant woman. Half of those who contract rubella during their first three months

of pregnancy will miscarry or deliver babies with heart disease, blindness, hearing loss, or learning problems. Any woman planning a pregnancy can be tested for immunity to rubella and receive the vaccine before getting pregnant. She should, however, wait three months after the immunization to get pregnant, however, because the vaccine can harm the fetus.

OPTIONAL VACCINES

Vaccines are also available for varicella-zoster virus (chicken pox), typhus, yellow fever, and influenza. The one-dose chicken pox vaccine is now available for children older than one year of age. While it is effective in preventing chicken pox, long-term studies have yet to be completed to determine if the vaccine will give lifelong immunity or whether it will protect against shingles, which is caused by the same virus, later in life. None of the other optional immunizations is yet recommended for children unless you're planning a trip overseas. Consult the doctor if you plan to travel.

KEEP A RECORD

Unfortunately, only about half of all insurance plans cover immunizations. However, many county health departments offer vaccinations free or at a reduced fee based on income. No matter where your child is vaccinated, you always should keep a record of when each vaccination was given and the name of the vaccine administered. Some brands have slightly different schedules than others and all of them have requirements for the spacing between doses. Ask for a copy of the immunization record to keep at home. If you have to cancel or postpone an immunization visit, your child can catch up at a later date. However, it is important to talk to your child's doctor about it first.

ACETAMINOPHEN

Administration Guidelines

• Usually given every 4 hours, but do not give more than 5 doses in a 24-hour period.

• Do not exceed recommended dosage or give for longer than 3 days without speaking to your child's doctor.

• Read the product label carefully and make sure you are giving your child the proper amount. It is easy to confuse the many different dosage forms and strengths.

Side Effects

Tell your child's doctor about any side effects that are persistent or particularly bothersome.

Less Common. Anemia, skin rashes. Contact the doctor if your child experiences fever or yellowing of eyes or skin.

Possible Drug Interactions

• Barbiturate drugs such as phenobarbital, carbamazepine (Tegretol), phenytoin (Dilantin), rifampin, and frequent alcohol use can increase the risk of liver damage.

Tell Your Child's Doctor If

• Your child has had allergic reactions to any medications, has any other diseases, or is taking any other medications.

• Your daughter is or becomes pregnant. This drug is generally safe for use during pregnancy.

• Your daughter is breast-feeding her baby. This drug passes into breast milk; however, the American Academy of Pediatrics considers it compatible with breast-feeding in most cases.

Symptoms of Overdose:
Nausea, vomiting, sweating, loss of appetite. If an overdose occurs, contact a poison control center immediately. An overdose of this drug can cause serious liver damage.

Special Notes

• Contact the doctor immediately if your child has a fever higher than 105°F. A fever this high may indicate serious illness.

• Can interfere with home blood glucose measurements in children with diabetes.

• Contact the doctor for any fever in infants younger than 4 months of age.

• There is no need to awaken a sleeping child simply to give this drug for a fever. It is important to allow the child to rest.

Brand Names: Feverall, Neopap, Acephen, Suppap, Anacin-3, Panadol, St. Joseph Aspirin-Free, Tempra, Tylenol, Phenaphen, Datril, Liquiprin. Also available in multiple combination products.

Generic Available: Yes

Type of Drug: Analgesic, antipyretic

Use: Relieves pain and reduces fever.

Time Required for Drug to Take Effect: 30 minutes to 2 hours

Dosage Forms and Strengths: Suppositories (120 mg, 125 mg, 300 mg, 325 mg, 650 mg); Tablets, chewable (80 mg); Tablets (160 mg, 325 mg, 500 mg, 650 mg); Capsules (500 mg); Liquid/Elixir (120 mg/mL, 130 mg/5 mL, 160 mg/5 mL, 325 mg/5 mL, and 500 mg/ 15 mL); Drops (48 mg/mL and 100 mg/mL)

Storage: Store at room temperature in tightly closed, light-resistant containers.

How This Drug Works: Decreases production of substances in the body that cause fever and pain.

Brand Names: Acetazolamide (various manufacturers), AK-Zol, Dazamide, Diamox, Diamox Sequels

Generic Available: Yes

Type of Drug: Carbonic anhydrase inhibitor

Use: Treats epilepsy, edema (fluid retention), and glaucoma, and may prevent the symptoms of mountain sickness.

Time Required for Drug to Take Effect: 2 hours for capsule; 1 to 1.5 hours for tablets. For mountain sickness prevention, therapy must begin 24 to 48 hours before the ascent and continue for 48 hours or longer while at high altitude.

Dosage Forms and Strengths: Capsules, sustained-release (500 mg); Tablets (125 mg, 250 mg)

Storage: Store at room temperature in tightly closed containers.

How This Drug Works: Lowers blood pressure in the eye; acts as a diuretic; decreases seizure activity.

ACETAZOLAMIDE

Administration Guidelines

• Give with food or a full glass of water or milk to avoid stomach irritation.

• Do not crush, break, or allow your child to chew sustained-release capsules. These actions destroy the sustained-release activity and may increase side effects.

• The pharmacist can crush the tablets and mix them into a suspension to disguise the taste.

• Missed doses: Give as soon as possible. However, if it is within 2 hours of the next dose, skip the missed dose and return to the regular dosing schedule. Do not give double doses.

Side Effects

Tell your child's doctor about any side effects that are persistent or particularly bothersome.

More Common. It is especially important to tell the doctor if your child experiences back pain; bloody or black, tarry stools; blurred vision; convulsions; difficult or painful urination; fever; rash; unusual bleeding or bruising; or yellowing of the eyes or skin.

Less Common. Confusion, drowsiness, increased urination, loss of appetite, or a tingling feeling. These side effects should disappear as your child's body adjusts to this drug.

Possible Drug Interactions

• Can decrease the excretion of amphetamines, ephedrine, flecainide, mexiletine, pseudoephedrine, tocainide, and quinidine. This can lead to an increased risk of side effects with these medications.

• Can cause increased softening of the bones, anemia, or abnormalities of the blood when used with carbamazepine, phenobarbital, phenytoin, and primidone.

• Dosage adjustments of insulin or oral antidiabetic medications may be necessary when this drug is started.

• May decrease the therapeutic benefits of lithium, methenamine, or methotrexate.

Tell Your Child's Doctor If

• Your child is taking any medications, especially any of those listed above.

• Your child has had unusual or allergic reactions to any medications, especially to this drug, methazolamide, sulfonamide antibiotics, diuretics, oral antidiabetics, dapsone, sulfone, or sulfoxone.

- Your child has or ever had acidosis, Addison disease (underactive adrenal gland), chronic lung disease, diabetes mellitus, electrolyte disorders, gout, kidney disease, or liver disease.

- Your daughter is breast-feeding her baby. It is not known whether this drug passes into breast milk.

Special Instructions

- Although several generic versions of this drug are available, do not switch from one brand to another without the doctor's or pharmacist's approval. These products are not all equivalent.

- Tolerance to this drug can develop quickly. Check with the doctor if you feel this drug is losing its effectiveness with your child.

Symptoms of Overdose: Drowsiness, abnormal tingling sensation

Special Notes

- This drug may cause drowsiness. Make sure your child has good body control before allowing participation in activities that require alertness, such as riding a bicycle.

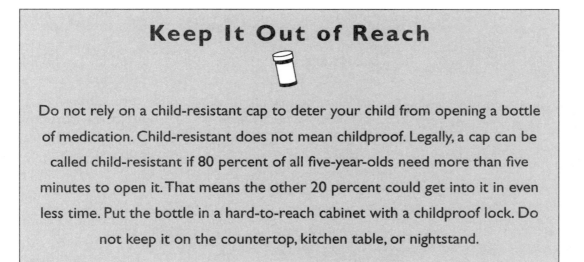

Keep It Out of Reach

Do not rely on a child-resistant cap to deter your child from opening a bottle of medication. Child-resistant does not mean childproof. Legally, a cap can be called child-resistant if 80 percent of all five-year-olds need more than five minutes to open it. That means the other 20 percent could get into it in even less time. Put the bottle in a hard-to-reach cabinet with a childproof lock. Do not keep it on the countertop, kitchen table, or nightstand.

Brand Name: Zovirax

Generic Available: No

Type of Drug: Antiviral

Use: Treats genital herpes and herpes infections of the skin, including chicken pox. May relieve pain and shorten duration of the infection.

Time Required for Drug to Take Effect: It may take a few days to affect the infection.

Dosage Forms and Strengths: Capsules (200 mg); Tablets (400 mg, 800 mg); Suspension, banana flavor (200 mg per 5 mL); Ointment (5 %)

Storage: Store ointment, capsules, and tablets in a cool, dry place. Keep suspension refrigerated.

How This Drug Works: Prevents the growth and multiplication of the herpes virus.

ACYCLOVIR

Administration Guidelines
- Usually given 2 to 5 times a day for 7 to 10 days, depending on the type of herpes infection.
- Apply ointment as soon as symptoms of a herpes infection appear. It is generally applied 6 times a day for 7 days.
- Wash infected area with soap and water; allow it to dry. Use a rubber glove or finger cot to apply the ointment to avoid spreading the infection. Apply enough to completely cover the infected area.
- Do not use ointment in or around the eyes.
- Missed doses: Give or apply as soon as possible. If it's time for the next dose, skip the missed dose. Do not give double doses.
- Your child should complete the full course of therapy, even if symptoms disappear sooner.

Side Effects
Tell your child's doctor about any side effects that are persistent or particularly bothersome.

More Common. Temporary pain, burning, stinging, itching, or rash when applied topically. Sore throat, diarrhea, difficulty sleeping, dizziness, fatigue, headache, rash, upset stomach, or vomiting after oral therapy. These side effects should disappear as the body adjusts to this drug.

Less Common. It is especially important to tell the doctor if your child experiences fever or muscle pain.

Tell Your Child's Doctor If
- Your child is taking any other medications or has had unusual or allergic reactions to any medications.
- Your child has or had kidney disease.
- Your daughter is or becomes pregnant or is breast-feeding her baby. This drug can pass into breast milk and cause side effects in the infant.

Special Instructions
- Avoid sexual activity while symptoms persist. This drug does not prevent the transmission of herpes or recurrences.
- Do not use this drug to treat a subsequent infection unless you consult the doctor.

Symptoms of Overdose: Severe forms of the side effects listed above.

ALBUTEROL

Administration Guidelines

- Give tablets and syrup with food to reduce stomach upset (unless your child's doctor directs you to do otherwise).

- Shake the inhaler well just before each use to distribute the ingredients and equalize the doses. If more than 1 inhalation is necessary, wait at least 1 full minute between doses to receive the full benefit of the first dose.

- Ask the doctor if you can give the last dose of this drug several hours before bedtime each day. This may help prevent difficulty in falling asleep.

- Missed doses: If you miss a dose and remember within 1 hour, give the missed dose immediately; then follow the regular dosing schedule. If more than 1 hour has passed, just wait until the next scheduled dose. Do not give double doses.

- Do not exceed the recommended dosage. Excessive use may lead to an increase in side effects or a loss of effectiveness.

- Do not spray aerosol in or near the eyes.

Side Effects

Tell your child's doctor about any side effects that are persistent or particularly bothersome.

More Common. It is especially important to tell the doctor if your child experiences chest pain, difficult or painful urination, itching, palpitations, or rash.

Less Common. Anxiety, dizziness, reddening of the face, headache, insomnia, irritability, loss of appetite, muscle cramps, nausea, nervousness, restlessness, sweating, tremors, vomiting, weakness, or dryness or irritation of the mouth or throat (from the inhalation aerosol). These side effects should disappear as your child's body adjusts to this drug.

Possible Drug Interactions

- Beta blockers (acebutolol, atenolol, labetalol, metoprolol, nadolol, pindolol, propranolol, timolol) decrease the effectiveness of this drug.

- Monoamine oxidase (MAO) inhibitors; tricyclic antidepressants; antihistamines; levothyroxine; and nonprescription cough, cold, asthma, allergy, diet, and sinus medications may increase the side effects of this drug.

- There may be a change in the dosage requirements of insulin or oral antidiabetic medications when this drug is started.

Brand Names: Proventil, Ventolin, Volmax

Generic Available: Yes

Type of Drug: Bronchodilator

Use: Relieves wheezing and shortness of breath caused by lung diseases such as asthma, bronchitis, and emphysema.

Time Required for Drug to Take Effect: 5 to 15 minutes for oral inhalation; up to 30 minutes for tablets

Dosage Forms and Strengths: Aerosol, for inhalation (90 mcg per spray, 200 inhalations); Capsules (Rotacaps), microfine, for inhalation (200 mcg); Solution, inhalation (0.83 mg per mL; 5 mg per mL); Syrup, strawberry flavor (2 mg per 5 mL); Tablets (2 mg, 4 mg); Tablets, extended-release (4 mg)

Storage: Store tablets and syrup at room temperature in tightly closed, light-resistant containers. Store the inhalation aerosol away from excessive heat—the contents are pressurized and can explode if heated.

How This Drug Works: Relaxes the smooth muscles of the bronchial airways.

- The use of this drug with other bronchodilators can increase side effects. Discuss this with the doctor.

Tell Your Child's Doctor If

- Your child is taking any medications, especially any listed above.

- Your child has or ever had diabetes mellitus, epilepsy, heart disease, high blood pressure, or thyroid disease.

- Your child has had unusual or allergic reactions to any medications, especially to this drug or any related medication (metaproterenol, terbutaline, amphetamines, ephedrine, epinephrine, isoproterenol, norepinephrine, phenylephrine, phenylpropanolamine, and pseudoephedrine).

- Your child does not respond to the usual dose.

- Your daughter is or becomes pregnant.

- Your daughter is breast-feeding her baby.

Symptoms of Overdose: Seizures, low blood pressure, high blood pressure, irregular heartbeats, awareness of a strong heartbeat, nervousness, dizziness, fatigue, insomnia, headache, lack of energy

Special Notes

- Before any medical or dental treatment, tell the doctor or dentist that your child is taking this drug.

- This drug can cause dizziness. Make sure your child has good body control before allowing participation in activities that require alertness, such as riding a bicycle.

Be Accurate

If you don't give medication correctly, it may be ineffective or even cause side effects. An estimated 10 to 30 percent of medications aren't effective because they have been given incorrectly. To do it right, you have to give the exact amount of medicine prescribed at the scheduled time, for the specified duration, and in the appropriate manner. Always read the label, follow the directions carefully, and use the appropriate equipment for measuring and administering the medication. Also, be sure to wash your hands before you give any medication to your child.

AMITRIPTYLINE

Administration Guidelines

• Give with food to decrease stomach upset.

• Give 2 or 3 times a day or as a single daily dose at bedtime.

• Doses are increased slowly to decrease the side effects.

• Missed doses: Give as soon as possible. However, if it's within 2 hours of the next dose, skip the missed dose. Do not give double doses. If a once-a-day bedtime dose is missed, do not give the missed dose in the morning because it may cause sedation.

Side Effects

Tell your child's doctor about any side effects that are persistent or particularly bothersome.

More Common. Drowsiness, dryness of mouth, dizziness, light-headedness, headache, nausea, increased appetite, weight gain, unpleasant taste, constipation, weakness

Less Common. Call the doctor if your child experiences blurred vision, confusion, difficulty in speaking or swallowing, eye pain, fainting, fast or irregular heartbeat, hallucinations, loss of balance, masklike face, nervousness or restlessness, problems urinating, shakiness, or slow movements.

Possible Drug Interactions

• Clonidine (Catapres) may lead to very high blood pressure when taken with this drug.

• Monoamine oxidase (MAO) inhibitors such as isocarboxazid (Marplan), phenelzine (Nardil), or tranylcypromine (Parnate) can cause very serious reactions and death when used with this drug.

• Central nervous system depressants such as alcohol, antihistamines, muscle relaxants, tranquilizers, sedatives, and some pain medications may cause extreme drowsiness when used with this drug.

• Cimetidine (Tagamet and Tagamet HB) and methylphenidate (Ritalin) may increase the effect of this drug.

• Phenobarbital may decrease the effect of this drug.

• Eyedrops and nasal sprays or drops that contain naphazoline, oxymetazoline, epinephrine, phenylephrine, or xylometazoline may cause an increase in heart rate and blood pressure.

Brand Names: Elavil, Emitrip, Endep

Generic Available: Yes

Type of Drug: Tricyclic antidepressant

Use: Treats mental depression, affective disorders, and some kinds of chronic pain; also prevents migraines.

Time Required for Drug to Take Effect: 7 to 21 days. Full benefit may not occur for 3 to 6 weeks.

Dosage Form and Strengths: Tablets (10 mg, 25 mg, 50 mg, 75 mg, 100 mg, 150 mg)

Storage: Store at room temperature in tightly closed, light-resistant containers.

How This Drug Works: Increases the concentration of serotonin and/or norepinephrine in the central nervous system.

Tell Your Child's Doctor If

- Your child has had an allergic reaction to this drug or any other medication.

- Your child has heart disease, seizures, glaucoma, thyroid disease, urinary retention, liver disease, kidney disease, or any other medical condition.

- Your child is or has been taking MAO inhibitors: isocarboxazid (Marplan), phenelzine (Nardil), or tranylcypromine (Parnate).

- Your child has taken or is taking any other prescription or nonprescription medicine.

- Your daughter is or becomes pregnant.

- Your daughter is breast-feeding her baby. This drug can pass into the milk and the American Academy of Pediatrics is concerned about its effect on the baby.

Special Instructions

- Do not suddenly stop giving this drug before speaking to the doctor.

- Your child should not drink alcohol or alcohol containing products while taking this drug.

- Do not give other medicines that may make your child sleepy.

- To avoid dizziness, have your child stand up slowly after sitting or lying down.

- Limit your child's caffeine intake.

- Your child should avoid exposure to sunlight and wear sunscreen when out-of-doors. This drug may cause a skin rash or severe sunburn with exposure to direct sunlight or ultraviolet light in tanning booths.

Symptoms of Overdose: Agitation; dry mouth; confusion; hallucinations; severe drowsiness; enlarged pupils; fever; vomiting; trouble breathing; urinary retention; low blood pressure; seizures; or fast, slow, or irregular heartbeat

Special Notes

- Drowsiness is common. Make sure you know how your child is reacting to this drug before allowing participation in activities that require alertness and coordination, such as riding a bicycle.

- The effects of this drug may last for 1 to 2 weeks after you stop giving it to your child.

- May cause urine to turn blue-green.

AMOXICILLIN

Administration Guidelines

- May be given either on an empty stomach or with food or milk (to prevent stomach upset).

- Generally given 3 times a day.

- Works best when blood concentrations are kept within a safe and effective range. Give doses at evenly spaced intervals around the clock. If you are to give 3 doses a day, space them approximately 8 hours apart.

- Shake suspension and drops well just before measuring each dose to distribute ingredients and equalize doses. The contents tend to settle on the bottom of the bottle.

- Missed doses: Give immediately. However, if you don't remember the missed dose until it is time for the next dose, give the missed dose and space the next dose about halfway through the regular interval between doses; then return to the regular schedule. Do not skip any doses.

- Give this drug for the entire time prescribed by your child's doctor (usually 7 to 14 days), even if symptoms disappear.

Side Effects

Tell your child's doctor about any side effects that are persistent or particularly bothersome.

More Common. Diarrhea, heartburn, nausea, or vomiting. These side effects should disappear as the body adjusts to this drug.

Less Common. It is especially important to tell the doctor if your child experiences bloating, chills, cough, darkened tongue, difficulty in breathing, fever, irritation of the mouth, muscle aches, rash, rectal or vaginal itching, severe or bloody diarrhea, or sore throat.

Possible Drug Interactions

- Probenecid can increase the blood concentration of this drug.

- May decrease the effectiveness of oral contraceptives (birth control pills). A different or additional form of birth control should be used to prevent pregnancy.

- Concurrent use of this drug and allopurinol can increase the risk of developing a rash.

Tell Your Child's Doctor If

- Your child is taking any other prescription or nonprescription medications.

Brand Names: Amoxil, Biomox, Olymox, Trimox, Utimox, Wymox (various manufacturers). Available in combination with clavulanic acid (Augmentin).

Generic Available: Yes

Type of Drug: Antibiotic

Use: Treats bacterial infections, especially those of the ear, nose, throat, lower respiratory tract, skin, and genitourinary tract.

Time Required for Drug to Take Effect: It may take a few days to affect the infection.

Dosage Forms and Strengths: Capsules (250 mg, 500 mg); Tablets, chewable (125 mg, 250 mg); Suspension (125 mg and 250 mg per 5 mL); Drops (50 mg per 1 mL)

Storage: Refrigerate liquids; do not freeze. Store capsules and tablets at room temperature in tightly closed, light-resistant containers. Discard after 14 days any unused portion of the suspension.

How This Drug Works: Kills susceptible bacteria but is not effective against viruses, parasites, or fungi.

- Your child has had allergic reactions to any medications, especially to this drug, ampicillin or penicillin, cephalosporin antibiotics, penicillamine, or griseofulvin.

- Your child has or ever had kidney disease or infectious mononucleosis.

- Symptoms of infection seem to be getting worse rather than improving.

- Your daughter is or becomes pregnant.

- Your daughter is breast-feeding her baby. Small amounts of this drug can pass into breast milk and temporarily cause diarrhea in the nursing infant.

Special Instructions
- Children with diabetes may have a false-positive sugar reaction with a Clinitest urine glucose test. To avoid this problem, switch to Clinistix™ or Tes-Tape during treatment.

- Do not use this drug to treat a subsequent infection unless you consult the doctor.

Symptoms of Overdose: Severe diarrhea, heartburn, nausea, or vomiting

To Each His Own

If one of your children has been prescribed an antibiotic and another child gets sick, it is not safe to give the antibiotic to the child for whom it was not prescribed. The medication may not be the appropriate one for the other child—even if the children's symptoms are similar. Treating an infection with the wrong drug may make the condition worse instead of better. What's more, children respond to the same drug differently and may need different dosages. The child who became ill first needs the drug in the amount prescribed for the time advised; otherwise, it may not be effective. If you think another child needs medication, consult the doctor.

AMOXICILLIN AND CLAVULANIC ACID COMBINATION

Administration Guidelines
• Give on an empty stomach or with food or milk (to prevent stomach upset).

• Generally given 3 times a day.

• Works best when blood concentrations are kept within a safe and effective range. Give doses at evenly spaced intervals around the clock.

• Missed doses: Give immediately. However, if it's time for the next dose, give the missed dose and space the next dose about halfway through the regular interval between doses; then return to the regular schedule. Do not skip any doses.

• Shake the suspension well just before measuring each dose to distribute ingredients and equalize doses. The contents tend to settle on the bottom of the bottle.

• Complete the full course of therapy, even if symptoms disappear sooner.

Side Effects
Tell your child's doctor about any side effects that are persistent or particularly bothersome.

More Common. Abdominal discomfort, bloating, diarrhea, gas, headache, heartburn, nausea, or vomiting. These side effects should disappear as the body adjusts to this drug.

Less Common. It is especially important to tell the doctor if your child experiences bloody or prolonged diarrhea, chills, cough, darkened tongue, difficulty in breathing, fever, irritation of the mouth, itching, muscle aches, rash, rectal or vaginal itching, sore throat, or unusual bleeding or bruising.

Possible Drug Interactions
• Probenecid can increase the blood concentration of amoxicillin.

• This drug may decrease the effectiveness of oral contraceptives. A different or additional form of birth control should be used to prevent pregnancy.

• This drug can increase the side effects of disulfiram (Antabuse).

• Concurrent use of this drug and allopurinol can increase the risk of developing a rash.

Brand Name: Augmentin

Generic Available: No

Type of Drug: Antibiotic

Use: Treats a wide variety of bacterial infections.

Time Required for Drug to Take Effect: It may take a few days to affect the infection.

Dosage Forms and Strengths: Tablets (250 mg amoxicillin and 125 mg clavulanic acid; 500 mg amoxicillin and 125 mg clavulanic acid); Tablets, chewable (125 mg amoxicillin and 31.25 mg clavulanic acid; 250 mg amoxicillin and 62.5 mg clavulanic acid); Suspension (125 mg amoxicillin and 31.25 mg clavulanic acid; 250 mg amoxicillin and 62.5 mg clavulanic acid per 5 mL)

Storage: Refrigerate suspension; do not freeze. Store tablets at room temperature in tightly closed containers. Discard after 10 days any unused portion of the suspension.

How This Drug Works: Kills susceptible bacteria, but is ineffective against viruses, parasites, or fungi. Clavulanic acid prevents the breakdown of amoxicillin, allowing higher amounts to get into the blood.

Tell Your Child's Doctor If

• Your child is currently taking any prescription or nonprescription medications.

• Your child has had unusual or allergic reactions to any medications, especially to penicillin, amoxicillin, ampicillin, cephalosporin antibiotics, penicillamine, griseofulvin, or clavulanic acid.

• Your child has or ever had kidney disease or infectious mononucleosis.

• Symptoms of infection seem to be getting worse rather than improving.

• Your daughter is or becomes pregnant.

• Your daughter is breast-feeding her baby. Small amounts of this drug pass into breast milk and may cause diarrhea in the nursing infant.

Special Instructions

• Children with diabetes may have a false-positive sugar reaction with a Clinitest urine glucose test. To avoid this problem, switch to Clinistix or Tes-Tape during treatment.

• Do not use this drug to treat a subsequent infection unless you consult the doctor.

Symptoms of Overdose: Severe diarrhea, vomiting, heartburn, or nausea

Measuring Up

Remember: Never use an ordinary tableware teaspoon to measure liquid doses. Instead, use a cylindrical dosing spoon, dosage cup, dropper, or syringe. These measuring devices can be found at your local drug store and sometimes at supermarkets, toy stores, and department stores.

AMPICILLIN
Administration Guidelines
- Best given on an empty stomach (1 hour before or 2 hours after a meal) with a full glass of water (not juice or soda pop).

- Generally given 4 times a day.

- Works best when blood concentrations are kept within a safe and effective range. Give doses at evenly spaced intervals around the clock. If you are to give 4 doses a day, they should be spaced approximately 6 hours apart.

- Missed doses: Give as soon as possible. However, if it is already time for the next dose, give the next dose only, spacing the next 2 doses at half the normal time interval (for example, if you were supposed to give 1 capsule every 6 hours, give the next 2 doses every 3 hours). Then resume the normal dosing schedule.

- Shake the suspension well just before measuring each dose to distribute ingredients and equalize doses. The contents tend to settle on the bottom of the bottle.

- Give this drug for the entire time prescribed by your child's doctor (usually 7 to 14 days), even if symptoms disappear.

Side Effects
Tell your child's doctor about any side effects that are persistent or particularly bothersome.

More Common. Diarrhea, nausea, or vomiting. These side effects should disappear as the body adjusts to this drug.

Less Common. It is especially important to tell the doctor if your child experiences a darkened tongue, difficulty in breathing, fever, joint pain, mouth sores, rash, rectal or vaginal itching, severe or bloody diarrhea, or sore throat.

Possible Drug Interactions
- Probenecid can increase the blood concentration of this drug.

- May decrease the effectiveness of oral contraceptives. A different or additional form of birth control should be used to prevent pregnancy.

- Concurrent use of this drug and allopurinol can increase the risk of developing a rash.

- Chloroquine may decrease the effectiveness of this drug.

Tell Your Child's Doctor If
- Your child is taking any other prescription or nonprescription medications.

Brand Names: D-Amp, Omnipen, Polycillin, Principen, Totacillin, Ampicillin (various manufacturers)

Generic Available: Yes

Type of Drug: Antibiotic

Use: Treats a wide variety of bacterial infections, especially middle ear infections and infections of the respiratory, urinary, and gastrointestinal tracts.

Time Required for Drug to Take Effect: It may take a few days to affect the infection.

Dosage Forms and Strengths: Capsules (250, 500 mg); Suspension (125 mg and 250 mg per 5 mL); Drops (100 mg per mL)

Storage: Refrigerate liquids; do not freeze. Store capsules at room temperature in tightly closed containers. Discard after the expiration date on the container.

How This Drug Works: Kills susceptible bacteria but is not effective against viruses, parasites, or fungi.

- Your child has had allergic reactions to any medications, especially to this drug, penicillin, amoxicillin, cephalosporin antibiotics, penicillamine, or griseofulvin.

- Your child has or has had liver or kidney disease or infectious mononucleosis.

- Your child's symptoms of infection seem to be getting worse.

- Your daughter is or becomes pregnant.

- Your daughter is breast-feeding her baby. Small amounts of this drug pass into breast milk and may temporarily cause diarrhea in the nursing infant.

Special Instructions

- Children with diabetes may have a false-positive sugar reaction with a Clinitest urine glucose test. To avoid this problem, switch to Clinistix or Tes-Tape during treatment.

- Do not use this drug to treat a subsequent infection unless you first consult the doctor.

Symptoms of Overdose: Severe diarrhea, vomiting, heartburn, and nausea

Outdated Doses

Safe and proper medication disposal is essential, especially when you have children in the house. Do not keep medication—whether prescription or nonprescription—past the expiration date, even if it appears normal. Expired medication may be ineffective and can even be dangerous. Make a habit of regularly checking the expiration date on all medicines in your home. Flush leftover medication down the toilet or pour it down the sink. Rinse the container before throwing it out. If your medication does not display an expiration date, throw it out after one year.

ASPIRIN

Administration Guidelines

- Do not give if your child has a fever or other symptoms of a viral infection, especially the flu or chicken pox. This drug can cause a serious illness called Reye syndrome if given to children or teenagers with these symptoms.

- Give with food or a full glass of water or milk to avoid stomach upset.

- Chewable tablets may be chewed, dissolved in fluid, or swallowed whole.

- Enteric-coated and controlled-release tablets should be swallowed whole. Do not crush.

- Unwrap and moisten suppositories before inserting in the rectum.

- Missed doses: Give as soon as you remember if it's within 2 hours of the missed dose. Otherwise, skip the missed dose and give the next dose at the scheduled time. Do not give double doses.

Side Effects

Tell your child's doctor about any side effects that are persistent or particularly bothersome.

More Common. Stomach pain, heartburn, nausea, vomiting

Less Common. Contact the doctor if your child experiences bloody or black, tarry stools; ringing in the ears; loss of hearing; confusion; difficult or painful urination; difficulty breathing; dizziness; severe stomach pain; skin rash; or unusual weakness.

Possible Drug Interactions

- Increases the effects of oral anticoagulants (blood thinners), leading to bleeding complications.

- May increase the stomach irritation experienced with nonsteroidal anti-inflammatory drugs, adrenocorticosteroids, and alcohol.

- Antacids and acetazolamide can decrease the effectiveness of this drug.

Tell Your Child's Doctor If

- Your child has a fever or other symptoms of a viral infection, especially the flu or chicken pox. Aspirin can cause a serious illness called Reye syndrome if given to children or teenagers with these symptoms.

- Your child has had an allergic reaction to any medications.

Brand Names: Anacin, Ascriptin, Bayer, Bufferin, Easprin, Ecotrin, Empirin, Measurin, ZORprin.

Generic Available: Yes

Type of Drug: Analgesic, anti-inflammatory

Use: Treats mild to moderate pain, inflammation, and arthritis. May be used to prevent blood clots. Do not use to treat fever in children unless specifically instructed by the doctor.

Time Required for Drug to Take Effect: In 30 to 60 minutes for mild pain relief. Full effect for other uses may take 2 to 3 weeks.

Dosage Forms and Strengths: Tablets (325 mg, 500 mg, 650 mg); Tablets, chewable (75 mg, 81 mg); Tablets, controlled-release (800 mg); Tablets, enteric-coated (80 mg, 165 mg, 325 mg, 500 mg, 650 mg, 975 mg); Suppositories (60 mg, 120 mg, 125 mg, 130 mg, 195 mg, 200 mg, 300 mg, 325 mg, 600 mg, 650 mg, 1200 mg); Chewing gum (227 mg)

Storage: Store at room temperature in tightly closed containers.

How This Drug Works: Inhibits the production of specific chemicals that are involved in inflammation and blood clotting.

- Your child has any diseases, especially asthma, bleeding disorders, diabetes, hemophilia, ulcers, or nasal polyps.

- Your child is taking any medications.

- Your daughter is or becomes pregnant.

- Your daughter is breast-feeding her baby. This drug can pass into breast milk and may cause significant adverse effects in infants.

Special Instructions

- Do not use if the container has a strong vinegar odor when opened.

- When taken for arthritis or to thin the blood, this drug must be given on a regular basis to be effective.

- Before your child has any medical or dental surgery, tell the doctor performing the procedure your child is taking this drug. The doctor may want to discontinue this drug 5 days before the surgery to prevent bleeding complications.

Symptoms of Overdose: Confusion, convulsions, ringing or buzzing in the ears, hearing loss, severe drowsiness, severe excitement, fast or deep breathing

Special Notes

- Check the labels of all nonprescription medications before giving them to your child. Some products such as Pepto-Bismol contain this drug or other salicylates and should not be given to a child with a fever or other symptoms of a viral infection, especially the flu or chicken pox, without first talking to the doctor.

Over-the-Counter Wisdom

Keep in mind that even a medication that is available without a doctor's prescription may still be harmful and should be given appropriately and only when necessary. Talk to your pediatrician about what to do if your child gets sick. Some illnesses can be treated at home, some require a call to the pediatrician's office, and some will require a visit to the doctor. In addition, ask the doctor what situations constitute an emergency. If you're not sure if it's safe or appropriate to give your child a particular over-the-counter medication, be sure to talk to the doctor first.

ASTEMIZOLE

Administration Guidelines
- Given once a day.
- Dosing guidelines for children younger than 12 years of age are not readily available
- Give on an empty stomach, 1 hour before or 2 hours after meals.
- Do not give more than 10 mg a day.
- Missed doses: Give immediately as long as the total daily dose does not exceed 1 tablet per day.
- Do not increase the dose in an attempt to accelerate the onset of action. Higher dosages may cause serious abnormal heartbeats or rhythms.
- Do not use this drug on an "as needed" basis; follow your child's doctor's directions.

Side Effects
Tell your child's doctor about any side effects that are persistent or particularly bothersome.

Most Common. It is especially important to tell the doctor if your child exhibits symptoms of a hypersensitivity reaction such as shortness of breath, rash, fainting, dizziness, or abnormal heartbeats.

Less Common. Abdominal pain, diarrhea, drowsiness, dry mouth, fainting, gas, headache, increased appetite, nervousness, increased sensitivity to sunlight, or weight gain

Possible Drug Interactions
- Erythromycin, ketoconazole, or itraconazole may cause an irregular heartbeat when used with this drug. Do not give these medications with this drug.
- Fluconazole, metronidazole, clarithromycin, azithromycin, and troleandomycin can increase the possibility of an irregular heart rate when taken with this drug.

Tell Your Child's Doctor If
- Your child has had unusual or allergic reactions to any medications.
- Your child is taking any medications.
- Your child has had an irregular heartbeat or any heart disease.
- Your child has liver disease, as it can decrease the elimination of this drug and lead to increased side effects.

Brand Name: Hismanal

Generic Available: No

Type of Drug: Antihistamine

Use: Treats or prevents symptoms of allergy. Also treats hives.

Time Required for Drug to Take Effect: Has a slow onset; it may take up to 2 days. Effects last up to 24 hours on 1 daily dose.

Dosage Form and Strength: Tablets (10 mg)

Storage: Store in tightly closed containers in a cool, dry place away from heat or direct light.

How This Drug Works: Blocks the action of histamine, a chemical released during an allergic reaction.

• Your daughter is or becomes pregnant or is breast-feeding her baby. The safety of this drug for the fetus or infant has not been established.

Symptoms of Overdose: Hallucinations, convulsions. May produce absurd excitation in the young child.

Special Notes

• This drug can diminish alertness, although it has less of a sedative effect than most other antihistamines.

• Consult the doctor before giving to a child younger than 12 years of age. Other antihistamines have been used for younger children and are known to be safe.

Keep a Lid on It

Pharmacists are required to put drugs in bottles that have child-resistant caps. Don't switch to a bottle that's easier for you to open—children may also find it easier to open. Remember, too, that child-resistant does not mean childproof. Children older than five years of age may be able to open most medicine bottles. That's why it's essential for you to teach them that drugs can be harmful if not taken correctly and that they need supervision before taking anything. And, just to be on the safe side, keep all medicines out of your child's reach.

ATENOLOL

Administration Guidelines
- Usually given once a day.

- May be given on an empty stomach or with meals, but be consistent.

- Give at approximately the same time each day.

- Missed doses: Give as soon as possible if you remember the same day. Otherwise, skip the missed dose. Do not give double doses.

- Do not stop giving this drug to your child without first speaking with the doctor.

Side Effects
Tell your child's doctor about any side effects that are persistent or particularly bothersome.

More Common. Constipation or diarrhea, upset stomach, difficulty sleeping, fatigue, dizziness, headache

Less Common. Allergic reactions, cold hands or feet, dry eyes or mouth. Call the doctor if your child experiences swelling of feet or legs, palpitations, difficulty breathing, hallucinations, confusion, unusual bleeding, tingling of hands or feet.

Possible Drug Interactions
- Aspirin and similar nonsteroidal, anti-inflammatory drugs may decrease the blood pressure-lowering activity of this drug.

- Cimetidine (Tagamet) and birth control pills can increase the side effects of this drug.

- Decongestants in cold and sinus medications can increase blood pressure when taken with this drug.

- Certain tranquilizers such as the phenothiazine group and the monoamine oxidase (MAO) inhibitors can cause excessively slow heart rate and low blood pressure when taken with this drug.

- Alcohol, barbiturate sedatives, and rifampin can decrease the effectiveness of this drug.

- This drug can decrease the therapeutic effect of asthma medications such as theophylline, albuterol, terbutaline, and metaproterenol.

- This drug can affect blood sugar levels in children with diabetes and mask symptoms of low blood sugar, such as fast heartbeat.

Brand Name: Tenormin

Generic Available: Yes

Type of Drug: Beta-adrenergic blocking agent (beta blocker)

Use: Treats abnormally fast heart rhythms (tachycardia), high blood pressure (hypertension), or chest pain in adults (angina). Also prevents migraine headaches.

Time Required for Drug to Take Effect: Several days to several weeks

Dosage Forms and Strengths: Tablets (25 mg, 50 mg, 100 mg); Injection (5 mg/10 mL)

Storage: Store at room temperature in tightly closed, light-resistant containers.

How This Drug Works: Controls nerve impulses that excite the heart, causing the heart to beat more slowly.

Tell Your Doctor If
• Your child is taking any other medications.

• Your child has allergies; asthma; wheezing; slow heartbeat; diabetes mellitus; heart or blood vessel disease; or liver, thyroid, or kidney disease.

• Your daughter is or becomes pregnant.

• Your daughter is breast-feeding her baby. This drug can pass into breast milk and may cause side effects in the baby.

Special Instructions
• Do not stop giving this drug to your child without first contacting the doctor.

Symptoms of Overdose: Excessively slow heartbeat, low blood pressure, difficulty breathing, unconsciousness

Be Accurate

If you don't give medication correctly, it may be ineffective or even cause side effects. An estimated 10 to 30 percent of medications aren't effective because they have been given incorrectly. To do it right, you have to give the exact amount of medicine prescribed at the scheduled time, for the specified duration, and in the appropriate manner. Always read the label, follow the directions carefully, and use the appropriate equipment for measuring and administering the medication. Also, be sure to wash your hands before you give any medication to your child.

ATTAPULGITE

Administration Guidelines

- Give after each loose bowel movement. Follow dosing directions on the package.

- Do not give to children younger than 3 years of age unless instructed to do so by your child's doctor.

- Do not exceed the maximum daily dose for your child's age as listed on the product dosing directions.

Side Effects

Tell your child's doctor about any side effects that are persistent or particularly bothersome.

More Common. Constipation

Possible Drug Interactions

- May interfere with the absorption of digoxin, clindamycin, promazine, tetracycline, and penicillamine.

Tell Your Child's Doctor If

- Your child has had allergic reactions to any medications.

- Your child has any diseases or is taking any other medications.

- Your daughter is or becomes pregnant.

- Your daughter is breast-feeding her baby.

Special Instructions

- Do not use if your child has a fever, bloody stools, or mucus in the stools. Contact the doctor.

- Do not give within 2 to 3 hours of any other medication. This drug may prevent the absorption of other medications.

- Contact the doctor if your child's diarrhea does not stop in 1 to 2 days.

Symptoms of Overdose: Severe constipation

Brand Names: Diasorb, Donnagel, Kaopectate, K-Pek, Parepectolin, Rheaban

Generic Available: No

Type of Drug: Antidiarrheal agent

Use: Treats diarrhea.

Time Required for Drug to Take Effect: 1 to 2 days

Dosage Forms and Strengths: Tablets (600 mg, 750 mg); Liquid (750 mg per 5 mL)

Storage: Store at room temperature in tightly closed, light-resistant containers.

How This Drug Works: Believed to work by adsorbing bacteria that may be causing the diarrhea.

Brand Name: Imuran

Generic Available: No

Type of Drug: Immunosuppressant

Use: Prevents rejection of kidney transplants and controls symptoms of severe rheumatoid arthritis.

Time Required for Drug to Take Effect: Can take up to 6 to 8 weeks.

Dosage Form and Strength: Tablets (50 mg)

Storage: Store at room temperature in tightly closed, light-resistant containers. Do not refrigerate.

How This Drug Works: The exact mechanism of action has not been well established.

AZATHIOPRINE

Administration Guidelines
• Give once a day.

• Give with food or after a meal to prevent nausea and vomiting.

• Missed doses: Give as soon as possible if it is between morning and bedtime of the same day. Otherwise, skip the missed dose and return to the regular dosing schedule. Do not give double doses. If you miss more than 1 dose, check with your child's doctor.

Side Effects
Tell your child's doctor about any side effects that are persistent or particularly bothersome.

More Common. It is especially important to tell the doctor if your child experiences darkened urine, fever, hair loss, joint pains, mouth sores, muscle aches, skin rash, sore throat, unusual bleeding or bruising, or yellowing of the eyes or skin. This drug may cause serious side effects months or years later, depending on the dose and duration of therapy. These delayed effects may include certain types of cancer. Be sure to discuss these possible effects with the doctor.

Less Common. Diarrhea, nausea, or vomiting. These side effects should disappear as your child's body adjusts to this drug.

Possible Drug Interactions
• Allopurinol can increase the blood levels of this drug, which can lead to serious side effects.

• May decrease the effect of anticoagulants (blood thinners) such as warfarin.

Tell Your Child's Doctor If
• Your child has had unusual or allergic reactions to any medications, especially those experienced when previously taking this drug.

• Your child has, or ever had, gout, kidney or liver disease, pancreatitis, or recurrent infections.

• Your child experiences unusual bleeding or bruising, fever, sore throat, mouth sores, signs of infection, stomach pain, pale stools, or darkened urine.

• Your child is taking allopurinol.

• Your daughter is or becomes pregnant. This drug is not recommended for use during pregnancy. Birth defects can occur if the mother or the father is taking this drug at the time of conception.

Special Instructions

• Do not stop giving this drug without first consulting the doctor. Stopping this drug abruptly may cause your child's condition to worsen.

• This drug can decrease your child's resistance to infection; contact the doctor at the first sign of infection.

Symptoms of Overdose: Nausea, vomiting, diarrhea. Very large doses may lead to marrow underdevelopment, bleeding, infection, and death.

Special Notes

• This drug is very potent; blood tests will be used occasionally to monitor the drug and to make sure the smallest dose possible is given.

• Females of child-bearing potential should be advised not to become pregnant.

☎ Just Call

If you have any concerns about any side effects, even minor ones, you should be sure to discuss them with your child's doctor. The doctor may be able to minimize or eliminate the side effects by prescribing a different medication or changing your child's dosage, dosing schedule, or the way the drug should be given. (Do not make adjustments on your own without discussing them with your doctor.) At the very least, the doctor can assure you that the medication's benefits far outweigh its side effects.

Brand Name: Zithromax

Generic Available: No

Type of Drug: Antibiotic

Use: Treats a wide variety of bacterial infections, such as those of the middle ear, upper and lower respiratory tracts, and skin, as well as certain sexually transmitted diseases.

Time Required for Drug to Take Effect: It may take a few days to affect the infection.

Dosage Forms and Strengths: Capsules (250 mg); Solution (100 mg and 200 mg per 5 mL); Suspension (1 gram single-dose pack)

Storage: Refrigerate liquids; store capsules at room temperature. Store both forms in tightly closed, light-resistant containers.

How This Drug Works: Prevents bacteria from manufacturing protein, thus preventing their growth. Kills certain bacteria but is not effective against viruses, parasites, or fungi.

AZITHROMYCIN

Administration Guidelines
- Works best if given on an empty stomach (1 hour before or 2 hours after a meal).

- Generally administered once a day. The initial dose is higher than the subsequent doses in order to achieve therapeutic blood concentrations.

- Works best when blood concentrations are kept within a safe and effective range. Give doses at the same time every day.

- Missed doses: Give immediately unless it is time for the next dose. Do not give double doses.

- Give this drug for the entire time prescribed by your child's doctor (usually 5 days), even if symptoms disappear.

Side Effects
Tell your child's doctor about any side effects that are persistent or particularly bothersome.

More Common. Diarrhea, nausea, vomiting, abdominal pain, headache, dizziness. These side effects should disappear as your child's body adjusts to this drug.

Less Common. It is especially important to tell the doctor if your child experiences fever, palpitations, chest pain, rash, shortness of breath, swelling of the face or neck, sore throat, rectal or vaginal itching, unusual bruising or bleeding, or yellowing of the eyes or skin.

Possible Drug Interactions
- This drug can increase blood levels of aminophylline, theophylline, carbamazepine, cyclosporin, phenytoin, digoxin, triazolam, phenobarbital, ergotamine, dihydroergotamine, or oral anticoagulants (blood thinners, such as warfarin), which may lead to serious side effects.

- Antacids containing aluminum and magnesium will decrease the efficacy of this drug. Give these antacids 1 hour before or 2 hours after a dose of this drug.

- Terfenadine, astemizole, and loratidine may cause an irregular heart rate when taken with this drug.

Tell Your Child's Doctor If
- Your child is taking any prescription or nonprescription medications.

- Your child has had unusual reactions to any medications, especially to this drug, erythromycin, or clarithromycin.

- Your child has or ever had kidney disease, liver disease, or heart disease.

- Your child's symptoms of infection seem to be getting worse.

- Your child is taking this drug before any surgery or any other medical or dental treatment.

- Your daughter is or becomes pregnant.

- Your daughter is breast-feeding her baby. It is not known if this drug passes into breast milk.

Special Instructions

- Can cause increased sensitivity to sunlight. Your child should avoid prolonged exposure to sunlight and sunlamps. Make sure your child wears protective clothing and uses an effective sunscreen when out-of-doors.

- Do not use this drug to treat a subsequent infection unless you consult the doctor.

Symptoms of Overdose: Severe diarrhea, heartburn, nausea, or vomiting

To Each His Own

If one of your children has been prescribed an antibiotic and another child gets sick, it is not safe to give the antibiotic to the child for whom it was not prescribed. The medication may not be the appropriate one for the other child—even if the children's symptoms are similar. Treating an infection with the wrong drug may make the condition worse instead of better. What's more, children respond to the same drug differently and may need different dosages. The child who became ill first needs the drug in the amount prescribed for the time advised; otherwise, it may not be effective. If you think another child needs medication, consult the doctor.

Brand Names: AK-Tracin Ophthalmic, Baciguent,* Bacitracin,* various manufacturers (*available over the counter)

Generic Available: Yes

Type of Drug: Antibiotic

Use: Prevents or treats superficial skin infections or infections of the eye.

Time Required for Drug to Take Effect: 4 to 7 days

Dosage Forms and Strengths: Ophthalmic ointment (500 units/g); Topical ointment (500 units/g)

Storage: Store at room temperature in tightly closed containers. Do not freeze.

How This Drug Works: Inhibits bacterial growth by inhibiting bacterial cell wall growth.

BACITRACIN

Administration Guidelines
• Do not use longer than 1 week unless directed to do so by your child's doctor.

• Do not use topical ointment in the eyes.

• Wash your hands with soap and water before applying.

• Do not touch the tip of the ophthalmic ointment tube or let it touch the eyes.

• See Chapter 5, page 14, for instructions for administering eye ointments.

Side Effects
Tell your child's doctor about any side effects that are persistent or particularly bothersome.

More Common. Rash, itching

Less Common. Nausea, vomiting, diarrhea, generalized itching, swelling of the lips and face

Tell Your Child's Doctor If
• Your child's eyes do not improve, or seem to be getting worse, after 1 to 2 days of treatment.

• Your child experiences redness, irritation, swelling, decreasing vision, or pain after 1 to 2 days of treatment.

Symptoms of Overdose: When applied topically or ophthalmically, it is difficult, if not impossible, to experience an overdose.

Special Notes
• Ophthalmic ointment may cause blurred vision temporarily.

BACLOFEN

Administration Guidelines
• Give on an empty stomach or with food or milk.

• Missed doses: Give as soon as you remember, then stagger subsequent doses evenly for the rest of the day. Do not give double doses.

Side Effects
Tell your child's doctor about any side effects that are persistent or particularly bothersome.

More Common. Dizziness, drowsiness, confusion, light-headedness, nausea, weakness

Less Common. Abdominal discomfort, clumsiness, trembling, constipation, diarrhea, frequent or painful urination, headache, loss of appetite, muscle pain, tingling of hands or feet, stuffy nose, trouble sleeping. Contact the doctor if your child experiences bloody or dark urine, chest pain, hallucinations, mood changes, ringing in the ears, skin rash, or itching.

Possible Drug Interactions
• Other central nervous system depressants (alcohol, antihistamines, muscle relaxants, tranquilizers, pain medications) can cause extreme drowsiness when used with this drug.

Tell Your Child's Doctor If
• Your child has had allergic reactions to any medications.

• Your child has any diseases or is taking any medications.

• Your daughter is or becomes pregnant.

• Your daughter is breast-feeding her baby. This drug may pass into breast milk; however, the American Academy of Pediatrics considers it compatible with breast-feeding in most cases.

Special Instructions
• Do not stop giving this drug before talking with the doctor. Abruptly stopping this drug could cause hallucinations, mood changes, or convulsions. Therefore, the doctor may want to gradually reduce your child's dose.

Symptoms of Overdose: Blurred or double vision, convulsions, severe muscle weakness, shortness of breath, slurred speech, vomiting

Brand Name: Lioresal

Generic Available: Yes

Type of Drug: Muscle relaxant

Use: Relieves muscle spasms.

Time Required for Drug to Take Effect: 3 to 4 days. It may take 1 week to achieve full effect.

Dosage Form and Strengths: Tablets (10 mg, 20 mg)

Storage: Store tablets at room temperature in tightly closed containers.

How This Drug Works: Acts on the central nervous system to relieve spasms.

Brand Names: Beclovent, Vanceril

Generic Available: No

Type of Drug: Inhalation corticosteroid

Use: Prevents asthma symptoms.

Time Required for Drug to Take Effect: May take as long as 4 weeks to begin to work. Several months may be needed for full effect.

Dosage Form and Strength: Aerosol (42 mcg/puff)

Storage: Store at room temperature in original container.

How This Drug Works: Acts locally in the lungs to decrease inflammation.

BECLOMETHASONE DIPROPIONATE (INHALATION)

Administration Guidelines

• Shake the canister at least 10 times before administering.

• Rinse your child's mouth with water after each dose. Make sure your child does not swallow the water after rinsing.

• Allow at least 1 minute between each puff.

• If your child also uses a bronchodilator inhaler such as isoproterenol, metaproterenol, or epinephrine, give it several minutes before giving this drug.

• This drug must be given regularly to be effective.

• Do not give more often than your child's doctor prescribed.

• Missed doses: Give as soon as you remember. However, if it is time for the next dose, skip the missed dose and give the next dose at the scheduled time. Do not give double doses.

Side Effects

Tell your child's doctor about any side effects that are persistent or particularly bothersome.

More Common. Cough, dry mouth, hoarseness, sore throat

Less Common. Dry throat, headache, nausea, unpleasant taste, skin bruising or thinning. Contact the doctor if your child has white patches in the mouth or throat, pain when swallowing, or experiences nervousness, restlessness, or behavior changes.

Tell Your Child's Doctor If

• Your child has had allergic reactions to or is taking any medications.

• Your child has a sore throat or mouth sores.

• Your child is taking this drug before surgery or any medical or dental procedure.

• Your daughter is or becomes pregnant.

• Your daughter is breast-feeding her baby.

Special Instructions

• Do not use this drug to relieve an asthma attack.

• Clean the inhaler, mouthpiece, and spacer (if your child uses one) at least 2 times a week to prevent blockage.

Symptoms of Overdose: Acne, rounding of the face, menstrual changes

BECLOMETHASONE DIPROPIONATE (NASAL)

Administration Guidelines
• Have your child blow the nose to clear the nasal passages before administering.

• Shake the canister at least 10 times before administering.

• Insert the nosepiece into your child's nostril and spray toward the inner corner of the eye.

• Do not give more often than your child's doctor prescribed.

• Missed doses: Give immediately. However, if it is time for the next scheduled dose, skip the missed dose and give the next dose at its scheduled time. Do not give double doses.

Side Effects
Tell your child's doctor about any side effects that are persistent or particularly bothersome.

More Common. Burning, irritation, or drying inside the nose; throat irritation; increased sneezing

Less Common. Contact the doctor if your child experiences bloody nose mucus; unexplained nosebleeds; white patches or sores in the nose; eye pain; gradual loss of vision; headache; hives; dizziness; loss of sense of taste or smell; nausea or vomiting; shortness of breath; wheezing; skin rash; sore throat; hoarseness; stomach pains; white patches in the throat; unusual fatigue or weakness; or swelling of the eyelids, lips, or face.

Tell Your Child's Doctor If
• Your child has had allergic reactions to any medications.

• Your child has any diseases or is taking any medications.

• Your child has symptoms of a nose or throat infection.

• Your daughter is or becomes pregnant.

• Your daughter is breast-feeding her baby.

Symptoms of Overdose: Rounding of the face, menstrual changes

Special Notes
• This drug must be given regularly to be effective.

Brand Names: Beconase, Beconase AQ, Vancenase, Vancenase AQ

Generic Available: No

Type of Drug: Nasal corticosteroid

Use: Relieves the stuffy nose and discomfort of hay fever and other allergies. Also prevents nasal polyps from growing back after surgical removal.

Time Required for Drug to Take Effect: Usually begins to work in about 1 week; 3 weeks may be needed to achieve full effect.

Dosage Form and Strength: Aerosol (42 mcg/puff)

Storage: Store at room temperature in original container.

How This Drug Works: Decreases inflammation in the nose.

Brand Names: Dulcolax, Carter's Little Pill, Fleet Bisacodyl Enema, Clysodrast

Generic Available: Yes

Type of Drug: Laxative, stimulant

Use: Treats constipation and cleans out the large bowel prior to surgery or medical tests.

Time Required for Drug to Take Effect: 15 to 60 minutes for rectal suppository; 6 to 10 hours for tablets

Dosage Forms and Strengths: Tablets (5 mg); Rectal suppository (10 mg); Enema (10 mg/30 mL); Powder for enema (1.5 mg with 2.5 mg tannic acid per packet). Also available in combination with other laxatives.

Storage: Store at room temperature in tightly closed, light-resistant containers. Store powder in a dry place.

How This Drug Works: Stimulates nerve endings in intestinal walls, which leads to increased movement of stool through the intestines.

BISACODYL

Administration Guidelines
• Give tablets on an empty stomach with plenty of water.

• Tablets should not be chewed, crushed, or given within 1 hour of milk, dairy products, or antacids. This will remove the special coating that prevents stomach irritation.

• Mix the powder in 1 liter of water and use the solution immediately after mixing.

• Do not give regularly for more than 1 week.

Side Effects
Tell your child's doctor about any side effects that are persistent or particularly bothersome.

Less Common. Mild abdominal cramps, nausea, vomiting, rectal burning, or skin irritation around rectal area. Contact the doctor if your child has rectal bleeding, blistering, burning, itching, or pain.

Possible Drug Interactions
• Milk, dairy products, and antacids decrease the effect and increase stomach irritation when used with the tablet form of this drug.

Tell Your Child's Doctor If
• Your child has had an allergic reaction to this drug or any other medication.

• Your child has taken or is taking any other medications.

• Your child experiences a sudden change in bowel movements that either lasts longer than 2 weeks or returns intermittently.

• Your daughter is or becomes pregnant. This drug generally is not used during pregnancy or while breast-feeding.

Special Instructions
• Do not use if your child has abdominal pain, appendicitis, intestinal blockage, nausea, vomiting, or rectal bleeding.

• Do not use this drug in children younger than 10 years of age.

• Do not give tablets to children younger than 6 years of age or to those children who cannot swallow tablets whole.

• Do not use suppositories in children younger than 6 years of age unless prescribed by the doctor.

• Do not give enemas to children younger than 2 years of age.

Symptoms of Overdose: Diarrhea, abdominal pain, or electrolyte and fluid disturbances

BISMUTH SUBSALICYLATE

Administration Guidelines

- Shake liquid well before measuring each dose.

- Have your child chew the tablets or let them dissolve in the mouth before swallowing.

- Missed doses: If giving this drug on a regular schedule, give the missed dose if you remember within 1 hour. Otherwise, skip the missed dose and go back to the regular schedule. Do not give double doses.

Side Effects

Tell your child's doctor about any side effects that are persistent or particularly bothersome.

More Common. Gray to black stools, darkening of the tongue

Less Common. Contact the doctor if your child experiences severe constipation, loss of hearing, ringing in ears, anxiety, confusion, slurred speech, headaches, mental depression, muscle spasms, uncontrolled body movements, severe diarrhea, fast or deep breathing, dizziness, light-headedness, severe drowsiness, increased sweating, increased thirst, severe nausea or vomiting, or severe stomach pain.

Possible Drug Interactions

- Aspirin and aspirin-containing products increase the risk of salicylate toxicity.

- Decreases the absorption of tetracycline.

- Increases the risk of bleeding when used with warfarin.

- Medications to control diabetes can cause problems with low blood sugar.

Tell Your Child's Doctor If

- Your child has had an allergic reaction to this drug; aspirin; salicylates; oil of wintergreen; ibuprofen or other nonsteroidal anti-inflammatory agents; or any other medication, foods, preservatives, or dyes.

- Your child has kidney disease, bleeding in the intestines or stomach, a bleeding disorder, dehydration, bloody diarrhea, or any other medical condition.

- Your child has symptoms of the flu or chicken pox.

- Your child's diarrhea continues for more than 2 days.

Brand Names: Pepto-Bismol, Bismatrol

Generic Available: Yes

Type of Drug: Antidiarrheal, gastrointestinal agent, antiulcer agent

Use: Treats mild, nonspecific diarrhea; prevents or treats traveler's diarrhea. Relieves the symptoms of upset stomach such as heartburn, indigestion, and nausea. Also used with other medications to treat ulcers caused by *Helicobacter pylori* bacteria.

Time Required for Drug to Take Effect: 30 minutes to 1 hour

Dosage Forms and Strengths: Liquid (262 mg/15 mL with 130 mg salicylate, 524 mg/15 mL with 236 mg salicylate); Tablets, chewable (262 mg, contains 102 mg of salicylate); Caplets (262 mg)

Storage: Store at room temperature in tightly closed containers. Do not freeze the liquid.

How This Drug Works: Absorbs extra water and toxins in the large intestine; forms a protective coating in the intestine.

• Your daughter is breast-feeding her baby. The American Academy of Pediatrics recommends caution when giving this drug to nursing mothers.

Special Instructions

• Do not give to children younger than 3 years of age unless prescribed by the doctor.

• This product contains salicylate. Do not give if your child has symptoms of the flu or chicken pox unless directed to do so by the doctor.

Symptoms of Overdose: Ringing in ears, fever, seizures

Special Notes

• Children with fever and dehydration are more susceptable to the toxic effects of salicylates.

• This drug is not recommended for the treatment of acute diarrhea in children, according to the American Academy of Pediatrics' 1996 guidelines.

Over-the-Counter Wisdom

Keep in mind that even a medication that is available without a doctor's prescription may still be harmful and should be given appropriately and only when necessary. Talk to your pediatrician about what to do if your child gets sick. Some illnesses can be treated at home, some require a call to the pediatrician's office, and some will require a visit to the doctor. In addition, ask the doctor what situations constitute an emergency. If you're not sure if it's safe or appropriate to give your child a particular over-the-counter medication, be sure to talk to the doctor first.

BROMPHENIRAMINE

Administration Guidelines
• Do not crush or allow your child to chew timed-release tablets.

• Give timed-release preparations only as directed by your child's doctor.

• Usually given every 4 to 6 hours; timed-release tablets usually given every 8 to 12 hours.

Side Effects
Tell your child's doctor about any side effects that are persistent or particularly bothersome.

More Common. It is especially important to tell the doctor if your child experiences a change in menstruation, clumsiness, feeling faint, flushing of the face, hallucinations, palpitations, rash, seizures, shortness of breath, sleeping disorders, sore throat, fever, tightness in the chest, unusual bleeding or bruising, or unusual fatigue or weakness. This drug may impair your child's ability to perform activities requiring alertness.

Less Common. Blurred vision; confusion; constipation; diarrhea; difficult or painful urination; dizziness; dry mouth, throat, or nose; headache; irritability; loss of appetite; nausea; restlessness; ringing or buzzing in the ears; stomach upset; or unusual increase in sweating. These side effects should disappear as your child's body adjusts to this drug. This drug also can cause increased sensitivity to sunlight.

Possible Drug Interactions
• Other central nervous system depressants, such as alcohol, barbiturates, benzodiazepine tranquilizers, muscle relaxants, narcotics, pain medications, and phenothiazine tranquilizers or tricyclic antidepressants can cause extreme drowsiness.

• Monoamine oxidase (MAO) inhibitors can increase the side effects of this drug. At least 14 days should separate the use of this drug and an MAO inhibitor.

• Can decrease the effectiveness of oral anticoagulants (blood thinners).

Tell Your Child's Doctor If
• Your child has high blood pressure, heart disease, diabetes, thyroid disease, asthma, or glaucoma.

• Your child has had unusual or allergic reactions to any medications, especially to this drug or to any other antihistamine such as carbinoxamine, chlorpheniramine, clemastine, and cyproheptadine.

Brand Names: Brompheniramine (various manufacturers), Bromarest,* Bromphen Elixir,* Chlorphed,* Codimal-A,* Cophene-B,* Dehist,* Diamine T.D.,* Dimetane Oral,* Veltane Tablet (*available over the counter)

Generic Available: Yes

Type of Drug: Antihistamine

Use: Treats or prevents symptoms of allergy.

Time Required for Drug to Take Effect: Begins working within 3 to 9 hours; can last up to 48 hours.

Dosage Forms and Strengths: Elixir (2 mg per 5 mL, contains 3% alcohol); Tablets (4 mg, 8 mg); Tablets, timed-release (8 mg, 12 mg)

Storage: Store at room temperature in tightly closed containers away from heat and other flammable agents.

How This Drug Works: Blocks the action of histamine, a chemical released by the body during an allergic reaction.

Special Instructions

• Your child should avoid prolonged exposure to sunlight. Have your child wear protective clothing and use an effective sunscreen when out-of-doors.

• Extended-release tablets are not recommended for children younger than 6 years of age. For children between 6 and 12 years of age, give only under the direction of the doctor.

• The elixir is flammable. Do not expose it to an open flame or ignited material such as a lighted cigarette.

• Be sure you know how your child is reacting to this drug before allowing participation in activities that require alertness, such as riding a bicycle.

Symptoms of Overdose: Toxic effects occur within 30 minutes to 2 hours. Effects may vary from symptoms of central nervous system depression (sedation, temporary cessation of breathing, diminished mental alertness) and cardiovascular collapse to stimulation (insomnia, hallucinations, tremors, or convulsions). Profound low blood pressure, respiratory depression, unconsciousness, coma, and death may occur.

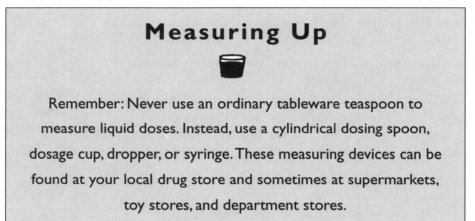

Measuring Up

Remember: Never use an ordinary tableware teaspoon to measure liquid doses. Instead, use a cylindrical dosing spoon, dosage cup, dropper, or syringe. These measuring devices can be found at your local drug store and sometimes at supermarkets, toy stores, and department stores.

BUDESONIDE

Administration Guidelines
- For nasal use only.

- Shake well just before each use to distribute ingredients evenly and equalize the doses.

- Have your child clear nasal passages by blowing the nose before using.

- Read package directions carefully before giving to your child. You may wish to consult your child's doctor or pharmacist about the proper administration of this drug.

- If more than 1 inhalation is necessary, wait at least 1 full minute between doses to obtain the full benefit of the first dose.

- Missed doses: Give immediately if you remember within 1 hour; then follow your regular dosing schedule. Otherwise, just wait until the next scheduled dose. Do not give double doses.

Side Effects
Tell your child's doctor about any side effects that are persistent or particularly bothersome.

More Common. Mild nose and throat irritation, nose irritation (burning, stinging, dryness)

Less Common. Inflammation of the throat, cough, dry mouth, indigestion, hoarseness, nasal pain, facial swelling, rash, itching, nervousness, hair loss

Tell Your Child's Doctor If
- Symptoms do not improve after 3 weeks of treatment.

- The condition worsens or sneezing or nasal irritation occurs.

- Your daughter is or becomes pregnant. The effects of this drug during pregnancy have not been thoroughly studied in humans.

- Your daughter is breast-feeding her baby. It is not known if this drug appears in breast milk.

Special Instructions
- Do not abruptly stop giving this drug. The doctor may want to gradually decrease the dose to avoid adverse side effects.

Symptoms of Overdose: Steroid-induced imbalances in the body, such as suppression of hypothalamic-pituitary-adrenal function, suppression of growth, or hypercorticism may occur.

Brand Name: Rhinocort

Generic Available: No

Type of Drug: Nasal corticosteroid

Use: Manages symptoms of seasonal or perennial rhinitis (inflammation of the mucous membranes of the nose).

Time Required for Drug to Take Effect: Symptoms may decrease in 24 hours, but it generally takes 3 to 7 days to achieve maximum benefit.

Dosage Form and Strength: Aerosol (50 mcg released per actuation, delivering approximately 32 mcg via nasal adaptor)

Storage: Store away from excessive heat. The contents are pressurized and can explode if heated.

How This Drug Works: Reduces inflammation of the nose and upper portion of the throat.

Brand Name: Kocaltrol

Generic Available: No

Type of Drug: Vitamin (a form of Vitamin D)

Use: Treats low calcium levels, especially in patients on long-term renal dialysis. Also used for elevated parathyroid hormone concentrations and for rickets.

Time Required for Drug to Take Effect: It may take up to 4 weeks to achieve maximum benefit.

Dosage Form and Strength: Capsules (0.25 and 0.5 mcg)

Storage: Store at room temperature in tightly closed, light-resistant containers.

How This Drug Works: Promotes the absorption of calcium in the intestines and prevents excessive calcium loss through the kidneys. Both these effects increase the level of calcium in the body.

CALCITRIOL

Administration Guidelines

• Give with food to avoid stomach upset. Can also be given on an empty stomach.

• Generally given once a day or once every other day.

• Works best when blood concentrations are kept within a safe and effective range. Give at the same time each day or every other day, depending on your child's dosing schedule.

• Do not stop giving this drug without first checking with your child's doctor.

• Missed doses: Give immediately. However, if it is time for the next dose, skip the missed dose and continue with the regular schedule. Do not give double doses.

Side Effects

Tell your child's doctor about any side effects that are persistent or particularly bothersome.

More Common. Weakness, drowsiness, headache, increased body temperature, itching, dry mouth, constipation, nausea, vomiting, loss of appetite, metallic taste, weight loss

Less Common. It is especially important to tell the doctor if your child experiences bone pain; frequent urination, especially at nighttime; difficulty with eyesight; and general weakness.

Possible Drug Interactions

• May reduce the effect of calcium channel-blocking drugs such as verapamil, nifedipine, isradipine, and diltiazem if blood calcium levels are increased too much.

• May increase the risk of digoxin toxicity.

• Thiazide diuretics such as chlorothiazide and hydrochlorothiazide may cause very high calcium levels when used with this drug.

Tell Your Child's Doctor If

• Your child is taking any prescription or nonprescription medications, especially any of those listed above.

• Your child has or ever had unusual or allergic reactions to any medications, especially to this drug.

• Your child has or ever had any diseases of the kidney, liver, or pancreas.

• Your daughter is or becomes pregnant. Studies in humans have not been conducted using high doses of this drug.

• Your daughter is breast-feeding her baby. A small amount of this drug will pass into breast milk.

Symptoms of Overdose: Severe nausea, vomiting, loss of consciousness, and convulsions

Special Notes

• The doctor may request frequent visits at the start of therapy to check calcium concentrations in the blood and to adjust the dose to suit your child's needs.

Keep a Lid on It

Pharmacists are required to put drugs in bottles that have child-resistant caps. Don't switch to a bottle that's easier for you to open—children may also find it easier to open. Remember, too, that child-resistant does not mean childproof. Children older than five years of age may be able to open most medicine bottles. That's why it's essential for you to teach them that drugs can be harmful if not taken correctly and that they need supervision before taking anything. And, just to be on the safe side, keep all medicines out of your child's reach.

Brand Names: Rolaids Calcium Rich, Tums, Tums 500, Tums E-X, Caltrate 600, Caltrate Chewable, Calcium 600, Calci-Chew, Os-Cal 250, Os-Cal 500, Titralac, Neo-Calglucon

Generic Available: Yes

Type of Drug: Calcium supplement, antacid

Use: Treats and prevents low calcium levels. Also treats heartburn and acid indigestion.

Time Required for Drug to Take Effect: Within minutes for heartburn relief.

Dosage Forms and Strengths: Tablets, chewable tablets, capsules, and liquids available in many different strengths.

Storage: Store at room temperature in tightly closed containers. Do not freeze the liquid.

How This Drug Works: Calcium carbonate neutralizes the acid in the stomach and provides additional calcium when insufficient amounts are consumed in the diet.

CALCIUM SUPPLEMENTS

Administration Guidelines
• Shake liquid well before measuring each dose.

• Give your child 4 to 8 ounces of water or juice to drink with each dose.

• Give 1 to 1½ hours after meals for best calcium absorption. Calcium glubionate syrup (Neo-Calglucon), however, should be given before meals for best absorption.

• Tablets should be chewed completely.

• Usually given 3 or 4 times a day.

• Do not give within 1 to 2 hours of other medications. This drug may decrease their absorption.

• Do not give within 1 to 2 hours of eating large amounts of fiber-containing foods such as whole-grain breads and cereals.

• Missed doses: If on a regular schedule, give the missed dose as soon as you remember; then go back to the regular schedule.

Side Effects
Tell your child's doctor about any side effects that are persistent or particularly bothersome.

More Common. Constipation, intestinal gas

Less Common. Contact the doctor if your child experiences difficult or painful urination, drowsiness, vomiting not associated with a virus, nausea or weakness, severe constipation, dry mouth, increased thirst, headache, irritability, mental depression, metallic taste.

Possible Drug Interactions
• Decreases the absorption of tetracycline, phenytoin, and iron.

• May cause abnormal heart rhythms when used with digoxin. Only use calcium with digoxin if prescribed by the doctor.

• Decreases the absorption of ciprofloxacin, norfloxacin, and ofloxacin. If possible, do not take calcium while taking these medications.

• Large amounts of alcohol or caffeine decreases calcium absorption.

• Tobacco use decreases calcium absorption.

Tell Your Child's Doctor If
• Your child has heart or parathyroid disease, kidney stones or disease, increased calcium levels, sarcoidosis, or any other medical condition.

- Your child has taken or is taking any other prescription or nonprescription medicine.

- Your child has had an allergic reaction to this drug, any other medication, foods, preservatives, or dyes.

- Your daughter is or becomes pregnant.

Special Instructions

- Children with kidney failure should drink the amount of water recommended by their doctor when taking calcium.

- Your child (teenagers included) should not drink large amounts of alcohol or caffeine-containing beverages while taking this drug.

- Your child should not smoke cigarettes or use other tobacco products while taking calcium.

- Do not give if your child is also taking other medications containing large amounts of calcium, magnesium, or vitamin D unless directed to do so by the doctor.

Symptoms of Overdose: Lethargy, nausea, vomiting, coma, or increased blood calcium level.

Special Notes

- Calcium products such as calcium carbonate and calcium glubionate are not 100 percent calcium. Read product labels carefully to make sure your child gets the correct amount of calcium. The Recommended Dietary Allowance (RDA) for elemental calcium is:

  6–12 months: 600 mg/day
  1–10 years: 800 mg/day
  11–24 years: 1200 mg/day

- Choose calcium carbonate products that say "U.S.P." on the label because these provide optimal calcium absorption. Some calcium carbonate products were shown to break up too slowly in the stomach, leading to decreased calcium absorption.

Keep It Out of Reach

Do not rely on a child-resistant cap to deter your child from opening a bottle of medication. Child-resistant does not mean childproof. Legally, a cap can be called child-resistant if 80 percent of all five-year-olds need more than five minutes to open it. That means the other 20 percent could get into it in even less time. Put the bottle in a hard-to-reach cabinet with a childproof lock. Do not keep it on the countertop, kitchen table, or nightstand.

Brand Name: Capoten

Generic Available: No

Type of Drug: Angiotensin converting enzyme (ACE) inhibitor

Use: Treats high blood pressure and congestive heart failure. Also manages kidney disease resulting from diabetes.

Time Required for Drug to Take Effect: Several days to several weeks

Dosage Forms and Strengths: Tablets (12.5 mg, 25 mg, 50 mg, 100 mg). The pharmacist can also prepare a special liquid if necessary.

Storage: Store tablets at room temperature in tightly closed, light-resistant containers. Refrigerate liquid.

How This Drug Works: Decreases production of compounds in the body that normally cause blood vessels to constrict. Dilated blood vessels lower blood pressure and allow the heart to pump blood more easily.

CAPTOPRIL

Administration Guidelines

- Give on an empty stomach at least 1 hour before meals.

- Usually given 1 to 4 times a day.

- Missed doses: Give as soon as possible. However, if it's almost time for the next dose, skip the missed dose. Do not give double doses. Call your child's doctor or the pharmacist for more specific instructions.

- Do not stop giving this drug abruptly without first speaking with the doctor.

Side Effects

Tell your child's doctor about any side effects that are persistent or particularly bothersome.

More Common. Difficulty sleeping, coughing, headache, tingling of hands and feet, fatigue, nausea, vomiting, diarrhea, taste disturbances, constipation, dry mouth, itching, increased sensitivity to sunlight. Call the doctor if your child has a skin rash.

Less Common. Palpitations. Call the doctor if your child experiences difficulty breathing, difficulty urinating, fever, or chills.

Possible Drug Interactions

- Phenothiazine-type drugs such as promethazine (Phenergan), prochlorperazine (Compazine), and chlorpromazine (Thorazine) can increase the side effects of this drug. Use with caution.

- Digoxin or lithium dosing may require adjustment when given with this drug.

- Spironolactone, triamterene, amiloride, potassium supplements, and salt substitutes can cause blood potassium levels to become elevated more than is desired when taken with this drug.

- Nonsteroidal anti-inflammatory agents (such as indomethacin and ibuprofen) can decrease the effectiveness of this drug in lowering blood pressure.

Tell Your Child's Doctor If

- Your child has kidney or liver disease, lupus, or any blood disorder.

- Your daughter is or becomes pregnant. This drug can harm the fetus, especially if given during the second and third trimesters.

- Your daughter is breast-feeding her baby. This drug can pass into breast milk.

Special Instructions

• Do not give your child any medications for coughs, colds, sinus problems, allergies, or asthma without first speaking with the doctor or pharmacist.

• Do not give antacids with this drug.

• Speak to the doctor about other treatment options if coughing becomes a continuing problem.

• Your child should wear an effective sunscreen and protective clothing when out-of-doors.

Symptoms of Overdose: Excessively low blood pressure, dizziness, fainting

Special Notes

• This drug can cause a false-positive urine test for acetone.

• Your child may become dizzy with the first few doses. Have your child lie down for a while if this occurs.

Just Call

If you have any concerns about any side effects, even minor ones, you should be sure to discuss them with your child's doctor. The doctor may be able to minimize or eliminate the side effects by prescribing a different medication or changing your child's dosage, dosing schedule, or the way the drug is given. (Do not make adjustments on your own without discussing them with your doctor.) At the very least, the doctor can assure you that the medication's benefits far outweigh its side effects.

Brand Names: Epitol, Tegretol, Carbamazepine (various manufacturers)

Generic Available: Yes

Type of Drug: Anticonvulsant

Use: Treats seizure disorders, neuralgia, and some mental disorders.

Time Required for Drug to Take Effect: May take about 1 week to achieve full effectiveness.

Dosage Forms and Strengths: Tablets (200 mg); Tablets, chewable (100 mg); Suspension (100 mg per 5 mL)

Storage: Store at room temperature in tightly closed containers.

How This Drug Works: It is not completely understood how this drug works in the central nervous system to prevent seizures.

CARBAMAZEPINE

Administration Guidelines

• Give with food to avoid stomach upset.

• Shake suspension well to distribute ingredients and equalize doses.

• Works best when blood concentrations are kept within a safe and effective range. Give doses at evenly spaced intervals around the clock. If you are to give 4 doses a day, space them approximately 6 hours apart.

• Missed doses: Give as soon as you remember, then stagger subsequent doses evenly for the rest of the day. Do not give double doses. If your child is taking this drug for a seizure disorder, contact your child's doctor if 2 or more doses are missed.

Side Effects

Tell your child's doctor about any side effects that are persistent or particularly bothersome.

More Common. Constipation, diarrhea, dizziness, drowsiness, dry mouth, headache, loss of appetite, muscle or joint pain, nausea, increased sensitivity of skin to sunlight, increased sweating

Less Common. Contact the doctor immediately if your child experiences abdominal pain; black, tarry stools; chills; depression; difficulty breathing; difficulty urinating; fainting; fever; hallucinations; loss of balance; mouth sores; numbness or tingling sensations; ringing in the ears; skin rash; sore throat; swelling of the hands and feet; twitching of the eyes; blurred or double vision; unusual bleeding or bruising; yellow eyes or skin; behavioral changes; vomiting; an increased number of seizures; difficulty speaking or slurred speech.

Possible Drug Interactions

• Increases drowsiness when used with alcohol or medications that cause drowsiness such as antihistamines, sedatives, tranquilizers, or muscle relaxants.

• Erythromycin, clarithromycin, isoniazid, cimetidine, verapamil, or diltiazem may cause increased effects of this drug.

• May decrease the effects of phenytoin, valproic acid, theophylline, warfarin, cyclosporin, or doxycycline.

• Decreases the effectiveness of oral contraceptives. Your child should use an additional form of birth control while taking this drug.

Tell Your Child's Doctor If

• Your child has had allergic reactions to any medications.

• Your child has any diseases.

• Your child is taking any prescription or nonprescription medications.

• Your daughter is or becomes pregnant. Seizure activity should be well controlled during pregnancy and your daughter should be under the doctor's care.

• Your daughter is breast-feeding her baby. This drug passes into breast milk; however, the American Academy of Pediatrics considers it compatible with breast-feeding in most cases.

Special Instructions

• Do not suddenly stop giving this drug if your child is taking it for a seizure disorder.

• If your child is taking this drug for nerve pain, only give it for that type of pain.

• Before your child has surgery or any medical or dental treatment, tell the doctor performing the treatment that your child is taking this drug.

• This drug may increase your child's sensitivity to sunlight. Make sure your child wears protective clothing and a sunblock with an SPF of 15 or more when out-of-doors. Your child should not use a sunlamp or tanning bed while taking this drug.

• There may be differences in how your child's body reacts to various products of this drug. Therefore, contact the doctor before switching from one brand to another.

Symptoms of Overdose: Severe dizziness or clumsiness, severe drowsiness, slow breathing, seizures or abnormal twitching, severe vomiting, abnormal eye movements, large pupils

Special Notes

• The doctor will routinely monitor the blood concentration of this drug to ensure its effectiveness.

Brand Name: Ceclor

Generic Available: No

Type of Drug:
Cephalosporin antibiotic

Use: Treats a wide variety of bacterial infections, particularly those of the middle ear, skin, upper and lower respiratory tract, and urinary tract.

Time Required for Drug to Take Effect: It may take a few days for this drug to affect the infection.

Dosage Forms and Strengths: Capsules (250 mg, 500 mg); Suspension (125 mg, 187 mg, 250 mg, and 375 mg per 5 mL)

Storage: Refrigerate suspension; do not freeze. Store capsules at room temperature. Store both forms in tightly closed containers. Discard any unused portion of the oral suspension after 14 days.

How This Drug Works: Kills susceptible bacteria but is not effective against viruses, parasites, or fungi.

CEFACLOR

Administration Guidelines

- May be given either on an empty stomach or with food or a glass of milk (in order to avoid an upset stomach).

- Generally given 3 times a day.

- Give doses at evenly spaced intervals around the clock. If you are to give 3 doses a day, space them approximately 8 hours apart.

- Missed doses: Give immediately. However, if you don't remember to give the missed dose until it is time for the next dose, give the missed dose and space the next dose halfway through the regular interval between doses; then return to the regular schedule. Do not skip any doses.

- Shake the suspension well just before measuring each dose to distribute ingredients and equalize doses. The contents tend to settle on the bottom of the bottle.

- Give this drug for the entire time prescribed by your child's doctor (usually 7 to 14 days), even if symptoms disappear.

Side Effects

Tell your child's doctor about any side effects that are persistent or particularly bothersome.

More Common. Abdominal pain, diarrhea, dizziness, fatigue, headache, heartburn, loss of appetite, nausea, or vomiting. These side effects should disappear as your child's body adjusts to this drug.

Less Common. It is especially important to tell the doctor if your child experiences darkened tongue, difficulty in breathing, fever, itching, joint or lower back pain, rash, rectal or vaginal itching, severe diarrhea (which can be watery or can contain pus or blood), sore mouth, stomach cramps, tingling in the hands or feet, unusual bleeding or bruising, or painful or difficulty urinating.

Possible Drug Interactions

- Probenecid can increase the blood concentrations and side effects of this drug.

- Furosemide, bumetanide, ethacrynic acid, colistin, vancomycin, and polymyxin B can increase side effects, especially those on the kidneys.

Tell Your Child's Doctor If

- Your child is currently taking any prescription or nonprescription medications.

• Your child has had unusual or allergic reactions to any medication, especially to this drug or other cephalosporin antibiotics (such as cefamandole, cephalexin, cephradine, cefadroxil, cefazolin, cefixime, cefoperazone, cefotaxime, cefpodoxime, cefprozil, ceftizoxime, cephalothin, cephapirin, and cefuroxime) or to penicillin antibiotics.

• Your child has or ever had kidney disease.

• Your child's symptoms of infection seem to be getting worse.

• Your daughter is or becomes pregnant.

• Your daughter is breast-feeding her baby. Small amounts of this drug can pass into breast milk and temporarily cause diarrhea or other gastrointestinal disturbances in the nursing infant.

Special Instructions

• Children with diabetes may have a false-positive sugar reaction with a Clinitest urine glucose test. To avoid this problem, switch to Clinistix or Tes-Tape during treatment.

• Do not use this drug to treat a subsequent infection unless you consult the doctor.

Symptoms of Overdose: Nausea, vomiting, stomach pain, and severe diarrhea

Special Notes

• With long-term use of this drug, your child may develop a second infection in addition to the one being treated. Bacteria and organisms that are not susceptible to this drug can grow unchecked, causing a second infection that may require treatment with a different drug.

Teach Your Children Well

Let's face it. Kids can be pretty stubborn when it comes to accepting medication. When appropriate, try giving your child information about his or her condition and how the medicine works. In a nonthreatening voice, talk about the consequences of not taking the medication, perhaps reminding the child of how uncomfortable he or she was before beginning the medication. Use reasoning when possible, but don't scare the child. Children who understand the importance of antibiotics for infection, insulin for diabetes, or inhalants for asthma are more likely to take the medication without objection.

Brand Names: Duricef, Ultracef, Cefadroxil (various manufacturers)

Generic Available: Yes

Type of Drug: Cephalosporin antibiotic

Use: Treats a wide variety of bacterial infections, including those of the middle ear, skin, upper and lower respiratory tract, and urinary tract.

Time Required for Drug to Take Effect: It may take a few days for this drug to affect the infection.

Dosage Forms and Strengths: Tablets (1 g); Capsules (500 mg); Suspension (125 mg, 250 mg, and 500 mg per 5 mL)

Storage: Refrigerate suspension; do not freeze. Store tablets and capsules at room temperature in tightly closed containers. Discard any unused portion of the suspension after 14 days.

How This Drug Works: Kills susceptible bacteria but is ineffective against viruses, parasites, or fungi.

CEFADROXIL

Administration Guidelines

• Give either on an empty stomach or, to avoid upset stomach, with food or a glass of milk.

• Usually given 2 times a day.

• Give doses at evenly spaced intervals around the clock. If you are to give 2 doses a day, space them 12 hours apart.

• Missed doses: Give the missed dose immediately. However, if you don't remember until it is time for the next dose, give the missed dose and space the next dose halfway through the regular interval between doses; then return to the regular schedule. Try not to skip any doses.

• Shake the suspension well just before measuring each dose to distribute ingredients and equalize doses. The contents tend to settle on the bottom of the bottle.

• Give this drug for the entire time prescribed by your child's doctor (usually 7 to 14 days), even if symptoms disappear.

Side Effects

Tell your child's doctor about any side effects that are persistent or particularly bothersome.

More Common. Abdominal pain, diarrhea, dizziness, fatigue, headache, heartburn, loss of appetite, nausea, or vomiting. These side effects should disappear as your child's body adjusts to this drug.

Less Common. It is especially important to tell the doctor if your child experiences darkened tongue, difficulty in breathing, fever, itching, joint or lower back pain, rash, rectal or vaginal itching, severe diarrhea (which can be watery, or contain pus or blood), sore mouth, stomach cramps, tingling in the hands or feet, unusual bleeding or bruising, or painful or difficulty urinating.

Possible Drug Interactions

• Probenecid can increase the blood concentrations and side effects of this drug.

• Furosemide, bumetanide, ethacrynic acid, colistin, vancomycin, and polymyxin B can increase side effects, especially those on the kidneys.

Tell Your Child's Doctor If

• Your child is taking any other prescription or nonprescription medications.

• Your child has had unusual or allergic reactions to any medication, especially to this drug or other cephalosporin antibiotics (such as cefamandole, cephalexin, cefaclor, cephradine, cefazolin, cefixime, cefoperazone, cefotaxime, cefpodoxime, cefprozil, ceftizoxime, cephalothin, cephapirin, cefoxitin, and cefuroxime) or to penicillin antibiotics.

• Your child has or ever had kidney disease.

• Your child's symptoms of infection seem to be getting worse.

• Your daughter is or becomes pregnant.

Special Instructions
• Children with diabetes may have a false-positive sugar reaction with a Clinitest urine glucose test. To avoid this problem, switch to Clinistix or Tes-Tape during treatment.

• Do not use this drug to treat a subsequent infection unless you consult the doctor.

Symptoms of Overdose: Severe diarrhea, heartburn, nausea, or vomiting

Special Notes
• With long-term use of this drug, your child may develop a second infection in addition to the one being treated. Bacteria and organisms that are not susceptible to this drug can grow unchecked, causing a second infection that may require treatment with a different drug.

To Each His Own

If one of your children has been prescribed an antibiotic and another child gets sick, it is not safe to give the antibiotic to the child for whom it was not prescribed. The medication may not be the appropriate one for the other child—even if the children's symptoms are similar. Treating an infection with the wrong drug may make the condition worse instead of better. What's more, children respond to the same drug differently and may need different dosages. The child who became ill first needs the drug in the amount prescribed for the time advised; otherwise, it may not be effective. If you think another child needs medication, consult the doctor.

Brand Name: Suprax

Generic Available: No

Type of Drug:
Cephalosporin antibiotic

Use: Treats a wide variety of bacterial infections, particularly those of the middle ear, skin, upper and lower respiratory tract, and urinary tract.

Time Required for Drug to Take Effect: It may take a few days to affect the infection.

Dosage Forms and Strengths: Tablets (200 mg, 400 mg); Suspension (100 mg per 5 mL)

Storage: Refrigerate suspension; do not freeze. Store tablets at room temperature. Store both forms in tightly closed containers. Discard after 14 days any unused portion of the suspension.

How This Drug Works: Severely injures the cell walls of the infecting bacteria, preventing them from growing and multiplying.

CEFIXIME

Administration Guidelines

• Give on an empty stomach or with food or milk (to avoid stomach upset).

• Generally given 1 or 2 times a day.

• Works best when blood concentrations are kept within a safe and effective range. Give doses at evenly spaced intervals around the clock. If you are to give 2 doses a day, space them 12 hours apart.

• Missed doses: Give the missed dose immediately. However, if you don't remember until it is time for the next dose, give the missed dose and space the next dose halfway through the regular interval between doses; then return to the regular schedule. Try not to skip any doses.

• Shake the suspension well just before measuring each dose to distribute ingredients and equalize doses. The contents tends to settle on the bottom of the bottle.

• Give this drug for the entire time prescribed by your child's doctor (usually 7 to 14 days), even if symptoms disappear.

Side Effects

Tell your child's doctor about any side effects that are persistent or particularly bothersome.

More Common. Abdominal pain, diarrhea, dizziness, fatigue, headache, heartburn, loss of appetite, nausea, or vomiting. These side effects should disappear as your child's body adjusts to this drug.

Less Common. It is especially important to tell the doctor if your child experiences darkened tongue, difficulty in breathing, fever, itching, joint or lower back pain, rash, rectal or vaginal itching, severe diarrhea (which can be watery or contain pus or blood), sore mouth, stomach cramps, tingling in the hands or feet, unusual bleeding or bruising, or difficulty urinating.

Possible Drug Interactions

• Probenecid can increase the blood concentrations and side effects of this drug.

• Furosemide, bumetanide, ethacrynic acid, colistin, vancomycin, and polymyxin B can increase side effects, especially those affecting the kidneys.

Tell Your Child's Doctor If

• Your child has had unusual or allergic reactions to any medication, especially to this drug or other cephalosporin antibiotics (such as cefoperazone, cefotaxime, cefpodoxime, ceftazidime, ceftizoxime, and ceftriaxone) or to penicillin antibiotics.

• Your child is currently taking any prescription or nonprescription medications.

• Your child has or ever had kidney disease.

• Your child has or ever had any type of gastrointestinal disease, particularly colitis.

• Your child's symptoms of infection seem to be getting worse.

• Your daughter is or becomes pregnant.

• Your daughter is breast-feeding her baby. Small amounts of this drug can pass into breast milk and temporarily cause diarrhea in the nursing infant.

Special Instructions

• Children with diabetes may have a false-positive sugar reaction with a Clinitest urine glucose test. To avoid this problem, switch to Clinistix or Tes-Tape during treatment.

• Do not use this drug to treat a subsequent infection unless you consult the doctor.

Symptoms of Overdose: Severe
diarrhea, nausea, heartburn, or vomiting

Special Notes

• May also cause a false-positive result for urinary ketones in tests using nitroprusside.

• With long-term use of this drug, your child may develop a second infection in addition to the one being treated. Bacteria and organisms that are not susceptible to this drug can grow unchecked, causing a second infection that may require treatment with a different drug.

Outdated Doses

Safe and proper medication disposal is essential, especially when you have children in the house. Do not keep medication—whether prescription or nonprescription—past the expiration date, even if it appears normal. Expired medication may be ineffective and can even be dangerous. Make a habit of regularly checking the expiration date on all medicines in your home. Flush leftover medication down the toilet or pour it down the sink. Rinse the container before throwing it out. If your medication does not display an expiration date, throw it out after one year.

Brand Name: Vantin

Generic Available: No

Type of Drug: Cephalosporin antibiotic

Use: Treats a wide variety of bacterial infections, particularly those of the middle ear, upper and lower respiratory tract, and urinary tract.

Time Required for Drug to Take Effect: It may take a few days to affect the infection.

Dosage Forms and Strengths: Tablets, film-coated (100 mg, 200 mg); Suspension (50 mg and 100 mg per 5 mL)

Storage: Refrigerate suspension; do not freeze. Store tablets at room temperature. Store both forms in tightly closed, light-resistant containers. Discard after 14 days any unused portion of the suspension.

How This Drug Works: Kills susceptible bacteria, but is ineffective against viruses, parasites, or fungi.

CEFPODOXIME

Administration Guidelines

• Give with food to improve absorption.

• Generally given 2 times a day.

• Give doses at evenly spaced intervals around the clock. If you are to give 2 doses a day, space them 12 hours apart.

• Missed doses: Give immediately. However, if you don't remember to give the missed dose until it is time for the next dose, give the missed dose and space the next dose halfway through the regular interval between doses; then return to the regular schedule. Try not to skip any doses.

• Shake the suspension well just before measuring each dose to distribute ingredients and equalize doses. The contents tend to settle on the bottom of the bottle.

• Give this drug for the entire time prescribed by your child's doctor (usually 7 to 14 days), even if symptoms disappear.

Side Effects

Tell your child's doctor about any side effects that are persistent or particularly bothersome.

More Common. Abdominal pain, diarrhea, dizziness, fatigue, headache, heartburn, loss of appetite, nausea, or vomiting

Less Common. It is especially important to tell the doctor if your child experiences darkened tongue, difficulty in breathing, fever, itching, joint or lower back pain, rash, rectal or vaginal itching, severe diarrhea (which may be watery or contain blood or pus), sore mouth, stomach cramps, tingling in the hands or feet, unusual bleeding or bruising, or difficulty urinating.

Possible Drug Interactions

• Probenecid can increase the blood concentrations of this drug.

• Furosemide, bumetanide, ethacrynic acid, colistin, vancomycin, and polymyxin B antibiotics can increase side effects, especially those on the kidneys.

Tell Your Child's Doctor If

• Your child has had unusual or allergic reactions to any medications, especially this drug or other cephalosporin antibiotics (such as cefamandole, cephalexin, cefaclor, cefadroxil, cefazolin, cefopera-zone, cefotaxime, ceftizoxime, cephalothin, cephradine, cephapirin, cefoxitin, or cefuroxime) or to penicillin antibiotics.

• Your child is currently taking any prescription or nonprescription medications.

- Your child has or ever had kidney disease.

- Your child's symptoms of infection seem to be getting worse.

- Your daughter is or becomes pregnant.

- Your daughter is breast-feeding her baby. Small amounts of this drug pass into breast milk and may temporarily cause diarrhea in the nursing infant.

Special Instructions

- Children with diabetes may have a false-positive sugar reaction with a Clinitest urine glucose test. To avoid this problem, switch to Clinistix or Tes-Tape during treatment.

- Do not use this drug to treat a subsequent infection unless you consult the doctor.

Symptoms of Overdose: Severe diarrhea, nausea, heartburn, or vomiting

Special Notes

- With long-term use of this drug, your child may develop a second infection in addition to the one being treated. Bacteria and organisms that are not susceptible to this drug can grow unchecked, causing a second infection that may require treatment with a different drug.

Measuring Up

Remember: Never use an ordinary tableware teaspoon to measure liquid doses. Instead, use a cylindrical dosing spoon, dosage cup, dropper, or syringe. These measuring devices can be found at your local drug store and sometimes at supermarkets, toy stores, and department stores.

Brand Names: Keflex, Keftab

Generic Available: Yes

Type of Drug: Antibiotic

Use: Treats bacterial infections, particularly those of the throat, skin, nose, and ear.

Time Required for Drug to Take Effect: 2 to 3 days

Dosage Forms and Strengths: Capsules (250 mg, 500 mg); Tablets (500 mg); Suspension (125 mg/5 mL, 250 mg/5 mL)

Storage: Keep suspension in the refrigerator; store capsules and tablets at room temperature. Store all forms in tightly closed containers. Do not freeze.

How This Drug Works: Destroys susceptible bacteria.

CEPHALEXIN

Administrative Guidelines
• Usually given 2 to 4 times a day.

• Usually given for 5 to 14 days.

• Shake suspension well just before measuring each dose.

• Missed doses: Give immediately. However, if it's less than 2 hours before the next scheduled dose, skip the missed dose and return to the regular dosing schedule. Do not give double doses.

Side Effects
Tell your child's doctor about any side effects that are persistent or particularly bothersome.

More Common. Abdominal pain, diarrhea, fatigue, headache

Less Common. Contact the doctor if your child develops hives, rash, intense itching, faintness soon after a dose (anaphylaxis), or has difficulty breathing.

Tell Your Child's Doctor If
• Your child has had an allergic reaction to a drug in the cephalosporin family or to penicillin antibiotics.

• Your child's symptoms persist or get worse.

Special Instructions
• Discard after 14 days any unused suspension that has been refrigerated.

Symptoms of Overdose: Severe nausea, vomiting, and/or diarrhea

Special Notes
• With long-term use of this drug, your child may develop a second infection in addition to the one being treated. Bacteria and organisms that are not susceptible to this drug can grow unchecked, causing a second infection that may require treatment with a different drug.

CHLORAL HYDRATE

Administration Guidelines
- Give capsules with a full glass of water to avoid stomach irritation.

- Mix syrup with at least ½ glass liquid to avoid stomach upset.

- Unwrap and moisten the suppository with water before placing in the rectum.

- When used to aid sleep, give 15 to 30 minutes before bedtime.

- Do not abruptly stop giving this drug. Your child's doctor may want to decrease the dose gradually to avoid side effects.

Side Effects
Tell your child's doctor about any side effects that are persistent or particularly bothersome.

More Common. Nausea, stomach pain, vomiting

Less Common. Clumsiness, confusion, diarrhea, dizziness, light-headedness, hallucinations, unusual excitement

Possible Drug Interactions
- Can cause extreme drowsiness when used with other central nervous system depressants (alcohol, antihistamines, muscle relaxants, tranquilizers, pain medications).

- Can increase the effects of blood thinners and lead to bleeding complications.

Tell Your Child's Doctor If
- Your child has had an allergic reaction to any medication.

- Your child has any diseases or is taking any other medication.

- Your daughter is or becomes pregnant.

- Your daughter is breast-feeding her baby. This drug passes into breast milk; however, the American Academy of Pediatrics considers it compatible with breast-feeding in most cases.

Symptoms of Overdose:
Convulsions, difficulty swallowing, severe drowsiness, low body temperature, severe stomach pain, shortness of breath, slurred speech, staggering, severe weakness

Special Notes
- Your child may develop a tolerance to this drug. Do not increase the dose unless you consult the doctor. This drug generally is not used for more than 2 weeks.

- May cause drowsiness. Be sure you know how your child is reacting to this drug before allowing participation in activities that require alertness, such as riding a bicycle.

Brand Names: Aquachloral Supprettes, Noctec

Generic Available: Yes

Type of Drug: Sedative, hypnotic

Use: Aids sleeping. Also used as an antianxiety drug.

Time Required for Drug to Take Effect: 10 to 20 minutes

Dosage Forms and Strengths: Capsules (250 mg, 500 mg); Syrup (250 mg and 500 mg per 5 mL); Suppository (324 mg, 500 mg, 648 mg)

Storage: Store at room temperature in tightly closed, light-resistant containers.

How This Drug Works: Depresses central nervous system activity.

Brand Names: Chloromycetin Kapseals, Chloramphenicol (various manufacturers)

Generic Available: Yes

Type of Drug: Antibiotic

Use: Treats a wide variety of bacterial infections.

Time Required for Drug to Take Effect: 2 to 3 days

Dosage Forms and Strengths: Capsules (250 mg); Suspension (150 mg per 5 mL)

Storage: Store at room temperature in tightly closed, light-resistant containers.

How This Drug Works: Destroys susceptible bacteria.

CHLORAMPHENICOL (SYSTEMIC)

Administrative Guidelines

• Give on an empty stomach 1 hour before or 2 hours after a meal.

• Shake suspension well just before measuring each dose.

• Usually given 4 times a day for 7 to 14 days.

• Missed doses: Give immediately. However, if it's within 2 hours of the next scheduled dose, skip the missed dose and return to the regular dosing schedule. Do not give double doses.

• Do not exceed prescribed dosage.

Side effects

Tell your child's doctor about any side effects that are persistent or particularly bothersome.

More Common. Diarrhea, headache, nausea, or vomiting

Less Common. Confusion, depression, fever, itching, mouth sores, skin rash, sores on the tongue, tingling sensations, unusual bleeding or bruising, or unusual weakness

Possible Drug Interactions

• This drug reduces the effectiveness of iron, vitamin B, and cyclophosphamide.

• Acetaminophen and penicillin may increase the blood concentrations and side effects of this drug.

• Phenobarbital and rifampin may decrease the blood concentration of this drug

• Phenytoin may increase the blood concentration of this drug.

Tell Your Child's Doctor If

• Your child is allergic to this drug.

• Your child has anemia, bleeding disorders, or kidney or liver disease.

• Your child has glucose-6-phosphate dehydrogenase deficiency.

• Your daughter is or becomes pregnant. This drug can cause serious side effects in the newborn baby if given to the mother late in pregnancy.

• Your daughter is breast-feeding her baby. The American Academy of Pediatrics is concerned about using this drug during breast-feeding.

Symptoms of Overdose:
Abdominal distension, severe vomiting, irregular breathing, loose green stools, difficulty breathing, fever, sore throat, bruising, gray baby syndrome.

Special Instructions

• Children with diabetes may have a false-positive sugar reaction with a Clinitest urine glucose test. To avoid this problem, switch to Clinistix or Tes-Tape during treatment with this drug.

Special Notes

• This drug should be reserved for use in patients who did not respond to less toxic therapy. This drug can cause 3 serious toxicities: aplastic anemia, bone marrow suppression, and gray baby syndrome (signs and symptoms include bluish color, poor circulation, coma, and abdominal distention).

• To ensure that a safe dose is given, blood concentrations of this drug may be monitored and tests to detect blood abnormalities may be performed.

Be Accurate

If you don't give medication correctly, it may be ineffective or even cause side effects. An estimated 10 to 30 percent of medications aren't effective because they have been given incorrectly. To do it right, you have to give the exact amount of medicine prescribed at the scheduled time, for the specified duration, and in the appropriate manner. Always read the label, follow the directions carefully, and use the appropriate equipment for measuring and administering the medication. Also, be sure to wash your hands before you give any medication to your child.

Brand Names: Aller-Chlor Oral,* Chlo-Amine Oral,* Chlorate Oral,* Chlor-Trimeton Oral,* Phenetron Oral, Telachlor Oral, Teldrin Oral*
(*available over the counter)

Generic Available: Yes

Type of Drug: Antihistamine

Use: Treats perennial and seasonal allergic rhinitis and other allergic symptoms, including itching.

Time Required for Drug to Take Effect: 15 to 30 minutes

Dosage Forms and Strengths: Capsules (12 mg); Capsules, timed-release (6 mg, 8 mg, 12 mg); Syrup (2 mg/5 mL); Tablets, chewable (2 mg); Tablets, timed-release (8 mg, 12 mg)

Storage: Store at room temperature in tightly closed, light-resistant containers.

How This Drug Works: Blocks the action of histamine, a chemical released from the body during an allergic reaction.

CHLORPHENIRAMINE

Administration Guidelines

• Give with food or a full glass of milk or water to avoid stomach upset, unless your child's doctor directs you to do otherwise.

• Timed-release tablets should be swallowed whole. Breaking, chewing, or crushing the tablets destroys the timed-release activity and may increase side effects.

• Missed doses: Give as soon as possible. However, if it's within 1 to 2 hours of the next dose (or 2 to 4 hours for timed-release forms) skip the missed dose and return to the regular dosing schedule. Do not give double doses.

Side Effects

Tell your child's doctor about any side effects that are persistent or particularly bothersome.

More Common. It is especially important to tell the doctor if your child experiences a change in menstruation, clumsiness, feeling faint, flushing or shortness of breath, sleeping disorders, sore throat or fever, tightness in the chest, unusual bleeding or bruising, or unusual fatigue or weakness.

Less Common. Blurred vision; confusion; constipation; diarrhea; difficult or painful urination; dizziness; dry mouth, throat, or nose; headache; irritability; loss of appetite; nausea; restlessness; ringing or buzzing in the ears; stomach upset; or unusual increase in sweating. These side effects should disappear as your child's body adjusts to this drug. This drug can also cause increased sensitivity to sunlight.

Possible Drug Interactions

• Can cause extreme drowsiness when used with tricyclic antidepressants or with central nervous system depressants such as alcohol, barbiturates, benzodiazepine tranquilizers, muscle relaxants, narcotics, pain medications, and phenothiazine tranquilizers.

• Monoamine oxidase (MAO) inhibitors such as isocarboxazid, pargyline, phenelzine, and tranylcypromine can increase the side effects of this drug. At least 14 days should separate the use of this drug and an MAO inhibitor.

Tell Your Child's Doctor If

• Your child has any unusual or allergic reactions to medications, especially to antihistamines such as brompheniramine, carbinoxamine, clemastine, cyproheptadine, dexchlorpheniramine dimenhydrinate, dimethindene, diphenhydramine, diphenylpyraline, doxylamine, hydroxyzine, promethazine, pyrilamine, terfenadine, trimeprazine, tripelennamine, and triprolidine.

- Your child has or ever had asthma, blood-vessel disease, high blood pressure, kidney disease, peptic ulcers, or thyroid disease.

- Your daughter is or becomes pregnant. The effects of this drug during pregnancy have not been thoroughly studied in humans.

- Your daughter is breast-feeding her baby. Small amounts of this drug pass into breast milk and may cause unusual excitement or irritability in nursing infants.

Special Instructions
- Make sure your child avoids prolonged exposure to sunlight. Apply an effective sunscreen and have your child wear protective clothing when out-of-doors.

- Remind your child to be careful on stairs when feeling light-headed or dizzy.

Symptoms of Overdose: Fixed, dilated pupils; flushed face; dry mouth; fever; excitation; hallucinations; incoordination; seizures; shaky movements; unsteady gait

Special Notes
- This drug can decrease your child's ability to perform tasks that require alertness, such as riding a bicycle.

Just Call

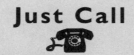

If you have any concerns about any side effects, even minor ones, you should be sure to discuss them with your child's doctor. The doctor may be able to minimize or eliminate the side effects by prescribing a different medication or changing your child's dosage, dosing schedule, or the way the drug is given. (Do not make adjustments on your own without discussing them with your doctor.) At the very least, the doctor can assure you that the medication's benefits far outweigh its side effects.

Brand Names: Thorazine, Ormazine, Thorazine Spansule, Thorazine Concentrate

Generic Available: Yes

Type of Drug: Antipsychotic agent, antiemetic

Use: Treats nervous, mental, emotional, and behavioral disorders such as psychoses, mania, and Tourette syndrome. Also treats severe nausea and vomiting.

Time Required for Drug to Take Effect: It may take 6 weeks to 6 months to achieve full benefit for mental and emotional disorders. Onset within 1 hour for nausea and vomiting.

Dosage Forms and Strengths: Tablets (10 mg, 25 mg, 50 mg, 100 mg, 200 mg); Capsule, extended-release (30 mg, 75 mg, 150 mg; 200 mg, 300 mg); Syrup (10 mg/5 mL); Suppository (25 mg, 100 mg); Concentrate (30 mg/mL, 100 mg/mL)

Storage: Store at room temperature in tightly closed, light-resistant containers. Do not freeze concentrate or syrup.

How This Drug Works: Causes complex changes in the central nervous system, producing tranquilizing effects.

CHLORPROMAZINE

Administration Guidelines

- Give with food or full glass of water or milk to decrease stomach upset.

- Dilute concentrate in juice, milk, water, soup, pudding, or carbonated beverage before giving. Syrup does not need to be diluted.

- Do not spill syrup or concentrate on skin or clothing. These forms can cause a skin rash.

- Do not break, crush, or allow your child to chew extended-release capsules.

- Do not give within 2 hours of giving antacids or medicine for diarrhea.

- Missed doses: Give as soon as you remember. Then give any remaining doses for that day at regularly spaced intervals. Do not give double doses.

- Do not stop giving this drug without first checking with the doctor, who may want to gradually reduce the dose before stopping it.

Side Effects

Tell your child's doctor about any side effects that are persistent or particularly bothersome.

More Common. Constipation, decreased sweating, dizziness, drowsiness, dry mouth, stuffy nose, low blood pressure, stomach upset, nausea, vomiting, weight gain, blurred vision, difficulty urinating, changes in menstrual period. Contact the doctor immediately if your child experiences lip smacking or puckering, puffing of cheeks, rapid or fine wormlike tongue movements, uncontrolled chewing movements, uncontrolled arm or leg movements, changes in color perception, difficulty seeing at night, difficulty in speaking or swallowing, fainting, inability to move eyes, loss of balance, mask-like face, muscle spasms, restlessness or need to keep moving, shuffling walk, stiffness of arms or legs, twitching movements, trembling and shaking, twisting movements of the body, weakness in the arms and legs, skin rash, or severe sunburn.

Less Common. Contact the doctor immediately if your child experiences seizures, difficult or fast breathing, fast or irregular heartbeat, fever, high or low blood pressure, increased sweating, loss of bladder control, severe muscle stiffness, pale skin, or unusual fatigue or weakness.

Possible Drug Interactions

- Central nervous system depressants such as alcohol, antihistamines, cold preparations, muscle relaxants, tranquilizers, and some pain medications may cause extreme drowsiness when used with this drug.

- Cough and cold products may increase the chance of heat stroke, dizziness, dry mouth, blurred vision, and constipation.

- Antidepressants, monoamine oxidase (MAO) inhibitors, and lithium cause an increase in side effects. These medications need to be dosed carefully when used together.

- Medications that lower blood pressure may lead to blood pressure that's too low when used with this drug.

- Antithyroid drugs lead to an increase in rare blood disorders when given with this drug.

- Epinephrine may cause low blood pressure.

Tell Your Child's Doctor If

- Your child has had allergic reactions to any medications.

- Your child has taken or is taking any other prescription or nonprescription medicine.

- Your child has lung or heart disease, seizures, glaucoma, liver or kidney disease, difficulty urinating, stomach ulcers, bone marrow or blood disorders, Reye syndrome, or any other medical condition.

- The blurred vision continues beyond the first few weeks or gets worse.

- Your child develops a new medical problem.

- Your child develops a rash from the sun.

- Your child continues to have dry mouth after 2 weeks. Continued dry mouth can lead to cavities.

- Your child develops side effects after this drug has been stopped.

- Your child abuses alcohol.

- Your daughter is or becomes pregnant.

- Your daughter is breast-feeding her baby. This drug can pass into breast milk, and the American Academy of Pediatrics is concerned about its effect on the baby.

Special Instructions

- Give this drug only as directed by the doctor. It is important that your child's progress is checked regularly by the doctor.

- Protect your child from overheating during exercise, play, or hot weather as this drug decreases sweating and can cause an increase in body temperature. Hot baths, hot tubs, or saunas may make your child dizzy or faint.

- Dress your child warmly as this drug increases sensitivity to cold weather.

- Your child should avoid exposure to sunlight and wear an effective sunscreen when out-of-doors. This drug may cause a skin rash or severe sunburn when your child is exposed to direct sunlight or ultraviolet light in tanning booths.

- Your child may need to wear sunglasses that block UV rays when outside because of an increased sensitivity to light.

- Do not give any other medication with this drug before talking to the pharmacist or doctor.

- Do not let your child have surgery or any medical treatment or dental work unless the doctor or dentist is aware that your child is taking this drug.

- Do not allow your child to drink alcohol while taking this drug.

- Do not give other medicines that may make your child sleepy.

- Do not give your child cough or cold products without first checking with the doctor.

Symptoms of Overdose: Deep sleep, coma, low blood pressure, increased severity of side effects

Special Notes

• Syrup and liquid may turn a light yellow color. If markedly discolored, do not use. Check with the pharmacy if you have any questions.

• Make sure you know how your child is reacting to this drug before allowing participation in an activity that requires alertness and coordination, such as riding a bicycle. This drug may cause your child to have blurred vision, dizziness, drowsiness, or to be less alert.

• This drug may cause serious side effects that do not go away after this drug is stopped. Discuss this with the doctor.

• Doses are increased slowly to decrease side effects.

• This drug can cause light-headedness and dizziness if your child gets up too quickly from a prone or sitting position. Have your child get up slowly to prevent these side effects.

• The effects of this drug may last up to 1 week after you stop giving it.

Keep It Out of Reach

Do not rely on a child-resistant cap to deter your child from opening a bottle of medication. Child-resistant does not mean childproof. Legally, a cap can be called child-resistant if 80 percent of all five-year-olds need more than five minutes to open it. That means the other 20 percent could get into it in even less time. Put the bottle in a hard-to-reach cabinet with a childproof lock. Do not keep it on the countertop, kitchen table, or nightstand.

CIMETIDINE

Administration Guidelines

- If giving 1 dose a day, give it at bedtime unless your child's doctor gives other directions.

- If giving 2 doses a day, give the first dose in the morning and the second dose at bedtime.

- For those taking several doses a day, give with meals and at bedtime.

- Missed doses: Give as soon as possible. However, if it's time for the next dose, skip the missed dose. Do not give double doses.

- Give 1 hour before or 2 hours after giving antacids.

- Give this drug for the entire time prescribed by the doctor even if your child feels better.

Side Effects

Tell your child's doctor about any side effects that are persistent or particularly bothersome.

More Common. Dizziness, agitation, headache, drowsiness, diarrhea, nausea, vomiting

Less Common. Contact the doctor if your child experiences burning or itching skin, skin rash, confusion, a fast or pounding heartbeat, fever, slow heartbeat, sore throat, swelling, tightness in the chest, unusual bleeding or bruising, or unusual fatigue or weakness.

Possible Drug Interactions

- Antacids decrease the absorption of this drug when given at the same time.

- Markedly decreases absorption of ketoconazole. Discuss this with the doctor or pharmacist.

- Increases the effect and/or side effects of theophylline, aminophylline, caffeine, diazepam, warfarin, antidepressants, metoprolol, phenytoin, procainamide, quinidine, propranolol, and metronidazole.

Tell Your Child's Doctor If

- Your child has taken or is taking any other prescription or nonprescription medicine.

- Your child has had allergic reactions to this drug, any other medications, foods, preservatives, or dyes.

- Your child has liver or kidney disease or any other medical condition.

- Your child's symptoms do not improve.

Brand Names: Tagamet, Tagamet HB

Generic Available: Yes

Type of Drug: Histamine H_2-receptor antagonist, H_2-blocker (antiulcer agent)

Use: Treats stomach and intestinal ulcers, gastric hypersecretory states, and gastric reflux. Prevents intestinal ulcer.

Time Required for Drug to Take Effect: 1 to 2 hours, but it may take a few days to relieve stomach pain. It takes a few weeks to heal an ulcer.

Dosage Forms and Strengths: Tablets (200 mg, 300 mg, 400 mg, 800 mg; 75 mg available without a prescription); Liquid (300 mg/5 mL)

Storage: Store at room temperature in tightly closed, light-resistant containers. Do not freeze liquid.

How This Drug Works: Blocks the H_2 receptors in the stomach so less acid is produced.

• Your daughter is or becomes pregnant. Alternative medications are preferred during pregnancy.

• Your daughter is breast-feeding her baby. This drug can pass into breast milk; however, the American Academy of Pediatrics considers it compatible with breast-feeding in most cases.

Special Instructions

• Do not give any other medications before talking to the doctor or pharmacist.

• Before your child undergoes skin tests for allergies, tell the doctor your child is taking this drug.

• To relieve stomach pain while waiting for this drug to begin working, give antacids after first consulting with the doctor.

• This drug is available over the counter; however, if your child is younger than 12 years of age, seek the doctor's advice before giving it. Your child's symptoms may require another type of care.

Symptoms of Overdose: Dry mouth, mild drowsiness, heartburn, slow heartbeat

Over-the-Counter Wisdom

Keep in mind that even a medication that is available without a doctor's prescription may still be harmful and should be given appropriately and only when necessary. Talk to your pediatrician about what to do if your child gets sick. Some illnesses can be treated at home, some require a call to the pediatrician's office, and some will require a visit to the doctor. In addition, ask the doctor what situations constitute an emergency. If you're not sure if it's safe or appropriate to give your child a particular over-the-counter medication, be sure to talk to the doctor first.

CIPROFLOXACIN

Administrative Guidelines

• Usually given 2 times a day

• Works best when given 2 hours after a meal with 8 ounces of water.

• Have your child drink 8 to 10 glasses of water per day.

• Missed doses: Give as soon as possible. However, if it's within 6 hours of the next scheduled dose, skip the missed dose and return to the regular dosing schedule. Do not give double doses.

• Give this drug for the entire time prescribed, even if symptoms disappear.

• Restrict your child's caffeine during treatment with this drug.

• Avoid giving dairy products at the same time as this drug. They decrease its absorption.

Side Effects

Tell your child's doctor about any side effects that are persistent or particularly bothersome.

More Common. Diarrhea, headache, light-headedness, nausea, stomach irritation, or vomiting

Less Common. Contact the doctor if your child experiences blood in the urine, changes in vision, confusion, seizures, agitation, hallucinations, lower back pain, muscle or joint pain, pain or difficulty in urinating, restlessness, skin rash, unusual bleeding or bruising, or yellowing of the eyes or skin.

Possible Drug Interactions

• Antacids decrease the absorption of this drug. Do not give antacids within 2 hours of giving this drug.

• Sucralfate can decrease the absorption of this drug. Do not give sucralfate within 2 hours of a dose of this drug unless the doctor tells you to do so.

• Can cause increased blood concentrations of theophylline and, as a result, an increased chance of nausea, vomiting, and headache.

• Can increase blood concentrations of cyclosporin and warfarin.

• Can exaggerate the effects of caffeine when large quantities of caffeinated drinks or foods are consumed.

Tell Your Child's Doctor If

• Your child has had an allergic reaction to this drug, enoxacin, ofloxacin, norfloxacin, cinoxacin, or nalidixic acid.

Brand Name: Cipro

Generic Available: No

Type of Drug: Antibiotic

Use: Treats a wide variety of bacterial infections such as those of the respiratory tract, skin and soft tissue, bone and joint, and eye and ear.

Time Required for Drug to Take Effect: Within 2 to 3 days in most cases.

Dosage Form and Strengths: Tablets (250 mg, 500 mg, and 750 mg)

Storage: Store at room temperature in tightly closed, light-resistant containers.

How This Drug Works: Destroys susceptible bacteria.

- Your child has had brain or spinal cord disease, seizures, kidney disease, or liver disease.

Special Instructions
- Do not give this drug to children younger than 18 years of age because of its effect on developing cartilage.

- This drug can make your child's skin more sensitive to the sun. Make sure your child wears sunscreen and protective clothing when out-of-doors.

- Children who are also taking theophylline or cyclosporin should have blood concentrations checked to ensure that a safe and effective dose is being given.

Symptoms of Overdose: Confusion, seizures, headache, severe nausea, vomiting

Special Notes
- With long-term use of this drug, your child may develop a second infection in addition to the one being treated. Bacteria and organisms that are not susceptible to this drug can grow unchecked, causing a second infection that may require treatment with a different drug.

To Each His Own

If one of your children has been prescribed an antibiotic and another child gets sick, it is not safe to give the antibiotic to the child for whom it was not prescribed. The medication may not be the appropriate one for the other child—even if the children's symptoms are similar. Treating an infection with the wrong drug may make the condition worse instead of better. What's more, children respond to the same drug differently and may need different dosages. The child who became ill first needs the drug in the amount prescribed for the time advised; otherwise, it may not be effective. If you think another child needs medication, consult the doctor.

CISAPRIDE

Administration Guidelines
• Give 15 minutes before meals and at bedtime.

• Missed doses: Give as soon as you remember if it's within 2 hours of the missed dose. Otherwise, skip the missed dose and give the next dose at its scheduled time. Do not give double doses.

Side Effects
Tell your child's doctor about any side effects that are persistent or particularly bothersome.

More Common. Side effects are not common.

Less Common. Diarrhea, nausea, constipation, abdominal cramping, headache, cough, stuffy nose, drowsiness. Contact the doctor immediately if your child experiences vision changes, severe stomach pain, or seizures.

Possible Drug Interactions
• Can cause extreme drowsiness when used with central nervous system depressants such as alcohol, antihistamines, cold preparations, muscle relaxants, tranquilizers, and pain relievers.

• May decrease the effectiveness of digoxin.

Tell Your Child's Doctor If
• Your child has had allergic reactions to any medications.

• Your child has any diseases, especially epilepsy, bleeding ulcers, or intestinal disorders.

• Your child is taking any other medications.

• Your daughter is or becomes pregnant.

• Your daughter is breast-feeding her baby. This drug can pass into breast milk; however, the American Academy of Pediatrics considers it compatible with breast-feeding in most cases.

Symptoms of Overdose: Severe nausea or vomiting, severe drowsiness, severe abdominal cramping, seizures

Brand Name: Propulsid

Generic Available: No

Type of Drug: Gastrointestinal agent

Use: Treats heartburn caused by stomach acid which backs up into the esophagus.

Time Required for Drug to Take Effect: 30 to 60 minutes

Dosage Form and Strengths: Tablets (10 mg, 20 mg)

Storage: Store at room temperature in tightly closed, light-resistant containers.

How This Drug Works: Increases the contractions of the stomach and intestines.

Brand Name: Biaxin

Generic Available: No

Type of Drug: Antibiotic

Use: Treats a wide variety of bacterial infections, particularly otitis media, infections in the upper and lower respiratory tract, and skin.

Time Required for Drug to Take Effect: 2 to 3 days

Dosage Forms and Strengths: Tablets (250 mg, 500 mg); Suspension (125 mg per 5 mL, 250 mg per 5 mL)

Storage: Store tablets and suspension at room temperature in tightly closed, light-resistant containers. Do not refrigerate the suspension; it is stable for 14 days at room temperature.

How This Drug Works: Destroys susceptible bacteria.

CLARITHROMYCIN

Administrative Guidelines
• Usually given 2 times a day.

• Give with food or milk.

• Give this drug for the entire time prescribed, usually 10 to 14 days, even if symptons subside.

• Missed doses: Give as soon as possible. However, if it's within 6 hours of the next scheduled dose, skip the missed dose and return to the regular dosing schedule. Do not give double doses.

• Shake suspension well before measuring each dose.

Side Effects
Tell your child's doctor about any side effects that are persistent or particularly bothersome.

More Common. Abdominal pain or discomfort, abnormal (metallic) taste, diarrhea, dyspepsia, headache, nausea

Less Common. Hearing loss, rash, rectal or vaginal itching, yellowing of the eyes or skin, persistent diarrhea

Possible Drug Interactions
• Can increase blood concentrations of carbamazepine, aminophylline, theophylline, and oxtriphylline.

• May increase blood concentrations of digoxin and anticoagulants.

• Can increase the possibility of irregular heart rate when taken with certain antihistamine drugs such as terfenadine, loratidine, and astemizole.

Tell Your Child's Doctor If
• Your child is taking any of the medications listed above.

• Your child is allergic to this drug, erythromycin, or azithromycin.

• Your child has kidney, heart, or liver disease.

Symptoms of Overdose:
Severe stomach upset, nausea, hearing loss

CLINDAMYCIN (SYSTEMIC)

Administration Guidelines
• Give with food or a full glass of water or milk.

• Shake suspension just before measuring each dose.

• Usually given every 6 to 8 hours.

• Usually given for 7 to 14 days.

• Missed doses: Give as soon as possible. However, if it's less than 4 hours before the next scheduled dose, skip the missed dose. Do not give double doses.

Side Effects
Tell your child's doctor about any side effects that are persistent or particularly bothersome.

More Common. Diarrhea, loss of appetite, nausea, stomach or throat irritation, or vomiting

Less Common. Bloody or pus-containing diarrhea, hives, itching, muscle or joint pain, skin rash, unusual bleeding or bruising, or yellowing of the eyes or skin

Tell Your Child's Doctor If
• Your child is allergic to this drug or lincomycin.

• Your child has colitis, kidney disease, or liver disease.

• Your child is sensitive to the color additive FD&C Yellow No. 5 (tartrazine).

• Your daughter is or becomes pregnant.

• Your daughter is breast-feeding her baby. This drug can pass into breast milk and cause side effects in the infant.

Special Instructions
• Stop giving this drug if your child experiences prolonged severe diarrhea. Contact the doctor immediately. Do not give anti-diarrheal medicine.

Symptoms of Overdose: Severe diarrhea, arrhythmias, renal dysfunction

Brand Names: Cleocin HCl, Cleocin Pediatric, Clindamycin (various manufacturers)

Generic Available: Yes

Type of Drug: Antibiotic

Use: Treats bacterial infections, such as those of the respiratory tract, skin and soft tissue, the female pelvis, and female genital tract, as well as intra-abdominal infections.

Time Required for Drug to Take Effect: 2 to 3 days

Dosage Forms and Strengths: Capsules (75 mg, 150 mg, and 300 mg); Suspension (75 mg per 5 mL); Vaginal cream (2%)

Storage: Store at room temperature in tightly closed containers. Suspension is stable for 14 days.

How This Drug Works: Destroys susceptible bacteria.

Brand Names: Cleocin T, Clina-Derm

Generic Available: Yes

Type of Drug: Antibiotic

Use: Treats acne vulgaris.

Time Required for Drug to Take Effect: An effect is usually seen in 3 to 4 days. However, effects may not be apparent for 12 weeks.

Dosage Forms and Strengths: Solution (10 mg per mL); Gel (1%); Lotion (10 mg per mL)

Storage: Store at room temperature in tightly closed containers. This drug contains alcohol and is flammable. Keep away from flames and heat.

How This Drug Works: Destroys susceptible bacteria. This drug does not cure acne, but will help to control it.

CLINDAMYCIN (TOPICAL)

Administration Guidelines

• Wash the affected area thoroughly with mild soap and warm water. Rinse and pat dry. Wait at least 30 minutes after washing or shaving before applying this drug.

• When applying the solution, press the applicator tip firmly against the skin and use a dabbing motion.

• Apply to entire area of skin affected by acne, not just the pimples.

• Missed doses: Apply as soon as possible. However, if it's less than 6 to 8 hours before the next scheduled dose, skip the missed dose. Do not give double doses.

Side Effects

Tell your child's doctor about any side effects that are persistent or particularly bothersome.

More Common. Diarrhea, dry skin, fatigue, headache, nausea, oily skin, skin irritation in sensitive areas

Less Common. Contact the doctor if your child experiences bloody or pus-containing diarrhea, increased urination, itching, sore throat, or swelling of the face.

Possible Drug Interactions

• Use of abrasive or medicated cleansers; medicated cosmetics; or any topical, alcohol-containing preparations (such as aftershave or perfume) with this drug can cause excessive skin dryness and irritation.

Tell Your Child's Doctor If

• Your child is allergic to this drug or lincomycin.

• Your child has ever had colitis.

• Your daughter is or becomes pregnant.

Special Notes

• Avoid getting this drug in the eyes, nose, or mouth, or in the areas surrounding scratches or burns.

• Your child should use water-based rather than oil-based cosmetics.

• Do not give any antidiarrheal medicine. If diarrhea occurs, contact the doctor immediately.

Symptoms of Overdose: Severe skin irritation may occur with excessive use. If ingested accidentally, contact your local poison control center.

CLONAZEPAM

Administration Guidelines
• May be given with food or water to decrease stomach upset.

• Usually given 2 or 3 times a day. Bedtime dosing may be possible for restless leg syndrome.

• Give every day and at the prescribed times to control seizures.

• Missed doses: Give immediately if you remember within 1 hour. Otherwise, skip the missed dose and go back to the regular dosing schedule. Do not give double doses.

• Doses usually are increased every 3 days to decrease the occurence of side effects from initial exposure to this drug.

• Discard suspension after 2 weeks.

Side Effects
Tell your child's doctor about any side effects that are persistent or particularly bothersome.

More Common. Clumsiness, unsteadiness, dizziness, lightheadedness, drowsiness, slurred speech, headache, dry mouth, constipation, diarrhea, nausea, change in appetite, vomiting

Less Common. Contact the doctor if your child experiences behavioral changes, difficulty concentrating, outbursts of anger, confusion, mental depression, seizures, hallucinations, impaired memory, muscle weakness, skin rash, itching, sore throat, fever, chills, sores in the mouth, uncontrolled body movements, unusual bleeding or bruising, unusual excitement or nervousness, irritability, unusual fatigue or weakness, or yellow skin.

Possible Drug Interactions
• Central nervous system depressants such as alcohol, antihistamines, muscle relaxants, tranquilizers, and some pain medications may cause extreme drowsiness when used with this drug.

Tell Your Child's Doctor If
• Your child has taken or is taking any other prescription or nonprescription medicine.

• Your child has had an allergic reaction to this drug, any other medications, foods, preservatives, or dyes.

• Your child has asthma, lung disease, seizures, glaucoma, liver or kidney disease, or any other medical condition.

• Your daughter is or becomes pregnant.

Brand Name: Klonopin

Generic Available: No

Type of Drug: Benzodiazepine anticonvulsant

Use: Treats seizures. Also treats restless leg syndrome as well as panic disorders and other mental disorders.

Time Required for Drug to Take Effect: 20 to 60 minutes. Depending on diagnosis, full benefit may not be achieved for a few weeks.

Dosage Forms and Strengths: Tablets (0.5 mg, 1 mg, 2 mg). A suspension can be made from the tablets by the pharmacist.

Storage: Store tablets at room temperature in tightly closed, light-resistant containers. Keep suspension in the refrigerator.

How This Drug Works: Depresses the central nervous system. Stops seizure activity by suppressing the spread of the seizure impulse in the brain.

- Your daughter is breast-feeding her baby. This drug can pass into breast milk, and the American Academy of Pediatrics is concerned about its effect on the baby.

Special Instructions

- Give this drug only as directed by the doctor.

- Do not give any other medication without first consulting the pharmacist or the doctor.

- Take your child to the doctor regularly to monitor progress.

- Do not suddenly stop giving this drug before speaking to the doctor. Stopping this drug abruptly can lead to seizures.

- Your child should not drink alcohol while taking this drug.

- Do not give other medicines that may make your child sleepy.

Symptoms of Overdose: Slurred speech, confusion, severe drowsiness, severe weakness, shakiness, trouble breathing, slow heartbeat, staggering, coma, or trouble walking

Special Notes

- Drowsiness is common. Make sure you know how your child is reacting to this drug before allowing participation in activities that require alertness and coordination, such as riding a bicycle.

- Children with preexisting brain damage experience more behavioral problems with this drug.

- Your child's body may take up to 3 weeks to adjust when this drug is stopped after long-term use.

Outdated Doses

Safe and proper medication disposal is essential, especially when you have children in the house. Do not keep medication—whether prescription or nonprescription—past the expiration date, even if it appears normal. Expired medication may be ineffective and can even be dangerous. Make a habit of regularly checking the expiration date on all medicines in your home. Flush leftover medication down the toilet or pour it down the sink. Rinse the container before throwing it out. If your medication does not display an expiration date, throw it out after one year.

CLONIDINE

Administration Guidelines
• Give with food or milk, but be consistent.

• Carefully follow instructions supplied with the skin patches.

• Missed oral doses: Give as soon as possible. However, if it's within 6 hours of the next dose, skip the missed dose and give the next regular dose. Do not give double doses. If 2 doses are missed in a row, call the doctor immediately.

Side Effects
Tell your child's doctor about any side effects that are persistent or particularly bothersome.

More Common. Nervousness, constipation, dry mouth, dizziness, fatigue, headache, difficulty sleeping, nausea and vomiting, stuffy nose. Patches can cause irritated skin at application site. These side effects may improve or disappear as your child's body adjusts to this drug. Contact the doctor if your child has a rash.

Less Common. Palpitations, vivid dreams or nightmares, itching (without rash), fever. Contact the doctor if your child experiences swelling of hands, feet, or face; yellowing of eyes or skin; chest pain; difficulty breathing; or difficulty urinating.

Possible Drug Interactions
• Other sedatives, such as antihistamines, tranquilizers, pain medications, and muscle relaxants, will intensify drowsiness.

• Tricyclic antidepressants such as amitriptyline, imipramine, and nortriptyline, and nonsteroidal anti-inflammatory agents such as ibuprofen and indomethacin can decrease the effectiveness of this drug in lowering blood pressure.

Tell Your Child's Doctor If
• Your child has had allergic reactions to any medications.

• Your child has any other diseases.

• Your child is taking any other medications.

• Your daughter is or becomes pregnant.

Special Instructions
• Dispose of patches by pressing the adhesive edges together and flushing them down the toilet. Any drug remaining in the patch can cause toxicity if handled by children.

• Do not give any medications for allergy, asthma, cough, cold, sinus problems, or weight control without first checking with the doctor or pharmacist.

Brand Names: Catapres, Catapres-TTS

Generic Available: Yes

Type of Drug: Antihypertensive

Use: Treats high blood pressure. Also treats Tourette syndrome, some forms of chronic diarrhea, and some withdrawal symptoms such as those associated with smoking cessation.

Time Required for Drug to Take Effect: Several days to weeks.

Dosage Forms and Strengths: Tablets (0.1 mg, 0.2 mg, 0.3 mg); Transdermal patch (releases 0.1 mg, 0.2 mg, or 0.3 mg per 24-hour period)

Storage: Store at room temperature in tightly closed, light-resistant containers. Do not remove patches from packaging until ready to use.

How This Drug Works: Works in the central nervous system to reduce nerve impulses that cause blood vessels to constrict, lowering blood pressure.

- Do not stop giving this drug without first speaking with the doctor.

Symptoms of Overdose: Excessively low blood pressure, dizziness, fainting, unconsciousness, difficulty breathing

Be Accurate

If you don't give medication correctly, it may be ineffective or even cause side effects. An estimated 10 to 30 percent of medications aren't effective because they have been given incorrectly. To do it right, you have to give the exact amount of medicine prescribed at the scheduled time, for the specified duration, and in the appropriate manner. Always read the label, follow the directions carefully, and use the appropriate equipment for measuring and administering the medication. Also, be sure to wash your hands before you give any medication to your child.

CLOTRIMAZOLE (TOPICAL)

Administrative Guidelines
• Wash your hands, cleanse the affected area with soap and water, pat skin dry, and then apply. Wash your hands again after applying.

• Do not bandage or cover the infection after applying.

• Missed doses: Apply as soon as possible. However, if it's less than 4 hours before the next scheduled dose, skip the missed dose. Do not give double doses.

• Do not apply to the eye area.

Side Effects
Tell your child's doctor about any side effects that are persistent or particularly bothersome.

More Common. Burning, itching, stinging, or redness

Less Common. Blistering, irritation, peeling of the skin, or swelling.

Tell Your Child's Doctor If
• Your child is allergic to this drug.

Special Instructions
• To avoid reinfection, keep the affected area clean and dry. Your child should wear freshly laundered clothes and avoid wearing tight-fitting clothing.

Symptoms of Overdose:
Severe skin irritation may occur if applied excessively. Contact your local poison control center if accidentally ingested.

Brand Names: Lotrimin, Lotrimin AF,* Mycelex, Mycelex OTC* (*Available without a prescription in 1% cream and 1% solution.)

Generic Available: Yes

Type of Drug: Antifungal

Use: Treats topical fungal and yeast infections of the skin.

Time Required for Drug to Take Effect: 5 to 7 days

Dosage Forms and Strengths: Cream (1%); Solution (1%); Lotion (1%)

Storage: Store at room temperature in tightly closed containers.

How This Drug Works: Prevents growth and multiplication of yeast and fungus.

Brand Names: Various manufacturers. Available in combination with other analgesics and antipyretics.

Generic Available: Yes

Type of Drug: Narcotic analgesic and cough suppressant

Use: Relieves mild to moderate pain. Also suppresses coughing.

Time Required for Drug to Take Effect: 30 to 60 minutes

Dosage Forms and Strengths: Tablets (15 mg, 30 mg, 60 mg); Solution (15 mg per 5 mL)

Storage: Store at room temperature in tightly closed, light-resistant containers.

How This Drug Works: Acts directly on the central nervous system to relieve pain.

CODEINE

Administration Guidelines

• May be given with food or milk to avoid stomach upset.

• Do not increase the dose or give it more often than your child's doctor prescribed.

• For best results, give at the onset of your child's pain. Do not wait until the pain increases.

• Do not give as a cough suppressant if your child has a productive cough (is coughing up phlegm).

Side Effects

Tell your child's doctor about any side effects that are persistent or particularly bothersome.

More Common. Constipation, dizziness, drowsiness, dry mouth, flushing, light-headedness

Less Common. Loss of appetite, nausea, painful or difficult urination, or sweating. Call the doctor immediately if your child has breathing difficulties, palpitations, tremors, excitation, rash, sore throat and fever, anxiety, or severe weakness.

Possible Drug Interactions

• Can cause extreme drowsiness when used with other central nervous system depressants such as alcohol, antihistamines, cold preparations, muscle relaxants, tranquilizers, or other pain medicines.

Tell Your Child's Doctor If

• Your child has had allergic reactions to any medications, especially to this drug or any other narcotic analgesics.

• Your child has any disease, especially respiratory diseases such as asthma.

• Your daughter is or becomes pregnant.

• Your daughter is breast-feeding her baby. This drug passes into breast milk; however, the American Academy of Pediatrics considers it compatible with breast-feeding in most cases.

Special Instructions

• Increase the fluid and fiber in your child's diet to avoid constipation.

• If you have been giving this drug to your child for several weeks, do not suddenly stop giving it without first talking with the doctor. The doctor may want to decrease the dose gradually to avoid withdrawal side effects.

Symptoms of Overdose: Convulsions or tremors, confusion, severe nervousness or restlessness, severe dizziness, severe drowsiness, slow or difficult breathing, or severe weakness

Special Notes
• Tolerance (decreased effectiveness) may be seen with long-term use of this drug.

• This drug can cause drowsiness. Make sure you know how your child is reacting to this drug before allowing participation in activities that require alertness, such as riding a bicycle.

Keep a Lid on It

Pharmacists are required to put drugs in bottles that have child-resistant caps. Don't switch to a bottle that's easier for you to open—children may also find it easier to open. Remember, too, that child-resistant does not mean childproof. Children older than five years of age may be able to open most medicine bottles. That's why it's essential for you to teach them that drugs can be harmful if not taken correctly and that they need supervision before taking anything. And, just to be on the safe side, keep all medicines out of your child's reach.

Brand Names: Intal, Intal Aerosol Spray, Intal Nebulizer Solution, Gastrocrom, Nasalcrom, Crolom, Opticrom

Generic Available: No

Type of Drug: Antiallergic, antiasthmatic

Use: Oral/Nasal: Prevents asthma attacks. Opthalmic: Treats conjunctivitis and allergic eye disorders.

Time Required for Drug to Take Effect: Oral/Nasal: Must be given at regular intervals for 2 to 4 weeks to be effective. Opthalmic: A few days to relieve symptoms; however, 6 weeks may be required in some patients.

Dosage Forms and Strengths: Capsules (100 mg), for inhalation (20 mg, to be used with Spinhaler); Drops, ophthalmic (4% solution); Inhalation (800 mg per spray); Solution for nebulization (20 mg/mL); Solution, nasal (40 mg/mL)

Storage: Store solution at room temperature in tightly closed, light-resistant containers. Store aerosol away from heat and sunlight; do not puncture or break.

How This Drug Works: Prevents the release of body chemicals responsible for the symptoms of asthma or allergy.

CROMOLYN SODIUM

Administration Guidelines

- Most effective when started before contact with allergens.
- Do not give powder for inhalation to patients with a lactase deficiency. Lactose-free preparations can be substituted.
- Works best when blood concentrations are kept within a safe and effective range. Give doses at evenly spaced intervals around the clock. If you are to give 4 doses a day, space them 6 hours apart.
- Use solution only with a power-operated nebulizer equipped with a face mask. Never use solution with a handheld nebulizer.
- Shake the aerosol well just before spraying each dose; the contents tend to settle to the bottom of the container.
- If another inhaler containing a bronchodilator is being used, have your child take it 20 to 30 minutes before using this drug.
- Nasal passages should be cleared before administering the nasal spray. Tell your child to inhale through the nose as you spray the solution.
- Missed doses: If you miss a dose of this drug and remember within 1 hour, give the missed dose immediately. If more than 1 hour has passed, do not take the missed dose at all; just return to the prescribed dosing schedule. Do not give double doses.

Side Effects

Tell your child's doctor about any side effects that are persistent or particularly bothersome.

More Common. It is especially important to tell the doctor about itching, joint swelling or pain, nosebleeds, nose burning, painful or increased urination, rash, swelling of the face or eyes, swollen glands, or wheezing. Those using the ophthalmic drops may experience a transient stinging or burning sensation following instillation. Other side effects include itchy or watery eyes, dryness around the eyes, and eye irritation. Those using the nasal spray may experience a bad taste in the mouth, headaches, irritation or stinging, nasal burning, postnasal drip, or sneezing. These side effects should stop as your child's body adjusts to this drug.

Less Common. Cough, dizziness, drowsiness, headache, increased urination, nasal congestion, nasal itching, nausea, sneezing, stomach irritation, or tearing. These side effects should disappear as your child's body adjusts to this drug.

Possible Drug Interactions

• This drug should not interact with other medications if it is used according to directions.

Tell Your Child's Doctor If

• Your child has had unusual or allergic reactions to any drugs.

• Your child has or ever had kidney or liver disease.

• Your daughter is or becomes pregnant. Asthma should be controlled during pregnancy.

• Your daughter is breast-feeding her baby. It is not known whether this drug passes into breast milk.

Special Instructions

• Do not stop giving this drug before you check with the doctor. Stopping this drug abruptly may make your child's condition worse.

• Your child should not wear soft contact lenses while being treated with the ophthalmic solution. Soft contact lenses can be worn within a few hours after discontinuing use of this drug.

Teach Your Children Well

Let's face it. Kids can be pretty stubborn when it comes to accepting medication. When appropriate, try giving your child information about his or her condition and how the medicine works. In a nonthreatening voice, talk about the consequences of not taking the medication, perhaps reminding the child of how uncomfortable he or she was before beginning the medication. Use reasoning when possible, but don't scare the child. Children who understand the importance of antibiotics for infection, insulin for diabetes, or inhalants for asthma are more likely to take the medication without objection.

Brand Names: Neoral (microemulsion), Sandimmune

Generic Available: No

Type of Drug: Immunosuppressant

Use: Prevents rejection after bone marrow transplant and solid organ transplant (kidney, liver, heart). Also treats severe psoriasis.

Time Required for Drug to Take Effect: The doctor will monitor your child's cyclosporine blood level routinely to ensure effectiveness.

Dosage Forms and Strengths: Capsules (25 mg, 100 mg); Solutions (100 mg per 1 mL)

Storage: Store at room temperature in original containers. Store out of direct light.

How This Drug Works: Interferes with the body's ability to reject the foreign transplanted marrow or tissue by reducing the body's natural immunity.

CYCLOSPORINE

Administration Guidelines

- Give at evenly spaced intervals around the clock to maintain a constant level of this drug in your child's bloodstream. If you are to give it 2 times a day, space the doses 12 hours apart.

- Give at the same time(s) each day.

- Give the same way each day to keep blood concentrations therapeutic. For instance, if your child prefers to take this drug with meals, always give it with meals.

- Solution can be mixed with milk, chocolate milk, orange juice, or apple juice. All should be at room temperature. Mix well in a glass (not plastic) container and give immediately; do not let it stand. Refill the glass with the same beverage and give this to your child to ensure the whole dose is taken.

- Wipe the dropper off with a clean towel after each use. Do not rinse the dropper with water or other cleaning solutions.

- Missed doses: Give as soon as you remember if it is within 2 hours of the missed dose. If more than 2 hours have passed, call your child's doctor for instructions.

- Discard the solution 2 months after opening the container.

Side Effects

Tell your child's doctor about any side effects that are persistent or particularly bothersome.

More Common. Abdominal discomfort, acne, diarrhea, flushing, headache, increased hair growth, leg cramps, nausea or vomiting, trembling of hands

Less Common. Contact the doctor immediately if your child experiences convulsions; difficult or painful urination; fever or chills; tingling of the hands or feet; unusual bleeding; shortness of breath; rapid weight gain (3 to 5 pounds in 1 week); yellowing of the eyes or skin; unusual weakness; or bleeding, tender, or enlarged gums.

Possible Drug Interactions

- This drug interacts with many other drugs. It is important to consult the doctor before your child is started on any other medications.

- Phenytoin, phenobarbital, carbamazepine, rifampin, and trimethoprim can decrease the effectiveness of this drug by decreasing its blood concentration.

- Erythromycin, fluconazole, ketoconazole, diltiazem, verapamil, and methylprednisolone can increase the side effects of cyclosporine by increasing its blood concentration.

Tell Your Child's Doctor If

- Your child experiences any new side effects.

- Your daughter is or becomes pregnant.

- Your daughter is breast-feeding her baby.

Special Instructions

- Do not have your child immunized without the doctor's approval.

- Other household members should not receive the oral polio vaccine while your child is taking this drug.

Symptoms of Overdose: Convulsions and severe trembling

Special Notes

- The doctor will want to see your child regularly to ensure the drug is working properly and to check for unwanted side effects.

Just Call

If you have any concerns about any side effects, even minor ones, you should be sure to discuss them with your child's doctor. The doctor may be able to minimize or eliminate the side effects by prescribing a different medication or changing your child's dosage, dosing schedule, or the way the drug is given. (Do not make adjustments on your own without discussing them with your doctor.) At the very least, the doctor can assure you that the medication's benefits far outweigh its side effects.

Brand Name: Periactin, various manufacturers

Generic Available: Yes

Type of Drug: Antihistamine

Use: Relieves year-round and seasonal allergic rhinitis, itching, and hives. Also treats anorexia nervosa.

Time Required for Drug to Take Effect: 15 to 30 minutes

Dosage Forms and Strengths: Syrup (2 mg per 5 mL, contains 5% alcohol); Tablets (4 mg)

Storage: Store at room temperature in tightly closed containers. Do not freeze the syrup. The syrup is flammable. Do not expose to an open flame or ignited material such as lighted cigarettes.

How This Drug Works: Blocks the action of histamine, a chemical released by the body during an allergic reaction.

CYPROHEPTADINE

Administration Guidelines
• Give with food or a full glass of milk or water to avoid stomach upset.

• Missed doses: Give as soon as possible. However, if it's within 2 hours of the next dose, do not take the missed dose at all; just return to your regular dosing schedule. Do not give double doses.

Side Effects
Tell your child's doctor about any side effects that are persistent or particularly bothersome.

More Common. It is especially important to tell the doctor if your child experiences a change in menstruation, clumsiness, feeling faint, flushing of the face, hallucinations, palpitations, rash, seizures, shortness of breath, sleeping disorders, sore throat or fever, tightness in the chest, unusual bleeding or bruising, or unusual fatigue or weakness.

Less Common. Blurred vision; confusion; constipation; diarrhea; difficult or painful urination; diminished alertness; dizziness; dry mouth, throat, or nose; headache; irritability; loss of appetite; nausea; restlessness; ringing or buzzing in the ears; stomach upset; increased sensitivity to sunlight; or unusual increase in sweating. These side effects should disappear as your child's body adjusts to this drug.

Possible Drug Interactions
• Other central nervous system depressants such as alcohol, barbiturates, benzodiazepine tranquilizers, muscle relaxants, narcotics, pain medications, and phenothiazine tranquilizers can cause extreme fatigue or drowsiness.

• Monoamine oxidase (MAO) inhibitors such as isocarboxazid, pargyline, phenelzine, and tranylcypromine can increase the side effects of this drug. At least 14 days should separate the use of this drug and a MAO inhibitor.

• Can decrease the activity of oral anticoagulants.

Tell Your Child's Doctor If
• Your daughter is breast-feeding her baby. This drug can pass into breast milk and cause serious adverse reactions in the nursing infant.

Special Instructions
• Your child should avoid prolonged exposure to sunlight and wear protective clothing and an effective sunscreen when out-of-doors.

Symptoms of Overdose: Hallucinations, convulsions

DESIPRAMINE

Administration Guidelines

• May be given with food to decrease stomach upset.

• Usually given 2 or 3 times a day or as a single daily dose at bedtime.

• Missed doses: Give the missed dose as soon as possible. However, if it's time for the next dose, skip the missed dose. Do not give double doses. If a once-a-day bedtime dose is missed, do not give the missed dose in the morning as it may cause sedation.

• Do not suddenly stop giving this drug before speaking to your child's doctor, who may want to gradually reduce the dose.

Side Effects

Tell your child's doctor about any side effects that are persistent or particularly bothersome.

More Common. Drowsiness, dry mouth, dizziness, light-headedness, headache, nausea, increased appetite, weight gain, unpleasant taste, constipation, weakness. May cause urine to turn a blue-green color.

Less Common. Contact the doctor if your child experiences blurred vision, confusion, difficulty in speaking or swallowing, eye pain, fainting, fast or irregular heartbeat, hallucinations, loss of balance, masklike face, nervousness or restlessness, problems urinating, shakiness, or slow movements.

Possible Drug Interactions

• Clonidine (Catapres) and this drug may lead to very high blood pressure.

• Monoamine oxidase (MAO) inhibitors such as isocarboxazid (Marplan), phenelzine (Nardil), or tranylcypromine (Parnate) and this drug can lead to very serious reactions and death.

• Central nervous system depressants such as alcohol, antihistamines, muscle relaxants, tranquilizers, and some pain medications may cause extreme drowsiness when used with this drug.

• Cimetidine (Tagamet, Tagamet HB) and methylphenidate (Ritalin) may increase the effect of this drug.

• Phenobarbital and carbamazepine may decrease the effect of this drug.

• Eyedrops and nasal sprays or drops containing naphazoline, oxymetazoline, epinephrine, phenylephrine, or xylometazoline may cause an increase in heart rate and blood pressure.

Brand Names: Norpramin, Pertofrane

Generic Available: Yes

Type of Drug: Antidepressant, tricyclic

Use: Treats mental depression. Also treats some kinds of chronic pain and attention deficit disorder with hyperactivity.

Time Required for Drug to Take Effect: Full benefit may not be achieved for more than 2 weeks.

Dosage Forms and Strengths: Capsules (25 mg, 50 mg); Tablets (10 mg, 25 mg, 50 mg, 75 mg, 100 mg, 150 mg)

Storage: Store at room temperature in tightly closed, light-resistant containers.

How This Drug Works: Increases the concentration of serotonin and norepinephrine in the central nervous system.

- Antithyroid drugs lead to an increase in rare blood disorders when given with this drug.

Tell Your Child's Doctor If
- Your child has heart disease, seizures, glaucoma, thyroid disease, urinary retention, liver disease, kidney disease, or any other medical condition.

- Your child is or has been taking MAO inhibitors such as isocarboxazid (Marplan), phenelzine (Nardil), or tranylcypromine (Parnate).

- Your child has had an allergic reaction to this drug or any other medication.

- Your child has taken or is taking any other prescription or nonprescription medicine.

- Your daughter is or becomes pregnant.

- Your daughter is breast-feeding her baby. This drug can pass into breast milk, and the American Academy of Pediatrics is concerned about its effect on the baby.

Special Instructions
- Give only as directed by the doctor. It is important that your child's progress is checked regularly by the doctor.

- Do not allow your child to drink alcohol while taking this drug.

- Do not give other drugs that may make your child sleepy.

- Limit your child's caffeine intake.

- Your child should avoid exposure to sunlight. Make sure your child wears sunscreen when out-of-doors. This drug may cause a skin rash or severe sunburn when your child is exposed to direct sunlight or ultraviolet light in tanning booths.

- Do not give any other medications before talking to the doctor or pharmacist.

Symptoms of Overdose: Agitation; dry mouth; confusion; hallucinations; severe drowsiness; enlarged pupils; fever; vomiting; trouble breathing; urinary retention; low blood pressure; seizures; or fast, slow, or irregular heartbeat

Special Notes
- Drowsiness is common. Make sure you know how your child is reacting to this drug before allowing participation in an activity that requires alertness and coordination, such as riding a bicycle. This drug may cause your child to have blurred vision, dizziness, drowsiness, or to be less alert.

- Some brands contain tartrazine dye. If your child is allergic to this dye, ask the pharmacist for a tartrazine-free product.

- The effects of this drug may last for 1 week after you stop giving this drug to your child.

- Doses are increased slowly to decrease side effects.

- This drug can cause light-headedness and dizziness if your child gets up too quickly from a prone or sitting position. Have your child get up slowly to prevent these side effects.

DEXAMETHASONE (SYSTEMIC)

Administration Guidelines
• May be given with food or milk to prevent stomach irritation.

• If your child is taking only 1 dose a day, try to give it before 9:00 A.M. This will mimic the body's normal production of similar cortisonelike chemicals.

• The concentrate may be mixed in juice, other liquids, or semisolid foods like applesauce.

• Missed doses: It is important not to miss a dose of this drug. If you miss a dose, follow these guidelines:

1. For those giving this drug more than once a day: Give the missed dose as soon as possible and then return to the regular schedule. If it is already time for the next dose, double it.

2. For those giving this drug once a day: Give the missed dose as soon as possible. If you do not remember until the next day, do not give the missed dose at all, just follow the regular dosing schedule. Do not give double doses.

3. For those giving this drug every other day: Give it as soon as you remember. If you missed the scheduled time by a whole day, give it when you remember, then skip a day before giving the next dose. Do not give double doses. If you miss more than one dose, contact your child's doctor.

Side Effects
Tell your child's doctor about any side effects that are persistent or particularly bothersome.

More Common. Dizziness, false sense of well-being, fatigue, increased appetite, increased sweating, indigestion, leg cramps, menstrual irregularities, muscle weakness, nausea, reddening of the skin on the face, restlessness, sleep disorders, thinning of the skin, or weight gain

Less Common. It is important to tell the doctor if your child experiences abdominal enlargement or pain; acne; back or rib pain; bloody or black, tarry stools; blurred vision; convulsions; eye pain; fever and sore throat; headaches; slow healing of wounds; increased thirst and urination; depression; mood changes; muscle wasting; nightmares; peptic ulcers; rapid weight gain (3 to 5 pounds in a week); rash; shortness of breath; unusual bleeding or bruising; or unusual weakness.

Possible Drug Interactions
• Decreases the effectiveness of vaccines and can lead to infection if a live virus vaccine is given.

Brand Names: Decadron, Dexone, Hexadrol, Dexamethasone (various manufacturers)

Generic Available: Yes

Type of Drug: Adrenocorticosteroid hormone

Use: Treats endocrine and rheumatic disorders, asthma, blood diseases, certain cancers, eye disorders, certain gastrointestinal disturbances, respiratory diseases, and inflammatory diseases such as arthritis and dermatitis.

Time Required for Drug to Take Effect: Varies depending on the illness being treated. It may be several days before an effect is achieved.

Dosage Forms and Strengths: Tablets (0.25 mg, 0.5 mg, 0.75 mg, 1 mg, 1.5 mg, 2 mg, 4 mg, 6 mg); Elixir (0.5 mg per 5 mL with 5% alcohol); Solution (0.5 mg per 5 mL); Concentrate (0.5 mg per 0.5 mL with 30% alcohol)

Storage: Store at room temperature in tightly closed containers.

How This Drug Works: How this drug works is not completely understood.

Tell Your Child's Doctor If
• Your child is taking any other medications.

• Your child has had an allergic reaction to this drug or other adrenocorticoids such as betamethasone, cortisone, fluocinolone, hydrocortisone, methylprednisolone, prednisolone, prednisone, and triamcinolone.

• Your child has recently been exposed to or currently has chicken pox or measles.

• Your child has any medical problems such as diabetes, glaucoma, fungal infections, heart disease, high blood pressure, peptic ulcers, thyroid disease, tuberculosis, ulcerative colitis, kidney disease, or liver disease.

• Your daughter is or becomes pregnant. This drug can have adverse effects on the fetus.

• Your daughter is breast-feeding her baby.

Special Instructions
• Your child should not be vaccinated or immunized while taking this drug.

Symptoms of Overdose: Severe restlessness

Special Notes
• With long-term use the doctor may want your child to be on a low-salt and potassium-rich diet. The doctor may also want your child's eyes examined periodically during treatment to detect glaucoma and cataracts.

• With long-term use, your child's dose may need to be increased during times of stress such as serious infection, injury, or surgery.

Measuring Up

Remember: Never use an ordinary tableware teaspoon to measure liquid doses. Instead, use a cylindrical dosing spoon, dosage cup, dropper, or syringe. These measuring devices can be found at your local drug store and sometimes at supermarkets, toy stores, and department stores.

DEXTROAMPHETAMINE

Administration Guidelines

• Give on an empty stomach 1 hour before or 2 hours after a meal for maximum benefit.

• For maximum absorption, do not give acidic foods, juices, or vitamin C for at least 1 hour before or 1 hour after you give this drug.

• Sustained-release capsules are usually given once a day before breakfast; tablets are usually given 1 to 3 times a day.

• Give the last dose of the day at least 6 hours before bedtime. The other doses should be divided equally during the daytime.

• Do not crush or allow your child to chew the sustained-release capsules.

• Missed doses: Give as soon as possible. However, if it is time for the next dose, skip the missed dose and return to the regular dosing schedule. Do not give double doses.

Side Effects

Tell your child's doctor about any side effects that are persistent or particularly bothersome.

More Common. Dizziness, depression, hyperirritability, insomnia, anorexia, nausea, vomiting, diarrhea, stomach cramps, metallic taste, dry mouth, movement disorder, tremor, difficulty focusing on objects, growth suppression, physical and psychological dependence with prolonged use

Less Common. It is especially important to tell the doctor if your child experiences fast heart rate, irritability, depression, or dizziness.

Possible Drug Interactions

• May decrease the effects of methyldopa.

• May increase the effects of tricyclic antidepressants such as amitriptyline, desipramine, doxepin, imipramine, and nortriptyline.

Tell Your Child's Doctor If

• Your child is taking any prescription or nonprescription medications, especially those listed above.

• Your child has or ever had unusual or allergic reactions to any medications, especially to any amphetaminelike drugs.

• Your child has or ever had any kidney, liver, or brain disease.

• Your child is allergic to tartrazine. Sustained-release capsules contain tartrazine, a dye to which many patients are allergic.

Brand Name: Dexedrine

Generic Available: No

Type of Drug: Central nervous system stimulant and anorexiant (appetite suppressant)

Use: As an adjunct in the treatment of attention deficit disorder with hyperactivity (ADHD); also treats narcolepsy and obesity.

Time Required for Drug to Take Effect: It may take a few days to achieve maximum effectiveness.

Dosage Forms and Strengths: Tablets (5 mg, 10 mg); Capsules, sustained-release (5 mg, 10 mg)

Storage: Store at room temperature in tightly closed, light-resistant containers.

How This Drug Works: Increases the levels of dopamine and norepinephrine in the brain.

- Your daughter is or becomes pregnant. This drug should not be used during pregnancy.

- Your daughter is breast-feeding her baby. This drug passes into breast milk and may lead to the side effects listed above and drug dependence.

Special Instructions

- Do not stop giving this drug abruptly. Abrupt discontinuation may lead to severe withdrawal and central nervous system crisis.

Symptoms of Overdose: Severe forms of the side effects listed above.

Special Notes

- The doctor may discontinue this drug periodically for a few days to assess the need for continuing treatment, to decrease drug dependence, and to limit suppression of growth and weight.

Keep It Out of Reach

Do not rely on a child-resistant cap to deter your child from opening a bottle of medication. Child-resistant does not mean childproof. Legally, a cap can be called child-resistant if 80 percent of all five-year-olds need more than five minutes to open it. That means the other 20 percent could get into it in even less time. Put the bottle in a hard-to-reach cabinet with a childproof lock. Do not keep it on the countertop, kitchen table, or nightstand.

DEXTROMETHORPHAN

Administration Guidelines
• Give either on an empty stomach or with food or milk.

• To loosen the mucus in the bronchi, your child should drink a glass of water after each dose.

• Missed doses: Give as soon as possible. However, if it's within 1 to 3 hours of the next dose, skip the missed dose and return to the regular dosing schedule. Do not give double doses.

Side Effects
Tell your child's doctor about any side effects that are persistent or particularly bothersome.

MORE COMMON. Side effects are not common.

LESS COMMON. Drowsiness or stomach upset. These side effects should disappear as your child's body adjusts to this drug.

Possible Drug Interactions
• Other central nervous system depressants such as alcohol, barbiturates, benzodiazepine tranquilizers, muscle relaxants, narcotics, pain medications, phenothiazine tranquilizers, and sleeping medications or tricyclic antidepressants can lead to drowsiness.

• Can cause high blood pressure and other side effects when used within 14 days of a monoamine oxidase (MAO) inhibitor such as isocarboxazid, pargyline, phenelzine, and tranylcypromine.

Tell Your Child's Doctor If
• Your child has had unusual or allergic reactions to any medications, especially to this drug.

• Your child is taking any medications, especially any of those listed above.

Special Instructions
• If this drug makes your child dizzy or drowsy, do not allow participation in activities that require alertness, such as riding a bicycle.

• Your child should drink several glasses of water a day to help loosen bronchial secretions while taking this drug.

Symptoms of Overdose: Shaky movements and unsteady gait, respiratory depression, convulsions

Special Notes
• Also available in combination with many other cough and cold products.

Brand Names: Benylin DM,* Children's Hold,* Delsym,* Dextromethorphan* (various suppliers), Hold DM,* Pertussin CS,* Pertussin ES,* Robitussin Cough Calmers,* Robitussin Pediatric,* Scot-Tussin DM Cough Chasers,* St. Joseph Cough Suppressant,* Sucrets Cough Control,* Suppress,* Trocal,* Vicks Formula 44,* Vicks Formula 44 Pediatric Formula* (*available over the counter)

Generic Available: Yes

Type of Drug: Cough suppressant

Use: Temporary control of cough due to minor throat and bronchial irritation.

Time Required for Drug to Take Effect: 15 to 30 minutes

Dosage Forms and Strengths: Lozenges (2.5 mg, 5 mg, 7.5 mg); Liquid (3.5 mg/5 mL, 7.5 mg/5 mL, 15 mg/5mL); Liquid, sustained-action (30 mg/5 mL); Syrup (10 mg/5 mL, 15 mg/15 mL)

Storage: Store at room temperature in tightly closed containers. Do not expose to high temperatures.

How This Drug Works: Reduces the activity of the cough center in the brain and depresses respiration.

Brand Names: Valium, Valrelease

Generic Available: Yes

Type of Drug: Benzodiazepine

Use: Treats general anxiety or panic disorders and some types of seizure disorders; provides sedation for test procedures; also relaxes skeletal muscles.

Time Required for Drug to Take Effect: 20 to 60 minutes. Depending on the diagnosis, full benefit may not be achieved for a few weeks. Onset within 2 to 10 minutes after rectal administration.

Dosage Forms and Strengths: Tablets (2 mg, 5 mg, 10 mg); Capsules, long-acting (15 mg); Solution (5 mg/5 mL, 5 mg/1 mL); Injection (5 mg/mL)

Storage: Store at room temperature in tightly closed, light-resistant containers. Do not freeze solution or injection.

How This Drug Works: Depresses the central nervous system. Stops seizure activity by suppressing the spread of the seizure impulse in the brain.

DIAZEPAM

Administration Guidelines

- May be given with food or water to decrease stomach upset.

- Usually given 2 to 4 times a day. Long-acting capsule is usually given once a day.

- Missed doses: Give immediately if you remember within 1 hour of missing the dose. Otherwise skip the missed dose and go back to the regular dosing schedule. Do not give double doses.

- Do not crush, break, or allow your child to chew the long-acting capsule. Have your child swallow it whole.

- For rectal administration, follow the directions given to you by your child's doctor. The dose may be drawn from the parenteral vial by using a needle and syringe. Remove the needle and administer the drug through tubing which has been inserted into the rectum. Flush tubing with normal saline solution and then remove tubing.

Side Effects

Tell your child's doctor about any side effects that are persistent or particularly bothersome.

More Common. Clumsiness, unsteadiness, dizziness, light-headedness, drowsiness, slurred speech, headache, dry mouth, constipation, diarrhea, nausea, change in appetite, vomiting

Less Common. Contact the doctor if your child experiences behavioral changes, difficulty concentrating, outbursts of anger, confusion, mental depression, seizures, hallucinations, impaired memory, muscle weakness, skin rash, itching, sore throat, fever, chills, sores in the mouth, uncontrolled body movements, unusual bleeding or bruising, unusual excitement or nervousness, irritability, unusual fatigue or weakness, or yellow skin.

Possible Drug Interactions

- Central nervous system depressants such as alcohol, antihistamines, muscle relaxants, tranquilizers, and some pain medications may cause extreme drowsiness when used with this drug.

Tell Your Child's Doctor If

- Your child has taken or is taking any other prescription or nonprescription medicine.

- Your child has had an allergic reaction to this drug or any other medications, foods, preservatives, or dyes.

- Your child has asthma, lung disease, seizures, glaucoma, liver or kidney disease, or any other medical condition.

• Your daughter is or becomes pregnant.

• Your daughter is breast-feeding her baby. This drug can pass into breast milk, and the American Academy of Pediatrics is concerned about its effect on the baby.

Special Instructions

• Give this drug only as directed by the doctor.

• Take your child to the doctor regularly to monitor progress.

• Do not suddenly stop giving this drug before speaking to the doctor. Stopping this drug abruptly can lead to seizures.

• Your child should not drink alcohol while taking this drug.

• Do not give other medicines that may make your child sleepy.

Symptoms of Overdose: Slurred speech, confusion, severe drowsiness, severe weakness, shakiness, low blood pressure, trouble breathing, slow heartbeat, staggering, coma, or trouble walking

Special Notes

• Drowsiness is common. Make sure you know how your child is reacting to this drug before allowing participation in activities that require alertness and coordination, such as riding a bicycle.

• Your child's body may take up to 3 weeks to adjust when this drug is stopped after long-term use.

Just Call

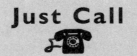

If you have any concerns about any side effects, even minor ones, you should be sure to discuss them with your child's doctor. The doctor may be able to minimize or eliminate the side effects by prescribing a different medication or changing your child's dosage, dosing schedule, or the way the drug is given. (Do not make adjustments on your own without discussing them with your doctor.) At the very least, the doctor can assure you that the medication's benefits far outweigh its side effects.

Brand Names: Dycill, Dynapen, Pathocil, Dicloxacillin Sodium (various manufacturers)

Generic Available: Yes

Type of Drug: Penicillin antibiotic

Use: Treats a wide variety of bacterial infections.

Time Required for Drug to Take Effect: 2 to 3 days

Dosage Forms and Strengths: Capsules (125 mg, 250 mg, and 500 mg); Suspension (62.5 mg per 5 mL)

Storage: Store capsules at room temperature in a tightly closed container. Refrigerate liquid.

How This Drug Works: Destroys susceptible bacteria.

DICLOXACILLIN

Administrative Guidelines

• Give on an empty stomach with a glass of water.

• Do not give with fruit juices or carbonated beverages.

• Usually given 4 times a day.

• Usually given for 7 to 14 days. Complete the prescribed course of therapy, even if symptoms subside.

• Shake the suspension before measuring each dose.

• Missed doses: Give as soon as possible. However, if it's less than 2 hours before the next scheduled dose, skip the missed dose. Do not give double doses.

Side Effects

Tell your child's doctor about any side effects that are persistent or particularly bothersome.

More Common. Diarrhea, heartburn, nausea, or vomiting

Less Common. Bloating, chills, cough, darkened tongue, difficulty breathing, irritation of the mouth, muscle aches, rash, rectal or vaginal itching, severe diarrhea, or sore throat

Possible Drug Interactions

• Decreases the effectiveness of oral contraceptives.

Tell Your Child's Doctor If

• Your child has had allergic reactions to this drug or other penicillins, or to cephalosporin antibiotics, penicillamine, or griseofulvin.

• Your child has kidney disease, asthma, or allergies.

• Your daughter is breast-feeding her baby.

Special Instructions

• Children with diabetes may have a false-positive sugar reaction with a Clinitest urine glucose test. To avoid this problem, switch to Clinistix or Tes-Tape during treatment with this drug.

Symptoms of Overdose: Severe nausea, vomiting, diarrhea, abdominal pain

DIDANOSINE (ddI; DIDEOXYINOSINE)

Administration Guidelines

- Give on an empty stomach, 1 hour before or 2 hours after a meal. Food significantly reduces the absorption of this drug.

- Usually given 2 times a day.

- Powder packets should be mixed only with water. Soda-pop or fruit juices may decrease the absorption of this drug.

- Your child should chew the tablets, or the tablets should be crushed or dispersed in water before you give them.

- Missed doses: Give as soon as possible. However, if it's within 6 hours of the next dose, skip the missed dose and give the next regular dose. Do not give double doses.

Side Effects

Tell your child's doctor about any side effects that are persistent or particularly bothersome.

More Common. Tingling of the hands or feet; pain in the hands, legs, or feet; headache; difficulty sleeping; depression; dizziness; diarrhea; nausea; vomiting; sore mouth; painful joints; chills; fever; runny nose. Contact the doctor if your child experiences difficulty breathing or unusual bleeding or bruising.

Less Common. Confusion, nervousness, anxiety, loss of memory, constipation, skin rash, anemia, hair loss. Contact the doctor if your child experiences symptoms of pancreatitis (stomach pain, nausea, vomiting), seizures, or yellowing of eyes or skin.

Possible Drug Interactions

- Antacids increase the absorption of this drug. This is a beneficial effect. Commercial products of this drug contain some acid-neutralizing compounds. The doctor may prescribe additional antacids.

- May decrease the absorption of dapsone, itraconazole, ketoconazole, quinolone antibiotics (such as ciprofloxacin), and tetracycline when taken at the same time.

- Zalcitabine can increase the risk of nerve damage when taken with this drug.

- Pentamidine or co-trimoxazole may increase the risk of pancreatitis.

Tell Your Child's Doctor If

- Your child has had allergic reactions to any medications.

Brand Names: Videx, Videx Pediatric

Generic Available: No

Type of Drug: Antiviral, antiretroviral

Use: Treats human immunodeficiency virus (HIV) infections which cause acquired immunodeficiency syndrome (AIDS).

Time Required for Drug to Take Effect: Must be given indefinitely.

Dosage Forms and Strengths: Tablets, chewable/dispersible (25 mg, 50 mg, 100 mg, 150 mg); Powder for solution (100 mg, 167 mg, 250 mg, 375 mg/packet); Powder for solution, pediatric (10 mg/mL final concentration)

Storage: Store at room temperature in tightly closed containers. Dispersible tablets added to water are stable for 1 hour. Powder packets added to water are stable for 4 hours. The pediatric solution is stable for 30 days in the refrigerator after mixing with water and antacid.

How This Drug Works: Slows the growth of HIV.

- Your child has any other diseases.

- Your child is taking any other medications.

- Your child has liver or kidney disease.

- Your daughter is or becomes pregnant.

- Your daughter is breast-feeding her baby. It is not known if this drug passes into breast milk. Mothers with HIV infections are generally advised not to breast-feed.

Symptoms of Overdose: Not well known, although nausea, vomiting, stomach pain, and pain in the hands, legs, or feet would be expected.

Special Notes

- This drug does not cure AIDS or prevent transmission of HIV.

- Tablets contain phenylalanine, which is important in phenylketonuria.

- Powder packets contain large amounts of sodium and should be used cautiously in children on sodium-restricted diets.

- Your child's doctor will perform several tests to ensure this drug is working and is safe.

Outdated Doses

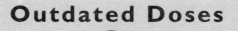

Safe and proper medication disposal is essential, especially when you have children in the house. Do not keep medication—whether prescription or nonprescription—past the expiration date, even if it appears normal. Expired medication may be ineffective and can even be dangerous. Make a habit of regularly checking the expiration date on all medicines in your home. Flush leftover medication down the toilet or pour it down the sink. Rinse the container before throwing it out. If your medication does not display an expiration date, throw it out after one year.

DIGOXIN

Administration Guidelines
• May be given with food or milk, but be consistent.

• Usually given 1 or 2 times a day.

• Missed doses: Give as soon as possible. However, if it's within 8 hours of the next dose, skip the missed dose and give the next scheduled dose. Do not give double doses.

• Use only the dropper provided with the elixir or an oral syringe to measure doses.

Side Effects
Tell your child's doctor about any side effects that are persistent or particularly bothersome.

More Common. Upset stomach, diarrhea, drowsiness, fatigue. Call the doctor if your child experiences prolonged nausea and vomiting, excessive fatigue, and palpitations.

Less Common. Dizziness, confusion, hallucinations, nausea and vomiting, blurred or yellow vision. Contact the doctor if your child experiences fainting and hallucinations.

Possible Drug Interactions
• Antacids may decrease the absorption of this drug from the intestinal tract.

• Penicillamine, anticonvulsants, and rifampin can decrease the effectiveness of this drug and may necessitate an adjustment of the dosage.

• Antibiotics, amiodarone, captopril, verapamil, diltiazem, quinidine, and spironolactone can increase the effectiveness of this drug and may require an adjustment of the dosage.

• Some asthma, allergy, cough, cold, or sinus medications can aggravate fast heart rhythms. Do not give this drug without first checking with the doctor.

Tell Your Child's Doctor If
• Your child has had allergic reactions to any medications.

• Your child has any diseases.

• Your child is taking any other medications.

• Your daughter is or becomes pregnant.

• Your daughter is breast-feeding her baby.

Brand Names: Lanoxin, Lanoxicaps

Generic Available: Yes

Type of Drug: Digitalis glycoside

Use: Treats congestive heart failure and abnormally fast heart rhythms (tachycardia).

Time Required for Drug to Take Effect: From several days to a week.

Dosage Forms and Strengths: Capsules (0.05 mg, 0.1 mg, 0.2 mg); Tablets (0.125 mg, 0.25 mg, 0.5 mg); Elixir (0.05 mg/mL)

Storage: Store at room temperature in tightly closed containers.

How This Drug Works: Acts on the heart muscle to strengthen heartbeat and control heart rhythm.

Special Instructions

• The doctor will periodically measure blood levels of this drug and other blood chemistries to help determine the proper dosage for your child.

• Make sure the pharmacist always dispenses the same brand of this drug. Switching between brands may require additional dosage adjustments.

• Always double-check doses to avoid giving your child an overdose.

Symptoms of Overdose: Excessively slow heart rate, nausea, and vomiting

Be Accurate

If you don't give medication correctly, it may be ineffective or even cause side effects. An estimated 10 to 30 percent of medications aren't effective because they have been given incorrectly. To do it right, you have to give the exact amount of medicine prescribed at the scheduled time, for the specified duration, and in the appropriate manner. Always read the label, follow the directions carefully, and use the appropriate equipment for measuring and administering the medication. Also, be sure to wash your hands before you give any medication to your child.

DILTIAZEM

Administration Guidelines

• May be given on an empty stomach or with meals, but be consistent.

• Give with a large glass of water.

• Cardizem SR is given 2 times a day; Cardizem CD and Dilacor-XR are given 1 time a day. Do not change brands without checking with your child's doctor.

• Do not crush or allow your child to chew long-acting capsules.

• Missed doses: Give as soon as possible. However, if it's time for the next dose, skip the missed dose. Do not give double doses.

• Tablets are usually given 3 or 4 times a day.

Side Effects

Tell your child's doctor about any side effects that are persistent or particularly bothersome.

More Common. Headache, slow heartbeat, dizziness, nausea, vomiting, fatigue, light-headedness, constipation, flushing

Less Common. Increased amount of gum tissue in the mouth. Contact the doctor immediately if your child experiences difficulty breathing, coughing, wheezing, irregular or fast heartbeat, skin rash, or swelling of ankles or legs.

Possible Drug Interactions

• Beta-adrenergic blocking agents (oral and eyedrops) such as propanol, atenolol, labetalol, metoprolol, and timolol lead to a low or dangerously low heart rate. These agents can be used with this drug but the doctor must carefully adjust the dosage and monitor your child closely.

• Diuretics, cardiac medications, and medications that lower blood pressure can lead to an increase in severe cardiac side effects. These drugs may be used together if the doctor carefully adjusts the dosage and monitors your child closely.

• Cough, cold, hay fever, sinus, and asthma medications; decongestants; and appetite control products may increase blood pressure.

• Increases the blood concentrations and side effects of carbamazepine, digoxin, quinidine, and cyclosporine.

Tell Your Child's Doctor If

• Your child has taken or is taking any other prescription or nonprescription medicine.

Brand Names: Cardizem, Cardizem CD, Cardizem SR, Dilacor XR

Generic Available: Yes

Type of Drug: Antihypertensive, antianginal, antiarrhythmic

Use: Treats high blood pressure, angina, and some abnormal heart rhythms.

Time Required for Drug to Take Effect: Within 1 hour for tablets; 2 to 3 hours for long-acting capsules. It may take up to 2 weeks to achieve full benefit for blood pressure control.

Dosage Forms and Strengths: Capsules, long-acting (60 mg, 90 mg, 120 mg, 180 mg, 240 mg, 300 mg); Tablets (30 mg, 60 mg, 90 mg, 120 mg)

Storage: Store at room temperature in tightly closed, light-resistant containers.

How This Drug Works: Blocks the movement of calcium into the cells of the heart and blood vessels. This relaxes blood vessels, lowers blood pressure, and increases the supply of oxygen to the heart.

- Your child has had an allergic reaction to this drug, any other medications, foods, preservatives, or dyes.

- Your child has heart, liver, or kidney disease; high blood pressure; any other medical condition; or suffers from depression.

- Your child's gums bleed, or are tender or swollen.

- Your daughter is or becomes pregnant.

- Your daughter is breast-feeding her baby. This drug can pass into breast milk; however, the American Academy of Pediatrics considers it compatible with breast-feeding in most cases.

Special Instructions

- Give this drug to your child only as directed by the doctor.

- Have your child's progress checked regularly by the doctor.

- Do not stop giving this drug without first checking with the doctor, who may want to gradually reduce the dosage before stopping it.

- Do not allow your child (teenagers included) to drink alcohol while taking this drug.

- Brush and floss your child's teeth daily and carefully massage the gums to decrease gum tissue overgrowth.

- Take your child to the dentist regularly.

- Limit your child's caffeine intake.

- Do not give any other medicines without first talking to the doctor.

Symptoms of Overdose: Low blood pressure, very low heart rate, confusion, nausea, vomiting, increase in blood sugar

Keep a Lid on It

Pharmacists are required to put drugs in bottles that have child-resistant caps. Don't switch to a bottle that's easier for you to open—children may also find it easier to open. Remember, too, that child-resistant does not mean childproof. Children older than five years of age may be able to open most medicine bottles. That's why it's essential for you to teach them that drugs can be harmful if not taken correctly and that they need supervision before taking anything. And, just to be on the safe side, keep all medicines out of your child's reach.

DIMENHYDRINATE

Administration Guidelines

- Give with food, milk, or water to avoid upset stomach unless your child's doctor directs you to do otherwise.
- Chewable tablets should be chewed for at least 2 minutes to obtain full therapeutic benefit.
- Take 1 hour before traveling to prevent motion sickness.
- Missed doses: Give as soon as possible. However, if it is 1 to 3 hours before your child's next dose, skip the missed dose and return to the regular dosing schedule. Do not give double doses.

Side Effects
Tell your child's doctor about any side effects that are persistent or particularly bothersome.

More Common. Confusion; constipation; diarrhea; dizziness; dry mouth, throat, or nose; headache; irritability; loss of appetite; nausea; restlessness; or stomach upset. These side effects should disappear as your child's body adjusts to this drug. Some children may experience unusual excitation.

Less Common. It is especially important to tell the doctor if your child experiences blurred vision, hallucinations, palpitations, ringing or buzzing in the ears, rash, seizures, sleeping disorders, or unusual fatigue or weakness.

Possible Drug Interactions
- Can cause extreme drowsiness when used with other central nervous system depressants such as alcohol, barbiturates, benzodiazepine tranquilizers, muscle relaxants, narcotics, pain medications, and phenothiazine tranquilizers or with tricyclic antidepressants.

Tell Your Child's Doctor If
- Your child is taking any medications, especially those listed above.
- Your child has had allergic or unusual reactions to any medications.
- Your child has or ever had asthma, blood-vessel disease, high blood pressure, kidney or thyroid disease, or peptic ulcers.
- Your child takes large amounts of aspirin on a regular basis in addition to this drug. This drug can mask the side effects of too much aspirin such as tinnitus (ringing in the ears).
- Your daughter is or becomes pregnant. The effects of this drug during pregnancy have not been thoroughly studied in humans.

Brand Names: Calm-X,* Dimetabs,* Dramamine,* Marmine,* Tega-Vert,* Triptone Caplets* (*available over the counter)

Generic Available: Yes

Type of Drug: Antiemetic (prevents nausea and vomiting due to motion sickness)

Use: Treats and prevents nausea, dizziness, and vomiting associated with motion sickness.

Time Required for Drug to Take Effect: 15 to 30 minutes

Dosage Forms and Strengths: Capsules (50 mg); Liquid (125 mg/4 mL, 15.62 mg/5 mL); Tablets (50 mg); Tablets, chewable (50 mg)

Storage: Store at room temperature in tightly closed, light-resistant containers.

How This Drug Works: The precise mode of action is not known. Antiemetic effects are believed to be due to diphenhydramine, an antihistamine also used as an antiemetic agent, that makes up half of this drug.

• Your daughter is breast-feeding her baby. Small amounts of this drug are excreted in breast milk. Your daughter should talk to the doctor about temporarily discontinuing nursing or discontinuing this drug.

Symptoms of Overdose: Most commonly, drowsiness. Convulsions, coma, and respiratory depression may occur with massive overdosage.

Special Notes

• Chewable tablets contain tartrazine dye which may cause allergic reactions in sensitive individuals, particularly those sensitive to aspirin.

• This drug can cause drowsiness or dizziness, decreasing your child's ability to perform tasks that require alertness, such as riding a bicycle. Take appropriate caution.

Teach Your Children Well

Let's face it. Kids can be pretty stubborn when it comes to accepting medication. When appropriate, try giving your child information about his or her condition and how the medicine works. In a nonthreatening voice, talk about the consequences of not taking the medication, perhaps reminding the child of how uncomfortable he or she was before beginning the medication. Use reasoning when possible, but don't scare the child. Children who understand the importance of antibiotics for infection, insulin for diabetes, or inhalants for asthma are more likely to take the medication without objection.

DIPHENHYDRAMINE

Administration Guidelines

• Give with food, milk, or water to avoid stomach upset.

• For motion sickness, give 30 minutes before anticipated motion. Give subsequent doses before meals and at bedtime.

• Missed doses: Give as soon as possible. However, if it is within 2 hours of the next dose, do not give the missed dose at all; just return to the prescribed dosing schedule. Do not give double doses.

Side Effects

Tell your child's doctor about any side effects that are persistent or particularly bothersome.

More Common. Confusion; constipation; diarrhea; dizziness; dry mouth, throat, or nose; headache; irritability; loss of appetite; nausea; restlessness; or stomach upset. These side effects should disappear as your child's body adjusts to this drug. Some children may experience unusual excitation.

Less Common. It is especially important to tell the doctor about blurred vision, hallucinations, palpitations, ringing or buzzing in the ears, rash, seizures, sleeping disorders, or unusual fatigue or weakness.

Possible Drug Interactions

• Other central nervous system depressants such as alcohol, barbiturates, benzodiazepine tranquilizers, muscle relaxants, narcotics, and pain medications can cause extreme fatigue or drowsiness.

Tell Your Child's Doctor If

• Your child has had unusual or allergic reactions to any medications, especially to this drug or any other antihistamine.

• Your child has or ever had asthma, blood vessel disease, high blood pressure, kidney or thyroid disease, or peptic ulcers.

• Your daughter is or becomes pregnant.

• Your daughter is breast-feeding her baby. Small amounts of this drug pass into breast milk and may cause unusual excitement or irritability in nursing infants.

Special Instructions

• Your child should avoid prolonged exposure to sunlight and sunlamps. When out-of-doors, your child should wear protective clothing and use an effective sunscreen.

Brand Names: AllerMax,* Banophen,* Belix,* Benadryl,* Benadryl Topical,* Benylin Cough Syrup,* Bydramine Cough Syrup,* Diphen Cough,* Dormin,* Genahist, Hydramyn Syrup,* Maximum Strength Nytol,* Nidryl,* Nordryl, Nytol,* Phendry,* Silphen Cough,* Sleepeze 3,* Sleepinal,* Sominex,* Tusstat Syrup, Twilite,* Uni-Bent Cough Syrup*
(*available over the counter)

Generic Available: Yes

Type of Drug: Antihistamine

Use: Treats or prevents allergy symptoms and treats motion sickness. Also used as a sleeping aid and nonnarcotic cough suppressant.

Time Required for Drug to Take Effect: 15 to 30 minutes

Dosage Forms and Strengths: Tablets (50 mg); Capsules (25 mg, 50 mg); Elixir (12.5 mg per 5 mL, with 14% alcohol); Syrup, for cough suppressant (12.5 mg per 5 mL, with 5% alcohol)

Storage: Store at room temperature in tightly closed containers, away from heat and direct sunlight.

How This Drug Works: Blocks the action of histamine, a chemical released during allergic reactions.

• The elixir is flammable. Do not expose it to an open flame or ignited material such as a lighted cigarette.

Symptoms of Overdose: Sleepiness, sedation, or coma. Sedation may be accompanied by profuse sweating, low blood pressure, or shock.

Special Notes

• This drug has a more sedative effect than the majority of other antihistamines.

Over-the-Counter Wisdom

Keep in mind that even a medication that is available without a doctor's prescription may still be harmful and should be given appropriately and only when necessary. Talk to your pediatrician about what to do if your child gets sick. Some illnesses can be treated at home, some require a call to the pediatrician's office, and some will require a visit to the doctor. In addition, ask the doctor what situations constitute an emergency. If you're not sure if it's safe or appropriate to give your child a particular over-the-counter medication, be sure to talk to the doctor first.

DIPHENOXYLATE AND ATROPINE

Administration Guidelines
• May be given with food to decrease stomach upset.

• Given in 2 to 4 doses a day.

• Missed doses: Give as soon as possible. However, if it's 4 hours or less before the next dose, skip the missed dose. Do not give double doses.

Side Effects
Tell your child's doctor about any side effects that are persistent or particularly bothersome.

More Common. Nervousness, restlessness, dizziness, drowsiness, headache, mental depression, intestinal blockage, dry mouth, difficulty urinating, blurred vision, and decreased breathing rate

Less Common. Contact the doctor if your child experiences bloating, constipation, loss of appetite, or severe stomach pain with nausea and vomiting.

Possible Drug Interactions
• Monoamine oxidase (MAO) inhibitors such as isocarboxazid (Marplan), phenelzine (Nardil), and tranylcypromine (Parnate) can lead to very serious reactions when given with this drug.

• Central nervous system depressants such as alcohol, antihistamines, muscle relaxants, tranquilizers, antidepressants, sleep medicine, narcotics, and some pain medications may cause extreme drowsiness when used with this drug.

Tell Your Child's Doctor If
• Your child has any signs of dehydration such as dry mouth, dizziness, light-headedness, increased thirst, decreased urination, wrinkled skin, or absence of tears when crying.

• Your child has diarrhea for more than 2 days.

• Your child has a fever.

• Your child is taking any other prescription or nonprescription medicine or has recently taken antibiotics.

• Your child has had an allergic reaction to this drug, any other medications, foods, preservatives, or dyes.

• Your child has heart, lung, thyroid, liver, or kidney disease; glaucoma; asthma; urinary retention; jaundice; an intestinal blockage or other intestinal problems; colitis; Down syndrome; or any other medical condition.

Brand Name: Lomotil

Generic Available: Yes

Type of Drug: Antidiarrheal

Use: Treats diarrhea.

Time Required for Drug to Take Effect: Onset within 1 hour

Dosage Forms and Strengths: Tablets (diphenoxylate 2.5 mg and atropine 0.025 mg); Liquid (diphenoxylate 2.5 mg and atropine 0.025 mg/5 mL)

Storage: Store at room temperature in tightly closed, light-resistant containers. Do not freeze liquid.

How This Drug Works: Slows down intestinal activity.

• Your child is younger than 2 years of age.

• Your child abuses alcohol or drugs.

• Your daughter is or becomes pregnant.

• Your daughter is breast-feeding her baby. This drug can pass into breast milk; however the American Academy of Pediatrics considers it compatible with breast-feeding in most cases.

Special Instructions

• Give your child plenty of fluids. Even if the stools look better after taking this drug, your child will continue to lose water into the intestine.

• Do not allow your child to drink alcohol while taking this drug.

• Do not give other medicines that may make your child sleepy.

Symptoms of Overdose: Drowsiness; low blood pressure; blurred vision; dry mouth; small pupils; shortness of breath; trouble breathing; fast heartbeat; unusual excitement; nervousness; restlessness; irritability; warm, dry, red skin

Special Notes

• Make sure you know how your child is reacting to this drug before allowing participation in an activity that requires alertness and coordination, such as riding a bicycle. This drug may cause your child to have blurred vision or to be dizzy, drowsy, or less alert.

• This drug is not recommended for the treatment of acute diarrhea in children, according to the American Academy of Pediatrics 1996 guidelines.

• Do not give this drug to children younger than 2 years of age.

• Children with Down syndrome may be particularly sensitive to this drug. If possible, avoid using it.

• This drug may be habit forming if used in larger doses than prescribed.

DIPIVEFRIN

Administration Guidelines
- For use in the eye(s) only.

- Usually instilled 2 times a day.

- Do not touch the tip of the dropper bottle while instilling the dose.

- Missed doses: Give as soon as possible. However, if it's within 6 hours of the next dose, skip the missed dose and give the next regular dose. Do not give double doses.

- Discard discolored solutions; they have deteriorated.

Side Effects
Tell your child's doctor about any side effects that are persistent or particularly bothersome.

More Common. Eye irritation (burning, stinging), bloodshot eyes, sensitivity to light

Less Common. Blurred vision, eye pain, headache, allergic reactions, palpitations. Contact the doctor if your child experiences difficulty breathing.

Possible Drug Interactions
- May have beneficial, increased effects when used with other antiglaucoma medications.

Tell Your Child's Doctor If
- Your child has had allergic reactions to any medications, has any other diseases, or is taking any other medications.

- Your daughter is or becomes pregnant.

- Your daughter is breast-feeding her baby. It is not known if this drug passes into breast milk. It should be used with caution in nursing mothers.

Special Notes
- Contains sulfite preservatives, which may cause allergic reactions in some individuals.

Brand Name: Propine

Generic Available: No

Type of Drug: Mydriatic, antiglaucoma agent

Use: Treats glaucoma.

Time Required for Drug to Take Effect: 1 hour

Dosage Form and Strength: Ophthalmic solution (0.1%)

Storage: Store at room temperature in tightly closed, light-resistant containers.

How This Drug Works: Decreases flow of intra-ocular fluid, which reduces pressure within the eye.

Brand Names: Colace, Disonate, D-S-S, Doss, DOK, Doxinate, Genasoft, Pro-Sof, Regutol, Regulax SS

Generic Available: Yes

Type of Drug: Stool softener, laxative

Use: Short-term relief of constipation. Also decreases straining during bowel movements.

Time Required for Drug to Take Effect: Begins working in 1 to 3 days. May take 3 to 5 days to achieve full effect.

Dosage Forms and Strengths: Tablets (50 mg, 100 mg); Capsules (50 mg, 60 mg, 100 mg, 240 mg, 250 mg, 300 mg); Syrup (50 mg and 60 mg per 15 mL); Liquid (150 mg per 15 mL); Solution (50 mg per 1 mL)

Storage: Store at room temperature in tightly closed, light-resistant containers.

How This Drug Works: Helps water mix with the stool in the intestine to soften the stool.

DOCUSATE SODIUM

Administration Guidelines

- Follow the age- or weight-appropriate dosage directions on the package if giving without a prescription.

- Do not give to children younger than 6 years of age unless prescribed by your child's doctor.

- Liquid forms may be given in milk or juice to improve the taste.

- Give plenty of fluids to make the stool softer.

- Do not give within 2 hours of giving another medication. This drug can reduce the effect of the other medication.

- Do not give for more than 1 week unless instructed to do so by the doctor.

- Do not give with mineral oil.

Side Effects

Tell your child's doctor about any side effects that are persistent or particularly bothersome.

More Common. Excessive bowel activity

Less Common. Stomach or intestinal cramping. Throat irritation may occur with liquid forms. Contact the doctor if your child develops a skin rash.

Tell Your Child's Doctor If

- Your child has had allergic reactions to any medications.

- Your child has any diseases or is taking any medications.

- Your daughter is or becomes pregnant. This drug generally is safe during pregnancy.

- Your daughter is breast-feeding her baby.

Special Instructions

- Do not give if your child has abdominal pain, nausea, or vomiting. Call the doctor.

- Notify the doctor if your child remains constipated after 1 week or if your child experiences rectal bleeding, muscle cramps or pain, dizziness, or weakness.

Symptoms of Overdose: Diarrhea, severe stomach or intestinal cramping

Special Notes

- Give only when needed. Laxatives are only a temporary measure. Frequent or excessive use can lead to dependence on laxatives.

DOXEPIN

Administration Guidelines
• May be given with food to decrease stomach upset.

• Mix solution with ½ cup water, milk, or juice (not grape juice or carbonated beverages) just before giving this drug.

• Given 2 or 3 times a day or as a single daily dose at bedtime.

• Doses are increased slowly to decrease the side effects.

• Missed doses: Give as soon as possible. However, if it's time for the next dose, skip the missed dose. Do not give double doses. If a once-a-day bedtime dose is missed, do not give the missed dose.

• Do not use the cream for more than 7 days.

• Do not use any type of dressing or bandage over the cream.

Side Effects
Tell your child's doctor about any side effects that are persistent or particularly bothersome.

More Common. Drowsiness, dry mouth, dizziness, light-headedness, headache, nausea, increased appetite, weight gain, unpleasant taste in the mouth, constipation, weakness

Less Common. Contact the doctor if your child experiences blurred vision, confusion, difficulty in speaking or swallowing, eye pain, fainting, fast or irregular heartbeat, hallucinations, loss of balance, masklike face, nervousness or restlessness, problems urinating, shakiness, or slow movements.

Possible Drug Interactions
• Clonidine (Catapres) may lead to very high blood pressure when used with this drug.

• Monoamine oxidase (MAO) inhibitors such as isocarboxazid (Marplan), phenelzine (Nardil), and tranylcypromine (Parnate) can lead to very serious reactions and death when used with this drug.

• Central nervous system depressants such as alcohol, antihistamines, muscle relaxants, tranquilizers, and some pain medications may cause extreme drowsiness when used with this drug.

• Cimetidine (Tagamet and Tagamet HB) may increase the effect and side effects of this drug.

• Phenobarbital and carbamazepine may decease the effectiveness of this drug.

Brand Names: Adapin, Sinequan, Zonalon Topical Cream

Generic Available: Yes

Type of Drug: Antidepressant, tricyclic

Use: Treats mental depression and anxiety disorders. Also treats some kinds of chronic pain. Cream is used for itching.

Time Required for Drug to Take Effect: Usually more than 2 weeks when used as an antidepressant. Antianxiety effect may occur sooner.

Dosage Forms and Strengths: Capsules (10 mg, 25 mg, 50 mg, 75 mg, 100 mg, 150 mg); Solution (10 mg/mL); Cream (5%)

Storage: Store at room temperature in tightly closed, light-resistant containers.

How This Drug Works: Increases the concentration of serotonin and/or norepinephrine in the central nervous system.

- Eyedrops and nasal sprays or drops that contain naphazoline, oxymetazoline, epinephrine, phenylephrine, or xylometazoline may increase heart rate and blood pressure.

- Antithyroid drugs lead to an increase in rare blood disorders.

Tell Your Child's Doctor If
- Your child has had an allergic reaction to this drug or any other medication.

- Your child has heart, thyroid, liver, or kidney disease; seizures; glaucoma; urinary retention; or any other medical condition.

- Your child is or has been taking MAO inhibitors such as isocarboxazid (Marplan), phenelzine (Nardil), or tranylcypromine (Parnate).

- Your child has taken or is taking any other prescription or nonprescription medicine.

- Your daughter is or becomes pregnant.

- Your daughter is breast-feeding her baby. This drug can pass into breast milk and the American Academy of Pediatrics is concerned about its effect on the baby.

Special Instructions
- Give this drug only as directed by the doctor. It is important that your child's progress is checked with regular visits to the doctor.

- Do not suddenly stop giving this drug before speaking to the doctor.

- The effects of this drug may last for a few days after you stop giving it.

- This drug can cause light-headedness and dizziness if your child gets up too quickly from a prone or sitting position. To prevent these side effects, have your child get up slowly.

- Do not allow your child to drink alcohol while taking this drug.

- Do not give other medicines that may make your child sleepy.

- Limit your child's caffeine intake.

- Your child should avoid exposure to sunlight. Make sure your child wears sunscreen when out-of-doors. This drug may cause a skin rash or severe sunburn when your child is exposed to direct sunlight or ultraviolet light.

- Ask the doctor or pharmacist before giving any other medication with this drug.

Symptoms of Overdose: Agitation; dry mouth; confusion; hallucinations; severe drowsiness; enlarged pupils; fever; vomiting; trouble breathing; urinary retention; low blood pressure; seizures; or fast, slow, or irregular heartbeat

Special Notes
- Drowsiness is common. Make sure you know how your child is reacting to this drug before allowing participation in an activity that requires alertness and coordination, such as riding a bicycle.

- The cream is not approved for use in children.

- The drug is absorbed through the skin from the cream and can cause the same side effects.

- May cause urine to turn blue-green.

DOXYCYCLINE

Administrative Guidelines

• Give with food.

• Do not give with milk as this may decrease the absorption of this drug.

• Do not mix syrup with food or drink.

• Shake suspension before measuring each dose.

• Discard suspension after 14 days. This drug can cause serious side effects, especially to the kidneys, after the expiration date.

• Do not give to children younger than 8 years of age.

• Missed doses: Give as soon as possible. However, if it's within 4 to 6 hours of the next dose, skip the missed dose. Do not give double doses.

Side Effects

Tell your child's doctor about any side effects that are persistent or particularly bothersome.

More Common. Discoloration of the nails, dizziness, loss of appetite, nausea, stomach cramps and upset, or vomiting

Less Common. Darkened tongue, difficulty in breathing, joint pain, mouth irritation, rash, rectal or vaginal itching, unusual bleeding or bruising, or yellowing of the eyes or skin

Possible Drug Interactions

• Increases the absorption of digoxin, which may lead to digoxin toxicity.

• May increase gastrointestinal side effects (nausea, vomiting, stomach upset) of theophylline.

• Adjustments may be necessary in the dosage of oral anticoagulants when this drug is started.

• Decreases the effectiveness of oral contraceptives.

• Barbiturates, carbamazepine, phenytoin, and antacids can lower the blood concentration of this drug, decreasing its effectiveness.

• Iron can decrease the absorption of this drug.

Tell Your Child's Doctor If

• Your child is allergic to this drug, oxytetracycline, tetracycline, or minocycline.

• Your child has kidney or liver disease.

Brand Names: Doryx, Doxy-Caps, Doxychel Hyclate, Doxycycline (various manufacturers), Vibramycin Hyclate, Vibra Tabs, Dynacin, Monodox

Generic Available: Yes

Type of Drug: Tetracycline antibiotic

Use: Treats a wide variety of bacterial infections; prevents or treats traveler's diarrhea.

Time Required for Drug to Take Effect: 2 to 3 days

Dosage Forms and Strengths: Tablets (50 mg, 100 mg); Capsules (50 mg, 100 mg); Capsules, coated pellets (100 mg); Suspension (25 mg per 5 mL); Syrup (50 mg per 5 mL)

Storage: Store all forms at room temperature in tightly closed containers.

How This Drug Works: Destroys susceptible bacteria.

• Your daughter is or becomes pregnant or is breast-feeding her baby. This drug can cause permanent discoloration of the teeth and can inhibit tooth and bone growth in the fetus and baby.

Special Instructions
• Your child should avoid unnecessary exposure to sunlight. Make sure your child wears an effective sunscreen when out-of-doors.

• Do not give at the same time as antacids or iron products.

Symptoms of Overdose: Severe nausea and vomiting

To Each His Own

If one of your children has been prescribed an antibiotic and another child gets sick, it is not safe to give the antibiotic to the child for whom it was not prescribed. The medication may not be the appropriate one for the other child—even if the children's symptoms are similar. Treating an infection with the wrong drug may make the condition worse instead of better. What's more, children respond to the same drug differently and may need different dosages. The child who became ill first needs the drug in the amount prescribed for the time advised; otherwise, it may not be effective. If you think another child needs medication, consult the doctor.

DROPERIDOL

Administration Guidelines
• Usually given every 4 to 6 hours for prevention or treatment of nausea and vomiting.

• Injected intramuscularly or intravenously. Intravenous injection should be given slowly over several minutes. Therefore it is not commonly given to ambulatory patients (those who can walk around).

Side Effects
Tell your child's doctor about any side effects that are persistent or particularly bothersome.

More Common. Drowsiness, dizziness, palpitations. Contact the doctor if your child experiences abnormal muscle or eye movements.

Less Common. Restlessness, nervousness, chills, shivering. Contact the doctor if your child experiences difficulty breathing, hallucinations, fainting, or chest pain.

Possible Drug Interactions
• Drugs which have depressant effects such as barbiturate sedatives (phenobarbital and others), antihistamines, and narcotic analgesics may increase the sedative effects of this drug.

Tell Your Child's Doctor If
• Your child has had allergic reactions to any medications.

• Your child has any other diseases.

• Your child is taking any other medications.

• Your child has liver or kidney damage.

• Your daughter is or becomes pregnant. Severe nausea and vomiting during pregnancy should be treated by the doctor.

• Your daughter is breast-feeding her baby. This drug can pass into breast milk and is not recommended for use by nursing mothers.

Symptoms of Overdose: Sedation, unconsciousness, low blood pressure

Brand Name: Inapsine

Generic Available: Yes

Type of Drug: Tranquilizer, antiemetic

Use: Reduces nausea and vomiting from chemotherapy and surgical procedures. Also may be used to cause sedation in preparation for surgery.

Time Required for Drug to Take Effect: Within 30 minutes of injection

Dosage Form and Strength: Injection (2.5 mg/mL)

Storage: Store at room temperature.

How This Drug Works: Blocks the effects of substances in the brain that cause the feeling of nausea.

Brand Name: Vasotec

Generic Available: No

Type of Drug: Angiotensin converting enzyme (ACE) inhibitor

Use: Treats high blood pressure and congestive heart failure. Treats kidney damage caused by diabetes.

Time Required for Drug to Take Effect: Several days to weeks

Dosage Forms and Strengths: Tablets (2.5 mg, 5 mg, 10 mg, 20 mg); Injection (1.25 mg/mL). Also available in combination products.

Storage: Store at room temperature in tightly closed, light-resistant containers.

How This Drug Works: Dilates blood vessels, decreasing blood pressure and allowing the heart to pump blood more easily.

ENALAPRIL

Administration Guidelines
• Can be given with food or on an empty stomach, but be consistent.

• Usually given 1 or 2 times a day. Try to give it at the same time(s) each day.

• Missed doses: Give as soon as possible. However, if it's within 8 hours of the next dose, skip the missed dose and give the next scheduled dose. Do not give double doses.

Side Effects
Tell your child's doctor about any side effects that are persistent or particularly bothersome.

More Common. Coughing (may be an ongoing side effect), drowsiness, dizziness (especially after the first few doses), headache, fatigue, nausea, diarrhea, low blood pressure. Contact the doctor if your child experiences chest pain, difficulty breathing, fainting, severe dizziness, or rash.

Less Common. Mouth sores, tingling fingers or toes, runny nose, sore throat, hoarseness, reddened eyes, tearing, hearing problems. Contact the doctor if your child experiences sore throat; fever; palpitations; swelling of face, lips, or tongue; or yellowing eyes or skin.

Possible Drug Interactions
• Spironolactone, triamterene, amiloride, potassium supplements, or salt substitutes can greatly increase blood potassium levels.

• Phenothiazine-type drugs such as prochlorperazine (Compazine), promethazine (Phenergan), and chlorpromazine (Thorazine) can increase the effects of this drug.

• If your child is also taking digoxin or lithium, a dosage adjustment of those drugs may be necessary.

Tell Your Child's Doctor If
• Your child has had allergic reactions to any medications.

• Your child has any other diseases.

• Your child is taking any other medications.

• Your child has a blood disorder, lupus, or liver or kidney disease.

• Your daughter is or becomes pregnant. Drugs similar to this drug can cause severe birth defects, especially if taken during the second and third trimesters.

• Your daughter is breast-feeding her baby. This drug can pass into breast milk.

Special Instructions

• Do not give your child medications for allergy, asthma, cough, cold, sinus problems, or weight control without first checking with the doctor or pharmacist.

• Do not give with antacids.

• Do not stop giving this drug to your child without first speaking with the doctor.

Symptoms of Overdose: Excessively low blood pressure, fainting

Special Notes

• May reduce blood sugar in children with diabetes.

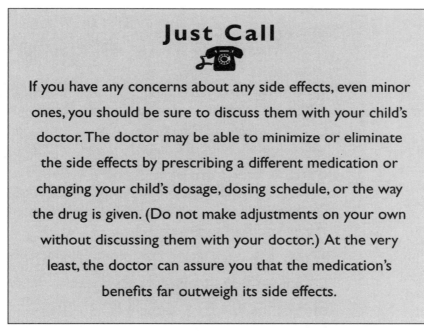

Just Call

If you have any concerns about any side effects, even minor ones, you should be sure to discuss them with your child's doctor. The doctor may be able to minimize or eliminate the side effects by prescribing a different medication or changing your child's dosage, dosing schedule, or the way the drug is given. (Do not make adjustments on your own without discussing them with your doctor.) At the very least, the doctor can assure you that the medication's benefits far outweigh its side effects.

Brand Names: E.E.S. 200 Liquid, E.E.S. 400 Filmtab, E-Mycin, ERYC, EryPed, Ery-Tab, Erythrocin Stearate Filmtabs, Erythromycin Base, Ilosone, Ilosone Pulvules, PCE Dispertab

Generic Available: Yes

Type of Drug: Antibiotic

Use: Treats a wide variety of bacterial infections such as otitis media, some pneumonias, skin infections, and respiratory tract infections.

Time Required for Drug to Take Effect: 2 to 3 days

Dosage Forms and Strengths: Tablets (250 mg, 333 mg, 500 mg); Tablets, chewable (200 mg); Tablets, enteric-coated (250 mg, 333 mg, 500 mg); Tablets, film-coated (250 mg, 400 mg, 500 mg); Tablets, polymer-coated (333 mg); Capsules (250 mg); Drops (100 mg per 2.5 ml); Suspension (125 mg, 200 mg, 250 mg, and 400 mg per 5 mL)

Storage: Store tablets and capsules at room temperature. Refrigerate drops and suspension. Store all forms in tightly closed, light-resistant containers.

How This Drug Works: Destroys susceptible bacteria.

ERYTHROMYCIN

Administration Guidelines
• Usually given 3 to 4 times a day.

• Discard liquid forms after 14 days.

• May be given with food to decrease stomach irritation if necessary.

• Do not mix liquid forms with food or drink.

• Shake suspension well before measuring each dose.

• Missed doses: Give as soon as possible. However, if it's within 4 hours of the next dose, skip the missed dose. Do not give double doses.

Side Effects
Tell your child's doctor about any side effects that are persistent or particularly bothersome.

More Common. Abdominal cramps, diarrhea, fatigue, irritation of the mouth, loss of appetite, nausea, sore tongue, or vomiting

Less Common. Hearing loss, hives, rash, rectal or vaginal itching, yellowing of the eyes or skin

Possible Drug Interactions
• Decreases the elimination of aminophylline, theophylline, digoxin, oral anticoagulants, and carbamazepine from the body. Can intensify side effects of those medications.

• Increases the effects of methylprednisolone.

• Do not use with astemizole or terfenadine.

Tell Your Child's Doctor If
• Your child is allergic to this drug, clarithromycin, or azithromycin.

• Your child has liver disease or develops severe nausea, vomiting, fever, colic, yellowing of the eyes or skin, or is extremely tired. These symptoms may indicate that the drug should be discontinued.

• Your daughter is breast-feeding her baby.

Special Instructions
• Some brands contain the color additive FD&C Yellow No. 5 (tartrazine), which can cause allergic reactions such as difficulty in breathing, rash, and fainting in susceptible individuals.

Symptoms of Overdose: Severe stomach upset, diarrhea, hearing loss

ERYTHROMYCIN AND SULFISOXAZOLE COMBINATION

Administrative Guidelines
• Give with food or milk.

• Usually given 3 to 4 times a day for 7 to 14 days.

• Shake well before measuring each dose.

• Missed doses: Give as soon as possible. However, if it's within 4 hours of the next dose, skip the missed dose. Do not give double doses.

• This product should not be used in children younger than 2 months of age.

Side Effects
Tell your child's doctor about any side effects that are persistent or particularly bothersome.

More Common. Diarrhea, dizziness, headache, loss of appetite, nausea, sleep disorders, sore mouth or tongue, vomiting, sensitivity to sunlight

Less Common. Rash, aching or painful joints or muscles, convulsions, difficult or painful urination, loss of hearing, redness, blistering or peeling of the skin, itching, uncoordinated movements, unusual bleeding or bruising, yellowing of the eyes or skin

Possible Drug Interactions
• Decreases the elimination and can intensify the side effects of aminophylline, theophylline, digoxin, oral anticoagulants (blood thinners), and carbamazepine.

• Increases the activity of oral anticoagulants, oral antidiabetic agents, methotrexate, and phenytoin, which can lead to serious side effects.

• Methenamine can increase the side effects to the kidneys caused by sulfisoxazole.

• Astemizole or terfenadine can cause serious effects on the heart when used with this drug. Neither should be given while your child is being treated with this drug.

• Probenecid and sulfinpyrazone can increase the blood concentrations of sulfisoxazole and intensify its side effects.

• Increases the effects of methylprednisolone.

Brand Names: Eryzole, Pediazole, Erythromycin and Sulfisoxazole (various manufacturers)

Generic Available: Yes

Type of Drug: Antibiotic

Use: Treats a wide variety of bacterial infections such as otitis media and infections of the upper and lower respiratory tract in children older than 2 months of age.

Time Required for Drug to Take Effect: 2 to 3 days

Dosage Form and Strength: Suspension (200 mg erythromycin and 600 mg sulfisoxazole per 5 mL)

Storage: Refrigerate in tightly closed containers. It is stable for 14 days.

How This Drug Works: Destroys susceptible bacteria.

Tell Your Child's Doctor If

• Your child is allergic to erythromycin, sulfisoxazole, any other sulfa medications (sulfonamide antibiotics, diuretics, dapsone, sulfoxone, oral antidiabetic medicines), or acetazolamide.

• Your child has glucose-6-phosphate dehydrogenase (G6PD) deficiency, kidney disease, or liver disease.

• Your daughter is or becomes pregnant.

• Your daughter is breast-feeding her baby.

Special Instructions

• Your child should avoid prolonged exposure to sunlight. Make sure your child wears a PABA-free sunscreen when out-of-doors.

Symptoms of Overdose: Severe diarrhea, stomach upset, hearing loss, vomiting

Measuring Up

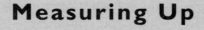

Remember: Never use an ordinary tableware teaspoon to measure liquid doses. Instead, use a cylindrical dosing spoon, dosage cup, dropper, or syringe. These measuring devices can be found at your local drug store and sometimes at supermarkets, toy stores, and department stores.

ETHAMBUTOL

Administration Guidelines

• May be given with food to avoid stomach upset.

• Give this drug for the full treatment course, which may be as long as 1 to 2 years, even if your child is feeling better.

• Missed doses: Give as soon as you remember, then stagger remaining doses evenly for the rest of the day. Do not give double doses.

Side Effects

Tell your child's doctor about any side effects that are persistent or particularly bothersome.

More Common. Nausea

Less Common. Confusion, headache, loss of appetite, stomach pain, vomiting. Contact the doctor if your child experiences chills; painful, hot, or swollen joints; blurred vision; eye pain; red-green color blindness; fever; skin rash; weakness, or numbness or tingling of the hands or feet.

Tell Your Child's Doctor If

• Your child has had allergic reactions to any medications.

• Your child has any eye problems.

• Your child has any diseases or is taking any other medications.

• Your daughter is or becomes pregnant.

• Your daughter is breast-feeding her baby. This drug can pass into breast milk; however, the American Academy of Pediatrics considers it compatible with breast-feeding in most cases.

Special Instructions

• If your child's symptoms do not improve in 2 to 3 weeks, contact the doctor. The doctor will want to check your child's progress regularly.

Symptoms of Overdose: Vomiting, confusion, severe stomach pain, severe headache

Special Notes

• This drug usually will be prescribed in combination with other antituberculosis medications. It should not be used alone.

• Not recommended for use in children younger than 13 years of age, although it has been used in children 6 years of age and older.

• In certain cases, monthly eye exams may be recommended.

Brand Name: Myambutol

Generic Available: No

Type of Drug: Antituberculosis agent

Use: Treats tuberculosis and other similar diseases.

Time Required for Drug to Take Effect: 2 to 3 weeks

Dosage Form and Strengths: Tablets (100 mg, 400 mg)

Storage: Store at room temperature in tightly closed, light-resistant containers.

How This Drug Works: Interferes with the multiplication of the tuberculosis organism.

Brand Name: Pepcid

Generic Available: No

Type of Drug: Histamine H$_2$ Receptor Antagonist, H$_2$ blocker (anti-ulcer agent)

Use: Treats duodenal, peptic, and gastric ulcers; relieves gastric acidity and heartburn.

Time Required for Drug to Take Effect: Provides immediate relief for heartburn and increased stomach acidity. May take a few days to achieve maximum benefit in treatment of ulcers and their associated pain.

Dosage Form and Strengths: Tablets, coated (20 mg, 40 mg)

Storage: Store tablets at room temperature in tightly closed containers.

How This Drug Works: Decreases the production of acid in the stomach.

FAMOTIDINE

Administration Guidelines

- Give with or without food. Food does not affect the absorption of this drug.

- Generally given 1 or 2 times a day.

- Give this drug at the same time each day.

- Missed doses: Give immediately. However, if it is time for the next dose, just give the next dose and continue with the regular schedule. Do not give double doses.

Side Effects

Tell your child's doctor about any side effects that are persistent or particularly bothersome.

More Common. Headache, vertigo, anxiety, fever, constipation, nausea, belching, altered taste in the mouth, weakness, joint pain

Less Common. It is especially important to tell the doctor about drowsiness, itching, rash, or difficulty breathing.

Possible Drug Interactions

- Can decrease the absorption of ketoconazole, triamterene, itraconazole, cefpodoxime, indomethacin, and melphalan from the stomach.

Tell Your Child's Doctor If

- Your child is currently taking any prescription or nonprescription medications, especially those listed above.

- Your child has or ever had unusual or allergic reactions to any medications, especially to this drug.

- Your child has any liver, kidney, or blood disease.

- Your child's symptoms of the underlying disease are getting worse rather than improving.

- Your daughter is or becomes pregnant. The safety of this drug during pregnancy has not been established.

- Your daughter is breast-feeding her baby. This drug is compatible with breast-feeding but should be used under the supervision of the doctor.

Special Instructions

- Do not give excessive amounts of other agents that stimulate stomach acid production or are irritating to the stomach (such as aspirin and coffee).

• This drug is available over the counter; however, if your child is younger than 12 years of age, seek the doctor's advice before giving it. Your child's symptoms may require another type of care.

Symptoms of Overdose: More severe forms of side effects listed above.

▯ Over-the-Counter Wisdom

Keep in mind that even a medication that is available without a doctor's prescription may still be harmful and should be given appropriately and only when necessary. Talk to your pediatrician about what to do if your child gets sick. Some illnesses can be treated at home, some require a call to the pediatrician's office, and some will require a visit to the doctor. In addition, ask the doctor what situations constitute an emergency. If you're not sure if it's safe or appropriate to give your child a particular over-the-counter medication, be sure to talk to the doctor first.

Brand Name: Felbatol

Generic Available: No

Type of Drug: Anticonvulsant

Use: Treats seizure disorders and Lennox-Gastaut syndrome.

Time Required for Drug to Take Effect: It may take about 1 week to achieve complete effectiveness when this drug is first started.

Dosage Forms and Strengths: Tablets (400 mg, 600 mg); Suspension (600 mg per 5 mL)

Storage: Store at room temperature in tightly closed containers.

How This Drug Works: It is not completely understood how this drug works in the central nervous system to prevent seizures.

FELBAMATE

Administration Guidelines
• May be given with food to prevent stomach upset.

• Shake the suspension well just before measuring each dose.

• Works best when blood concentrations are kept within a safe and effective range. Give doses at evenly spaced intervals around the clock. If you are to give 3 doses a day, space them approximately 8 hours apart.

• Missed doses: Give as soon as you remember, then stagger remaining doses evenly for the rest of the day. Do not give double doses. Contact your child's doctor if 2 or more doses are missed.

Side Effects
Tell your child's doctor about any side effects that are persistent or particularly bothersome.

More Common. Constipation, diarrhea, dizziness, drowsiness, headache, nausea, rash, vomiting, change in sense of taste, difficulty in sleeping, loss of appetite, blurred vision, increased skin sensitivity to sunlight

Less Common. Contact the doctor immediately if your child has abnormal gait; blurred vision; chest pain; depression; difficulty breathing; double vision; fever; numbness or tingling in the hands or feet; palpitations; rash; sleepiness; tremors; black, tarry stools; unusual bleeding or bruising; vomiting; sore throat; mouth sores; yellowing of eyes or skin; or dark urine.

Possible Drug Interactions
• The levels of this drug and other anticonvulsants such as phenytoin, valproic acid, or carbamazepine may be altered if taken together.

Tell Your Child's Doctor If
• Your child has had allergic reactions to any medications.

• Your child has any diseases or is taking any medications.

• Your daughter is or becomes pregnant.

• Your daughter is breast-feeding her baby.

Special Instructions
• Before your child has any medical or dental treatment or surgery, tell the doctor your child is taking this drug.

• Do not suddenly stop giving this drug to your child.

Symptoms of Overdose: Severe dizziness or clumsiness, severe drowsiness, slow breathing, seizures or abnormal twitching, severe vomiting

Special Notes

• Aplastic anemia, a severe form of bone marrow failure, has been reported with the use of this drug. The doctor, therefore, will frequently and routinely monitor your child.

• This drug is generally reserved for patients who have not responded to other anti-seizure medications.

• Some symptoms of toxicity may not occur until several months after starting this drug. Be sure to monitor your child for side effects for the entire time you are giving this drug.

Be Accurate

If you don't give medication correctly, it may be ineffective or even cause side effects. An estimated 10 to 30 percent of medications aren't effective because they have been given incorrectly. To do it right, you have to give the exact amount of medicine prescribed at the scheduled time, for the specified duration, and in the appropriate manner. Always read the label, follow the directions carefully, and use the appropriate equipment for measuring and administering the medication. Also, be sure to wash your hands before you give any medication to your child.

Brand Name: Diflucan

Generic Available: No

Type of Drug: Antifungal agent

Use: Treats fungal infections such as those of the mouth, throat, kidney, and liver.

Time Required for Drug to Take Effect: 2 to 3 days. In some cases, it may take longer.

Dosage Forms and Strengths: Tablets (50 mg, 100 mg, 200 mg); Suspension (50 mg and 200 mg per 5 mL)

Storage: Store at room temperature in tightly closed, light-resistant containers.

How This Drug Works: Destroys susceptible fungus.

FLUCONAZOLE

Administration Guidelines

• Give with food or milk

• Shake suspension well before measuring each dose.

• Usually given once a day.

• Discard suspension after 14 days

• Missed doses: If it's within 6 to 8 hours of the next dose, skip the missed dose. Otherwise, give the missed dose as soon as possible. Do not give double doses.

Side Effects

Tell your child's doctor about any side effects that are persistent or particularly bothersome.

More Common. Abdominal pain or cramps, diarrhea, nausea, vomiting, dizziness, headache, skin rash, or itching

Less Common. Call the doctor if your child experiences unusual bleeding or bruising, yellowing of the skin or eyes, dark urine, or pale stools.

Possible Drug Interactions

• May increase the effectiveness of warfarin, phenytoin, cyclosporine, and oral antidiabetic agents.

• Rifampin decreases the effectiveness of this drug.

Tell Your Child's Doctor If

• Your child is allergic to this drug.

• Your child has liver disease.

• Your daughter is or becomes pregnant or is breast-feeding her baby. This drug should not be given to pregnant women or nursing mothers.

FLUNISOLIDE (NASAL)

Administration Guidelines
• Shake well before using.

• Your child should clear nasal passages before using the spray.

• Insert the nosepiece into each nostril and aim the spray toward the inner corner of the eye.

• Missed doses: Give as soon as you remember. However, if it is time for the next scheduled dose, skip the missed dose and give the next dose at its scheduled time. Do not give double doses.

Side Effects
Tell your child's doctor about any side effects that are persistent or particularly bothersome.

More Common. Burning, dryness or irritation of the nose, sneezing, throat irritation, bitter taste in mouth

Less Common. Bloody mucus or unexplained nosebleeds; crusting, white patches or sores inside the nose; headache; hives; dizziness; light-headedness; loss of sense of smell; nausea; sore throat; hoarseness; watery eyes. Contact the doctor if your child has white patches in the nose or throat.

Tell Your Child's Doctor If
• Your child has had allergic reactions to any medications.

• Your child has any diseases or is taking any medications.

• Your daughter is or becomes pregnant.

• Your daughter is breast-feeding her baby.

Symptoms of Overdose: Acne, rounding of the face

Special Notes
• To be effective, this drug must be given regularly.

• Do not stop giving this drug abruptly. The doctor may want to gradually reduce the dosage before stopping it.

Brand Name: Nasalide

Generic Available: No

Type of Drug: Adrenocorticosteroid hormone

Use: Relieves symptoms of rhinitis (inflammation of the nasal passages).

Time Required for Drug to Take Effect: Effects may not be apparent for up to 3 weeks.

Dosage Form and Strength: Nasal solution (25 mcg per spray)

Storage: Store at room temperature in tightly closed containers. Discard opened containers after 3 months.

How This Drug Works: How this drug works is not completely understood. This drug is similar to the cortisonelike chemicals naturally produced by the adrenal gland. These chemicals are involved in various regulatory processes in the body such as fluid balance, temperature, and reaction to inflammation.

Brand Name: Prozac

Generic Available: No

Type of Drug:
Antidepressant

Use: Treats mental depression and obsessive-compulsive disorder.

Time Required for Drug to Take Effect: Full benefit may not be achieved for 4 weeks or longer.

Dosage Forms and Strengths: Capsules (10 mg, 20 mg); Liquid (20 mg/5 mL)

Storage: Store at room temperature in tightly closed, light-resistant containers. Do not freeze liquid.

How This Drug Works: Increases the concentration of serotonin in the central nervous system.

FLUOXETINE

Administration Guidelines

• May be given with food to decrease stomach upset.

• Given as a single dose in the morning or 2 times a day in the morning and at noon.

• Missed doses: Skip the missed dose and continue with the next dose. Do not give double doses.

• Give the last dose of the day before 4 P.M. to avoid trouble sleeping.

Side Effects

Tell your child's doctor about any side effects that are persistent or particularly bothersome.

More Common. Headache, nervousness, drowsiness, dry mouth, nausea, diarrhea, anxiety, increased sweating, trouble sleeping, dizziness, fatigue, sedation, constipation, decreased appetite

Less Common. Abnormal dreams, change in taste, changes in vision, cough, dizziness, light-headedness, feeling of warmth, flushing, frequent urination, stuffy nose, tremors, fatigue, weakness. Contact the doctor if your child experiences chest pain; chills; fever; joint or muscle pain; skin rash, hives, or itching; trouble breathing; burning or tingling in the fingers, hands, or arms; cold sweats; confusion; seizures; excessive hunger; fast heartbeat; shakiness or unsteady walk; swelling of feet or lower legs; swollen glands; unusual fatigue.

Possible Drug Interactions

• Monoamine oxidase (MAO) inhibitors such as isocarboxazid (Marplan), phenelzine (Nardil), or tranylcypromine (Parnate) can lead to very serious reactions and death when used with this drug.

• Central nervous system depressants such as alcohol, antihistamines, cold preparations, muscle relaxants, tranquilizers, sleeping medications, sedatives, narcotics, and some pain medications may cause extreme drowsiness when used with this drug.

• Increases the effect and side effects of tricyclic antidepressants such as amitriptyline, imipramine, desipramine, and doxepin.

• The effect of lithium may increase or decrease and requires close supervision by the doctor when given with this drug.

• The effect of phenytoin is increased when given with this drug.

Tell Your Child's Doctor If

• Your child has had an allergic reaction to this drug, any other medications, foods, preservatives, or dyes.

• Your child has seizures; diabetes mellitus; cardiac, liver, or kidney disease; or any other medical condition.

• Your child is or has been taking MAO inhibitors such as isocarboxazid (Marplan), phenelzine (Nardil), or tranylcypromine (Parnate).

• Your child is or has been taking other antidepressants.

• Your child is taking any other prescription or nonprescription medicine.

• Your child has a dry mouth after taking this drug for 2 weeks.

• Your daughter is or becomes pregnant.

• Your daughter is breast-feeding her baby. This drug can pass into breast milk, and the American Academy of Pediatrics is concerned about its effect on the infant.

Special Instructions

• Give this drug only as directed by the doctor. It is important that your child's progress is checked with regular visits to the doctor.

• If your child develops a skin rash or hives, stop giving this drug and check with the doctor as soon as possible.

• Do not give tryptophan supplements to your child. Dangerous side effects can occur.

• Do not allow your child to drink alcohol while taking this drug.

• Do not give other medicines that may make your child sleepy.

• Do not give any other medications without first asking the pharmacist or doctor.

Symptoms of Overdose: Agitation, restlessness, unusual excitement, nausea, vomiting, ataxia, sedation, coma, decreased breathing effort, seizures

Special Notes

• Doses are increased slowly to decrease side effects.

• Make sure you know how your child is reacting to this drug before allowing participation in an activity that requires alertness and coordination, such as riding a bicycle. This drug may cause your child to feel dizzy, drowsy, or less alert.

• The effects of this drug may last for a few weeks after you stop giving it to your child.

Brand Name: Lasix

Generic Available: Yes

Type of Drug: Loop diuretic

Use: Treats congestive heart failure, liver disease, kidney disease, and high blood pressure.

Time Required for Drug to Take Effect: Several days to several weeks for full effect.

Dosage Forms and Strengths: Tablets (20 mg, 40 mg, 80 mg); Solution (10 mg/mL and 40 mg/5 mL); Injection (10 mg/mL)

Storage: Store tablets at room temperature in tightly closed, light-resistant containers. Refrigerate the solution.

How This Drug Works: Removes excess fluid from the body by eliminating salt and water through the kidneys.

FUROSEMIDE

Administration Guidelines

• Give on an empty stomach or with meals, but be consistent.

• Usually given 1 or 2 times a day.

• Give doses at the same time(s) each day. Avoid giving doses after 6 P.M. so your child won't have to get up at night to urinate.

• Missed doses: Give as soon as possible and space remaining doses for that day at regular intervals. However, if it's within 6 hours of the next dose, skip the missed dose and take the next regular dose. Do not give double doses.

• Use only the dropper provided with the solution or an oral syringe to measure doses.

Side Effects

Tell your child's doctor about any side effects that are persistent or particularly bothersome.

More Common. Increased sensitivity to sunlight, upset stomach, vomiting, diarrhea, dizziness. Contact the doctor if your child experiences weakness, muscle cramps, difficulty breathing, rash, or tingling fingers or toes.

Less Common. Ringing in the ears, deafness, blurred vision, anemia. Contact the doctor if your child experiences confusion, fainting, joint pain, palpitations, stomach pain, sore throat, unusual bleeding or bruising, or yellowing of eyes or skin.

Possible Drug Interactions

• Dosage adjustment of lithium, warfarin, and antidiabetic drugs may be required.

• Phenytoin (Dilantin) and nonsteroidal anti-inflammatory agents (such as ibuprofen or indomethacin) may decrease the effectiveness of this drug.

• May increase risk of salicylate toxicity with high-dose aspirin therapy.

Tell Your Child's Doctor If

• Your child has had allergic reactions to any medications, especially to sulfa drugs.

• Your child has any other diseases.

• Your child is taking any other medications.

• Your child has had liver or kidney disease, diabetes, gout, asthma, pancreatic disease, or lupus.

• Your daughter is or becomes pregnant.

• Your daughter is breast-feeding her baby. This drug passes into the breast milk and can cause side effects in the infant.

Special Instructions
• Do not give your child medications for coughs, colds, asthma, allergies, sinus problems, or weight control without first checking with the doctor or pharmacist.

Symptoms of Overdose: Excessive urination and dehydration

Special Notes
• Solution formulations contain varying amounts of alcohol and sorbitol, which can cause diarrhea.

• Can cause loss of potassium from your child's body. The doctor will use blood tests to measure potassium levels.

• Can raise blood sugar levels in children with diabetes.

Teach Your Children Well

Let's face it. Kids can be pretty stubborn when it comes to accepting medication. When appropriate, try giving your child information about his or her condition and how the medicine works. In a nonthreatening voice, talk about the consequences of not taking the medication, perhaps reminding the child of how uncomfortable he or she was before beginning the medication. Use reasoning when possible, but don't scare the child. Children who understand the importance of antibiotics for infection, insulin for diabetes, or inhalants for asthma are more likely to take the medication without objection.

Brand Name: Neurontin

Generic Available: No

Type of Drug: Anticonvulsant

Use: Treats convulsions or seizures.

Time Required for Drug to Take Effect: It may take 1 week to achieve full benefit.

Dosage Form and Strengths: Capsules (100 mg, 300 mg, 400 mg)

Storage: Store at room temperature in tightly closed, light-resistant containers.

How This Drug Works: It is not completely understood how this drug works in the central nervous system to reduce the number and severity of seizures.

GABAPENTIN

Administration Guidelines
• May be given with food to avoid stomach upset.

• Give at evenly spaced intervals around the clock to keep blood concentrations of this drug within a safe and effective range. If this drug is to be given 3 times a day, the doses should be spaced 8 hours apart.

• Missed doses: Give as soon as you remember, then stagger remaining doses evenly for the rest of the day. Do not give double doses. Contact your child's doctor if you miss 2 or more doses.

• Do not increase the dose or give more frequently than the doctor prescribed.

Side Effects
Tell your child's doctor about any side effects that are persistent or particularly bothersome.

More Common. Dizziness, drowsiness, stomach upset, constipation, headache

Less Common. Fatigue, blurred vision, tremor, anxiety, weight gain. Contact the doctor if your child experiences skin rash, flulike symptoms, itching, difficulty breathing, clumsiness, seizures, or rapid or irregular heartbeat.

Possible Drug Interactions
• Antacids may decrease the absorption of this drug from the stomach. Do not give this drug within 2 to 3 hours of taking an antacid.

• Alcohol, antidepressants, or tranquilizers can increase drowsiness.

Tell Your Child's Doctor If
• Your child has had allergic reactions to any medications.

• Your child has any diseases.

• Your child is taking any medications.

• Your daughter is or becomes pregnant. Seizure disorders should be controlled by the doctor during pregnancy.

• Your daughter is breast-feeding her baby.

Special Instructions
• Before your child has surgery or any medical or dental treatment, tell the doctor performing the treatment that your child is taking this drug.

• Do not suddenly stop giving this drug. Abruptly stopping this drug could cause seizures. The doctor may slowly decrease the dosage over a 1 to 2 week period.

Symptoms of Overdose: Severe dizziness or clumsiness, severe drowsiness, blurred or double vision, seizures or abnormal twitching, severe vomiting, abnormal eye movements, staggered walk, slurred speech

Special Notes

• Initially, the doctor may gradually increase the dose to determine the proper amount for your child.

• The doctor will want to follow your child's progress with regular office visits.

Keep It Out of Reach

Do not rely on a child-resistant cap to deter your child from opening a bottle of medication. Child-resistant does not mean childproof. Legally, a cap can be called child-resistant if 80 percent of all five-year-olds need more than five minutes to open it. That means the other 20 percent could get into it in even less time. Put the bottle in a hard-to-reach cabinet with a childproof lock. Do not keep it on the countertop, kitchen table, or nightstand.

Brand Names: Garamycin, Genoptic, Genoptic SOP, Gentacidin, Gentak, Gentamicin (various manufacturers), Gentamicin Ophthalmic, G-Myticin

Generic Available: Yes

Type of Drug: Antibiotic

Use: Treats superficial infections of the skin caused by susceptible bacteria.

Time Required for Drug to Take Effect: About 2 days

Dosage Forms and Strengths: Cream, topical (0.1%); Ointment, ophthalmic, as sulfate (0.3%); Ointment, topical (0.1% g); Solution, ophthalmic (0.3%)

Storage: Store at room temperature in tightly closed containers. Do not freeze. Discard any eyedrops that are no longer needed.

How This Drug Works: Kills susceptible bacteria.

GENTAMICIN (TOPICAL/OPHTHALMIC)

Administration Guidelines
- Do not use cream or topical ointment in the eyes. Use only the ophthalmic preparation.
- Wash your hands with soap and water before applying this drug.
- Do not touch the tip of the ointment tube or let it touch the eyes.

Side Effects
Tell your child's doctor about any side effects that are persistent or particularly bothersome.

More Common. Ocular burning and irritation when used in the eye, itching

Less Common. Hallucinations

Tell Your Child's Doctor If
- Your child's eyes are not improving, or seem to be getting worse, after 1 to 2 days.
- Your child experiences increased redness, irritation, swelling, decreasing vision, or pain after application of ophthalmic solution or ointment.

Special Notes
- Ophthalmic ointment may cause temporary blurred vision.

GLYCERIN

Side Effects

Tell your child's doctor about any side effects that are persistent or particularly bothersome.

More Common. Rectal discomfort or irritation

Less Common. Skin irritation around the anus. Contact the doctor for rectal bleeding, blistering, burning, itching, or pain.

Tell Your Child's Doctor If

• Your child has had allergic reactions to this drug or any other medication.

• Your child has taken or is taking any other prescription or nonprescription medicine.

• Your child experiences a sudden change in bowel movements that either lasts longer than 2 weeks or returns intermittently.

• Your daughter is or becomes pregnant.

Special Instructions

• Do not use if your child has abdominal pain, appendicitis, intestinal blockage, nausea, vomiting, or rectal bleeding.

• Do not use suppositories in children younger than 6 years of age unless prescribed by the doctor.

Symptoms of Overdose: Nausea, vomiting, diarrhea

Special Notes

• Frequent or continued use may cause in dependence on laxatives. Do not give regularly for more than 1 week.

Brand Names: Fleet Babylax Rectal, Sani-Supp, Glycerin Laxative Rectal Applicator

Generic Available: Yes

Type of Drug: Laxative, osmotic

Use: Treats occasional constipation.

Time Required for Drug to Take Effect: 15 to 60 minutes

Dosage Forms and Strengths: Suppository (adult, pediatric/infant); Rectal liquid (4 mL and 7.6 mL per applicator)

Storage: Store at room temperature in tightly closed containers. Do not freeze.

How This Drug Works: Draws fluid into the colon, causing a bowel movement. Also lubricates and softens the stool. Sodium stearate causes a local irritation leading to a bowel movement.

Brand Name: Kytril

Generic Available: No

Type of Drug: Antiemetic

Use: Prevents (does not treat) nausea and vomiting.

Time Required for Drug to Take Effect: Up to 1 hour

Dosage Form and Strength: Tablets (1 mg)

Storage: Store at room temperature in tightly closed, light-resistant containers.

How This Drug Works: Blocks the release of certain chemicals in the body and brain that stimulate the impulse to vomit.

GRANISETRON

Administration Guidelines

• Typically used to treat nausea and vomiting due to drugs that treat cancer (chemotherapy).

• Give at least 1 hour before chemotherapy. Usually repeated in 12 hours.

• Missed doses: Give as soon as possible. However, if it's within a couple hours of the next dose, skip the missed dose. Do not give double doses.

Side Effects

Tell your child's doctor about any side effects that are persistent or particularly bothersome.

More Common. Abdominal pain, constipation, diarrhea, headache, unusual fatigue or weakness

Less Common. Call the doctor if your child experiences fever, chest pain, skin rash, hives, itching, or shortness of breath.

Tell Your Child's Doctor If

• Your child is allergic to this drug.

• Your daughter is or becomes pregnant.

Special Notes

• Use only to prevent symptoms.

GRISEOFULVIN

Administration Guidelines
• Give with food or milk.

• Give this drug for the entire time prescribed by your child's doctor even if the infection seems better.

• Shake the suspension well for several minutes before measuring each dose.

• Missed doses: Give as soon as possible. However, if it's within 6 hours of the next dose, skip the missed dose and take the next regular dose. Do not give double doses.

Side Effects
Tell your child's doctor about any side effects that are persistent or particularly bothersome.

More Common. Increased sensitivity to sunlight, allergic reactions including skin rashes, headache, upset stomach, nausea, vomiting. Contact the doctor if your child experiences itching or skin rash.

Less Common. Fatigue, weakness, difficulty sleeping. Contact the doctor if your child experiences confusion, sore throat, or tingling hands or feet.

Possible Drug Interactions
• Can increase the side effects of alcohol, such as drowsiness.

• Barbiturate drugs (such as phenobarbital) can decrease the effectiveness of this drug.

• Can decrease the effectiveness of oral contraceptives and oral anticoagulants such as warfarin.

• Cyclosporin dosages may need adjustment.

Tell Your Child's Doctor If
• Your child has had allergic reactions to any medications, has any other diseases, or is taking any other medications.

• Your child has had liver disease, porphyria, or lupus.

• Your child is allergic to penicillin or cephalosporin antibiotics.

• Your daughter is or becomes pregnant.

Special Instructions
• This drug may cause increased sensitivity to the sun. Your child should avoid exposure to the sun and wear sunscreen to prevent severe sunburn.

Brand Names: Fulvicin U/F, Fulvicin P/G, Grifulvin V, Grisactin, Grisactin Ultra, Gris-PEG

Generic Available: Yes

Type of Drug: Antifungal

Use: Treats fungal infections of the hair, skin, and nails such as ringworm.

Time Required for Drug to Take Effect: Several weeks to several months

Dosage Forms and Strengths: Tablets (125 mg, 165 mg, 250 mg, 330 mg, 500 mg); Capsules (125 mg, 250 mg); Suspension (125 mg/5 mL)

Storage: Store at room temperature in tightly closed, light-resistant containers.

How This Drug Works: Slows the growth of fungus and makes normal tissue less likely to be infected with it.

Brand Names: Amonidrin,* Anti-Tuss,* Breonesin,* Fenesin, Guaifenesin* (various manufacturers), Gee-Gee,* Genatuss, GG-Cen,* Glyate,* Glytuss,* Glycotuss,* Guiatuss,* Glyate,* Halotussin,* Humibid L.A., Humibid Sprinkle, Hytuss* (sf), Hytuss 2X*(sf), Malotuss, Mytussin,* Robitussin,* Scot-tussin Expectorant*(sf), Sinumist-SR Capsulets, Uni-tussin* (*available over the counter, sf=sugar free.)

Generic Available: Yes

Type of Drug: Expectorant

Use: Helps nonproductive coughs become more productive and less frequent.

Time Required for Drug to Take Effect: 15 to 30 minutes

Dosage Forms and Strengths: Syrup (100 mg/ 5 mL); Liquid (200 mg/5 mL); Capsules (200 mg); Capsules, sustained-release (300 mg); Tablets (100 mg, 200 mg); Tablets, sustained-release (600 mg)

Storage: Store at room temperature in tightly closed, light-resistant containers.

How This Drug Works: Stimulates respiratory tract secretions.

GUAIFENESIN

Administration Guidelines
• Give with a large quantity of fluid.

Side Effects
Tell your child's doctor about any side effects that are persistent or particularly bothersome.

More Common. Nausea

Less Common. Drowsiness, headache, rash, vomiting

Tell Your Child's Doctor If
• Your child's cough persists for more than 1 week, is recurrent, or is accompanied by fever, rash, or persistent headache.

• Your child is taking this drug. It may interact with selected laboratory tests.

Special Instructions
• Do not give for persistent or chronic cough such as that occurring with smoking, asthma, chronic bronchitis, or for cough accompanied by excessive mucus or sputum.

Symptoms of Overdose: Gastrointestinal upset, vomiting

Special Notes
• Available in several combination products over the counter.

• Can cause drowsiness. Make sure you know how your child is reacting to this drug before allowing participation in activities that require alertness, such as riding a bicycle.

HALOPERIDOL

Administration Guidelines

• May be given with food or milk to decrease stomach upset.

• Usually given 2 or 3 times a day.

• Doses are increased slowly to decrease side effects.

• Give the liquid plain or dilute it in water and give immediately.

• Do not spill liquid on skin or clothing as a skin rash may develop.

• Missed doses: Give as soon as you remember, then give any remaining doses for that day at regularly spaced intervals. Do not give double doses.

Side Effects

Tell your child's doctor about any side effects that are persistent or particularly bothersome.

More Common. Blurred vision, constipation, dry mouth, drowsiness, nausea, vomiting. Contact the doctor if your child experiences trouble speaking or swallowing, loss of balance, masklike face, inability to move eyes, muscle spasms, restlessness or the need to keep moving, shuffling walk, stiff arms and legs, trembling, or twisting movements.

Less Common. Contact the doctor immediately if your child has seizures, difficult or fast breathing, fast or irregular heartbeat, fever, high or low blood pressure, increased sweating, loss of bladder control, severe muscle stiffness, pale skin, unusual fatigue or weakness, decreased thirst, difficulty urinating, dizziness, fainting, light-headedness, hallucinations, lip smacking or puckering, puffing of cheeks, rapid or wormlike movements of the tongue, skin rash, uncontrolled chewing movements, or uncontrolled arm or leg movements.

Possible Drug Interactions

• Central nervous system depressants such as alcohol, antihistamines, muscle relaxants, tranquilizers, sedatives, sleeping medications, narcotics, and some pain medications may cause extreme drowsiness, low blood pressure, and a decrease in breathing when used with this drug.

• Cough and cold products may increase the chance of dizziness, dry mouth, blurred vision, and constipation.

• Antidepressants, monoamine oxidase (MAO) inhibitors, and lithium lead to increased side effects. These medications need to be dosed carefully when used together.

Brand Name: Haldol

Generic Available: Yes

Type of Drug: Antipsychotic agent

Use: Treats nervous, mental, emotional, and behavioral disorders such as psychoses, mania, and Tourette syndrome.

Time Required for Drug to Take Effect: Full benefit for mental and emotional disorders may take 6 weeks to 6 months.

Dosage Forms and Strengths: Tablets (0.5 mg, 1 mg, 2 mg, 5 mg, 10 mg, 20 mg); Liquid, concentrate (2 mg/mL)

Storage: Store at room temperature in tightly closed, light-resistant containers. Do not freeze liquid.

How This Drug Works: Produces complex changes in the central nervous system.

- Phenobarbital and carbamazepine may decease the effect of this drug.

- Epinephrine may cause low blood pressure.

Tell Your Child's Doctor If
- Your child has had an allergic reaction to this drug, any other medications, foods, preservatives, or dyes.

- Your child has taken or is taking any other prescription or nonprescription medicine.

- Your child abuses alcohol or has lung, heart, liver, kidney, or thyroid disease; seizures; glaucoma; difficult urination; bone marrow disease; or any other medical condition.

- Your child continues to have a dry mouth after 2 weeks. Continued dry mouth can lead to cavities.

- Your child develops a rash from the sun.

- The blurred vision continues beyond the first few weeks or gets worse.

- Your daughter is or becomes pregnant.

- Your daughter is breast-feeding her baby. This drug can pass into breast milk, and the American Academy of Pediatrics is concerned about its effect on the baby.

Special Instructions
- Give this drug only as directed by the doctor. Your child's progress should be checked with regular visits to the doctor.

- Do not stop giving this drug without first checking with the doctor, who may gradually reduce the dosage before stopping it.

- Do not allow your child to drink alcohol while taking this drug.

- Do not give other medicines that may make your child sleepy.

- Your child should avoid exposure to sunlight. Make sure your child wears sunscreen when out-of-doors. This drug may cause a skin rash or severe sunburn with exposure to direct sunlight or ultraviolet light in tanning booths.

- Monitor your child often during exercise, play, or hot weather to prevent overheating. This drug decreases sweating, causing body temperature to rise. Hot baths, hot tubs, or saunas may make your child dizzy or faint.

- Do not let your child have surgery or any medical or dental treatment unless you tell the doctor or dentist your child is taking this drug.

- Do not give any other medication without first asking the pharmacist or the doctor.

Symptoms of Overdose: Severe breathing difficulty, dizziness, deep sleep, severe drowsiness, coma, decreased breathing, low blood pressure, agitation, irregular heartbeat, muscle trembling, jerking, stiffness, uncontrolled movement, severe fatigue, weakness

Special Notes
- This drug may cause side effects that are serious or may not go away after treatment is stopped. Discuss this with the doctor.

- Make sure you know how your child is reacting to this drug before allowing participation in an activity that requires alertness and coordination, such as riding a bicycle. This drug may cause your child to have blurred vision, dizziness, or drowsiness, or to be less alert.

- Some brands contain tartrazine dye. If your child is allergic to this dye, ask the pharmacist for a tartrazine-free product.

- Your child may need to wear sunglasses because of an increased sensitivity to light.

- The safety and efficacy of this drug has not been established for children younger than 3 years of age.

- This drug can cause light-headedness and dizziness if your child gets up too quickly from a prone or sitting position. Have your child get up slowly to prevent these side effects.

HYDROCHLOROTHIAZIDE

Administration Guidelines
• Give with food or milk.

• Usually given 1 or 2 times a day. Try to give it at the same time(s) each day.

• Don't give doses after 6 P.M. or your child may have to get up at night to urinate.

• Missed doses: Give as soon as possible and space remaining doses for the day at equal intervals. However, if it's within 6 hours of the next dose, skip the missed dose. Do not give double doses.

Side Effects
Tell your child's doctor about any side effects that are persistent or particularly bothersome.

More Common. Constipation, diarrhea, upset stomach, increased sensitivity to sunlight. Contact the doctor if your child experiences muscle cramps or tingling fingers or toes.

Less Common. Dizziness, fatigue. Contact the doctor if your child experiences blurred vision, confusion, difficulty breathing, dry mouth or excessive thirst, excessive weakness, fever, itching, joint pain, palpitations, or yellowing of the eyes or skin.

Possible Drug Interactions
• Can decrease the effectiveness of oral anticoagulants, insulin, oral antidiabetic medications, and methenamine.

• Nonsteroidal anti-inflammatory medications (NSAIDS, such as ibuprofen) can decrease the effectiveness of this drug. Some patients may exhibit increased toxicity of NSAIDS.

• Can increase the side effects of calcium supplements and cortisonelike drugs such as prednisone.

• Lithium dosage may require adjustment when taking this drug.

Tell Your Child's Doctor If
• Your child has had allergic reactions to any medications.

• Your child has any other diseases.

• Your child is taking any other medications.

• Your child is allergic to sulfa drugs.

• Your child has kidney disease, diabetes mellitus, liver disease, asthma, pancreatic disease, or lupus.

• Your daughter is or becomes pregnant.

Brand Names: Esidrix, HydroDIURIL, Oretic, Hydro-par, Ezide

Generic Available: Yes

Type of Drug: Thiazide diuretic

Use: Treats hypertension and edema due to congestive heart failure, liver disease, and nephrotic syndrome. Also treats nephrogenic diabetes insipidus.

Time Required for Drug to Take Effect: Several days to several weeks

Dosage Forms and Strengths: Tablets (25 mg, 50 mg, and 100 mg); Solution (50 mg/5 mL and 100 mg/mL)

Storage: Store at room temperature in tightly closed, light-resistant containers.

How This Drug Works: Removes excess fluid from the body by increasing the elimination of salt and water through the kidneys.

• Your daughter is breast-feeding her baby. This drug can pass into breast milk.

Symptoms of Overdose: Excessive urination, dehydration, lethargy, and severe dizziness or fainting

Special Notes

• This drug may cause your child's body to lose too much potassium, causing muscle cramps and weakness. The doctor will do blood tests to check the levels of minerals, including potassium, in your child's blood. Potassium supplements may be necessary.

• Blood glucose levels may be increased in children with diabetes.

Measuring Up

Remember: Never use an ordinary tableware teaspoon to measure liquid doses. Instead, use a cylindrical dosing spoon, dosage cup, dropper, or syringe. These measuring devices can be found at your local drug store and sometimes at supermarkets, toy stores, and department stores.

HYDROCODONE

Administration Guidelines

- May be given with food or milk to avoid stomach upset.

- Do not increase the dose or give it more often than your child's doctor prescribed.

- Works best if given at the onset of your child's pain, rather than after the pain increases.

- Missed doses: Give as soon as you remember if it's within 2 hours of the missed dose. Otherwise skip the missed dose and give the next dose at the scheduled time. Do not give double doses.

Side Effects

Tell your child's doctor about any side effects that are persistent or particularly bothersome.

More Common. Constipation, dizziness, drowsiness, dry mouth, flushing, light-headedness, loss of appetite, nausea, or sweating

Less Common. Blurred vision, nightmares or unusual dreams, trouble sleeping. Call the doctor immediately if your child experiences breathing difficulties, palpitations, tremors, excitation, rash, sore throat and fever, anxiety, severe weakness, or difficult or painful urination.

Possible Drug Interactions

- Other central nervous system depressants such as alcohol, antihistamines, cold preparations, muscle relaxants, tranquilizers, and other pain medicines can cause extreme drowsiness.

Tell Your Child's Doctor If

- Your child has had an allergic reaction to this drug or to other narcotic analgesics.

- Your child has any diseases, such as asthma.

- Your child is taking any other medications.

- Your daughter is or becomes pregnant.

- Your daughter is breast-feeding her baby.

Special Instructions

- Do not give to suppress a productive cough.

- Do not give as a cough suppressant to children younger than 2 years of age without first speaking to the doctor.

- Increase the fluid and fiber in your child's diet to avoid constipation.

Brand Names: Hycodan, Hydropane (in combination with acetaminophen: Anexsia, Co-Gesic, Duocet, Hydrocet, Hydrogesic, Lorcet, Vicodin)

Generic Available: Yes

Type of Drug: Narcotic analgesic and cough suppressant

Use: Relieves moderate to severe pain. Also used to suppress coughing.

Time Required for Drug to Take Effect: 10 to 20 minutes

Dosage Forms and Strengths: Tablets, with acetaminophen (2.5 mg, 5 mg, 7.5 mg, 10 mg); Capsules, with acetaminophen (5 mg); Solution (5 mg per 5 mL); Solution, with acetaminophen (2.5 mg)

Storage: Store at room temperature in tightly closed, light-resistant containers.

How This Drug Works: Acts directly on the central nervous system to relieve pain.

- Do not suddenly stop giving this drug without talking to the doctor if you have been giving it for several weeks. The doctor may want to decrease the dose gradually to avoid withdrawal side effects.

Symptoms of Overdose: Convulsions (tremors), confusion, severe nervousness or restlessness, severe dizziness, severe drowsiness, slow or difficult breathing, severe weakness, pinpoint pupils of the eyes

Special Notes

- Tolerance (decreased effectiveness) may be seen with long-term use.

- This drug may cause drowsiness. Be sure you know how your child is reacting to this drug before allowing participation in activities that require alertness, such as riding a bicycle.

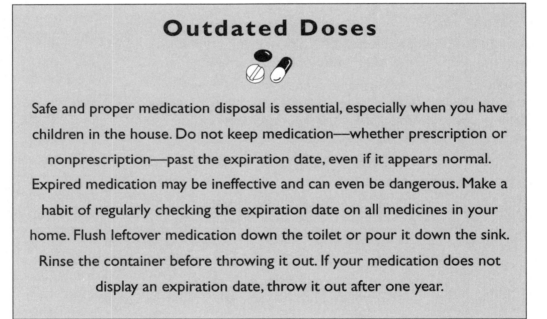

Outdated Doses

Safe and proper medication disposal is essential, especially when you have children in the house. Do not keep medication—whether prescription or nonprescription—past the expiration date, even if it appears normal. Expired medication may be ineffective and can even be dangerous. Make a habit of regularly checking the expiration date on all medicines in your home. Flush leftover medication down the toilet or pour it down the sink. Rinse the container before throwing it out. If your medication does not display an expiration date, throw it out after one year.

HYDROCORTISONE (SYSTEMIC)

Administration Guidelines

• May be given with food or milk to prevent stomach irritation.

• If your child is taking only 1 dose of this drug a day, try to give it before 9:00 A.M. This will mimic the body's normal production of this chemical.

• Shake the suspension well before measuring each dose.

• Missed doses: It is important not to miss a dose of this drug. If you miss a dose, follow these guidelines:

1. For those giving this drug more than once a day: Give the missed dose as soon as possible, and then return to the regular schedule. However, if it is already time for the next dose, double the dose.

2. For those giving this drug once a day: Give the missed dose as soon as possible. If you do not remember until the next day, do not give the missed dose at all, just follow the regular dosing schedule. Do not double the next dose.

3. For those giving this drug every other day: Give it as soon as you remember. If the scheduled time was missed by a whole day, give it when you remember, then skip a day before you give the next dose. Do not give double doses. If more than 1 dose is missed, contact your child's doctor.

Side Effects

Tell your child's doctor about any side effects that are persistent or particularly bothersome.

More Common. Dizziness, false sense of well-being, fatigue, increased appetite, increased sweating, indigestion, leg cramps, menstrual irregularities, muscle weakness, nausea, swelling of the skin on the face, restlessness, sleep disorders, or weight gain

Less Common. It is important to tell the doctor if your child experiences abdominal enlargement or pain; acne; back or rib pain; bloody or black, tarry stools; blurred vision; convulsions; eye pain; fever and sore throat; headaches; slow healing of wounds; increased thirst and urination; mental depression; mood changes; muscle wasting; nightmares; peptic ulcers; rapid weight gain (3 to 5 pounds in a week); rash; shortness of breath; unusual bleeding or bruising; or unusual weakness.

Brand Names: Cortef, Hydrocortone

Generic Available: Yes

Type of Drug: Adrenocorticosteroid hormone

Use: Treats endocrine and rheumatic disorders; asthma; blood diseases; certain cancers; eye disorders; gastrointestinal disturbances such as ulcerative colitis; respiratory diseases; and inflammatory diseases such as arthritis, dermatitis, and poison ivy.

Time Required for Drug to Take Effect: Varies depending on the illness being treated. It may be several days before it takes effect.

Dosage Forms and Strengths: Tablets (5 mg, 10 mg, 20 mg); Suspension (10 mg per 5 mL)

Storage: Store at room temperature in tightly closed containers.

How This Drug Works: How this drug works is not completely understood. This drug is similar to the cortisonelike chemicals naturally produced by the adrenal gland. These chemicals are involved in various regulatory processes in the body such as fluid balance, temperature, and reaction to inflammation.

Possible Drug Interactions
• Decreases the effectiveness of vaccines and can lead to infection if a live virus vaccine is given.

Tell Your Child's Doctor If
• Your child is taking any medications.

• Your child has had allergic reactions to this drug or other adrenocorticosteroids such as betamethasone, cortisone, dexamethasone, fluocinolone, methylprednisolone, prednisolone, prednisone, and triamcinolone.

• Your child has recently been exposed to or currently has chicken pox or measles.

• Your child has any medical problems such as diabetes, glaucoma, fungal infections, heart disease, high blood pressure, peptic ulcers, thyroid disease, tuberculosis, ulcerative colitis, kidney disease, or liver disease.

• Your daughter is or becomes pregnant. This drug can have adverse effects on the fetus.

• Your daughter is breast-feeding her baby.

Special Instructions
• Your child should not be vaccinated or immunized while taking this drug.

Symptoms of Overdose: Severe restlessness

Special Notes
• With long-term use, the doctor may want your child to be on a low-salt and potassium-rich diet. The doctor may also want your child's eyes examined periodically during treatment to detect glaucoma and cataracts.

• With long-term use, your child's dosage may need to be increased during times of stress such as serious infection, injury, or surgery.

• Do not abruptly stop giving this drug, especially if giving high doses over a long period of time. The doctor probably will want to decrease the dose slowly.

Just Call
If you have any concerns about any side effects, even minor ones, you should be sure to discuss them with your child's doctor. The doctor may be able to minimize or eliminate the side effects by prescribing a different medication or changing your child's dosage, dosing schedule, or the way the drug is given. (Do not make adjustments on your own without discussing them with your doctor.) At the very least, the doctor can assure you that the medication's benefits far outweigh its side effects.

HYDROXYZINE

Administration Guidelines

• May be given with food or a full glass of milk or water to avoid stomach upset.

• Shake the suspension well just before measuring each dose.

• Missed doses: Give as soon as possible. However, if it is time for the next dose, skip the missed dose and return to the regular dosing schedule. Do not give double doses.

Side Effects

Tell your child's doctor about any side effects that are persistent or particularly bothersome.

More Common. It is especially important to tell the doctor if your child experiences convulsions, feeling faint, irritability, confusion, rash, trembling, or shakiness.

Less Common. Drowsiness, dizziness, dry mouth, unsteady walk, and urinary retention. These side effects should disappear as your child's body adjusts to this drug. Tremors and convulsions are rare.

Possible Drug Interactions

• May increase the effect of alcohol and other central nervous system depressants such as narcotics and barbiturates.

Tell Your Child's Doctor If

• Your daughter is or becomes pregnant.

• Your daughter is breast-feeding her baby. It is not known if this drug passes into breast milk.

Symptoms of Overdose: Oversedation

Special Notes

• This drug can cause drowsiness or dizziness. Your child's ability to perform tasks that require alertness, such as riding a bicycle, may be decreased.

• Syrup may contain sucrose or sorbitol, which may cause diarrhea.

Brand Names: Anxanil, Atarax, Atozine, Durrax, Hy-Pam, Vamate, Vistaril; Hydroxyzine Hydrochloride, Hydroxyzine Pamoate (various manufacturers)

Generic Available: Yes

Type of Drug: Antihistamine, sedative/hypnotic, antiemetic

Use: Treats or prevents symptoms of allergy; also used as a sleeping aid and to relieve the symptoms of anxiety and tension. Has been used to treat nausea and vomiting.

Time Required for Drug to Take Effect: 15 to 30 minutes

Dosage Forms and Strengths: Hydroxyzine hydrochloride syrup (10 mg/5 mL); Tablets (10 mg, 25 mg, 50 mg, 100 mg); Hydroxyzine pamoate capsules (25 mg, 50 mg, 100 mg); Suspension (25 mg/5 mL)

Storage: Store at room temperature in tightly closed, light-resistant containers. Do not freeze.

How This Drug Works: Blocks the action of histamine, a chemical released by the body during an allergic reaction.

Brand Names: Advil, Genpril, Haltran, Ibuprin, Medipren, Midol 200, Motrin, Motrin IB, Nuprin, Pamprin-IB, PediaProfen, Rufen, Trendar

Generic Available: Yes

Type of Drug: Nonsteroidal anti-inflammatory analgesic

Use: Relieves mild to moderate pain, inflammation of arthritis, and fever.

Time Required for Drug to Take Effect: 1 to 2 hours for relief of pain and fever; 1 to 2 weeks for relief of arthritis inflammation

Dosage Forms and Strengths: Tablets (200 mg, 300 mg, 400 mg, 600 mg, 800 mg); Suspension (100 mg per 5 mL).

Storage: Store at room temperature in tightly closed, light-resistant containers.

How This Drug Works: Decreases the production of the chemical prostaglandin.

IBUPROFEN

Administration Guidelines

- Give with a full glass of water.

- Give with food to avoid stomach upset.

- Shake the suspension well before each dose.

- Give on a regular basis if your child is taking this drug for arthritis.

- Missed doses: Give as soon as you remember if it is within 2 hours of the missed dose. Otherwise, skip the missed dose and give the next dose at the scheduled time. Do not give double doses.

- Do not give for more than 3 days for fever unless you contact the doctor.

Side Effects

Tell your child's doctor about any side effects that are persistent or particularly bothersome.

More Common. Heartburn, nausea, vomiting, stomach pain, dizziness, drowsiness, light-headedness, indigestion

Less Common. Bitter taste, constipation, decreased appetite, flushing. Contact the doctor if your child experiences bloody or black, tarry stools; changes in vision; spitting up or vomiting of blood; severe stomach upset; skin rash; hives; trouble breathing; wheezing; ringing in the ears; or difficult or painful urination.

Possible Drug Interactions

- Other anti-inflammatory medications (indomethacin) and aspirin can increase stomach upset.

- May decrease the effect of diuretics.

Special Notes

- Available over the counter.

- Do not give to children who have recently been exposed to chicken pox and have a fever without first calling the doctor.

IMIPRAMINE

Administration Guidelines

• May be given with food to decrease stomach upset.

• Given 2 or 3 times a day or as a single daily dose at bedtime.

• Doses are increased slowly to decrease the side effects.

• Give 1 hour before bedtime if used for bed-wetting. However, give children with early night bed-wetting a split dose, half in the mid-afternoon and half at bedtime.

• Missed doses: Give as soon as possible. However, if it's within 2 hours of the next dose, skip the missed dose. Do not give double doses. If you miss a once-a-day bedtime dose, do not give the missed dose in the morning because it may cause sedation.

• Do not use for bed-wetting in children younger than 6 years of age.

Side Effects

Tell your child's doctor about any side effects that are persistent or particularly bothersome.

More Common. Drowsiness, dry mouth, dizziness, light-headedness, headache, nausea, increased appetite, weight gain, unpleasant taste, constipation, weakness

Less Common. Contact the doctor if your child experiences blurred vision, confusion, difficulty in speaking or swallowing, eye pain, fainting, fast or irregular heartbeat, hallucinations, loss of balance, a masklike face, nervousness or restlessness, problems urinating, shakiness, or slow movements.

Possible Drug Interactions

• Ask the pharmacist or doctor before giving any other medication with this drug.

• Clonidine (Catapres) may lead to very high blood pressures.

• Monoamine oxidase (MAO) inhibitors, isocarboxazid (Marplan), phenelzine (Nardil), or tranylcypromine (Parnate) can lead to very serious reactions and death.

• Central nervous system depressants such as alcohol, antihistamines, cold preparations, muscle relaxants, tranquilizers, and some pain medications may cause extreme drowsiness when used with this drug.

• Cimetidine (Tagamet and Tagamet HB) and methylphenidate (Ritalin) may increase the effect of this drug.

• Phenobarbital and carbamazepine may decrease the effect of this drug.

Brand Names: Tofranil, Tofranil-PM, Janimine

Generic Available: Yes

Type of Drug: Anti-depressant, tricyclic

Use: Treats depression, some kinds of chronic pain, and bed-wetting. Relieves symptoms of Attention Deficit Hyperactivity Disorder (ADHD).

Time Required for Drug to Take Effect: Full anti-depressant benefit may not be achieved for more than 2 weeks. If satisfactory effect is not seen for bed-wetting within 1 week, the dosage should be increased.

Dosage Forms and Strengths: Capsule (75 mg, 100 mg, 125 mg, 150 mg of pamoate); Tablets (10 mg, 25 mg, 50 mg of hydrochloride)

Storage: Store at room temperature in tightly closed, light-resistant containers.

How This Drug Works: Increases the concentration of serotonin and norepinephrine in the central nervous system.

- Eyedrops and nasal sprays or drops that contain naphazoline, oxymetazoline, epinephrine, phenylephrine, or xylometazoline may cause an increase in heart rate and blood pressure.

- Antithyroid drugs lead to an increase in rare blood disorders.

Tell Your Child's Doctor If
- Your child has had an allergic reaction to this drug or to any other medication.

- Your child has heart disease, seizures, glaucoma, thyroid disease, urinary retention, liver or kidney disease, or any other medical condition.

- Your child is or has been taking MAO inhibitors such as isocarboxazid (Marplan), phenelzine (Nardil), or tranylcypromine (Parnate).

- Your child has taken or is taking any other prescription or nonprescription medicine.

- Your daughter is or becomes pregnant.

- Your daughter is breast-feeding her baby. This drug can pass into breast milk, and the American Academy of Pediatrics is concerned about its effect on the infant.

Special Instructions
- Only use the hydrochloride form of this drug for bed-wetting.

- Give this drug to your child only as directed by the doctor.

- Take your child to the doctor regularly to monitor progress.

- Do not stop giving this drug without first speaking to the doctor, who may want to gradually reduce the dosage.

- The effects of this drug may last for up to 1 week after you stop giving it to your child.

- Your child should not drink alcohol while taking this drug.

- Do not give other medicines that may make your child sleepy.

- Limit your child's intake of caffeine.

- Protect your child's skin with sunscreen when out-of-doors. This drug may cause a skin rash or a severe sunburn with exposure to direct sunlight or ultraviolet light in tanning booths.

Symptoms of Overdose: Agitation; dry mouth; confusion; hallucinations; severe drowsiness; enlarged pupils; fever; vomiting; trouble breathing; urinary retention; low blood pressure; seizures; or fast, slow, or irregular heartbeat.

Special Notes
- Drowsiness is common. Make sure you know how your child is reacting to this drug before allowing participation in activities that require alertness and coordination, such as riding a bicycle.

- Some products contain tartrazine dye. If your child is allergic to it, ask the pharmacist for a tartrazine-free product.

- May cause urine to turn blue-green.

INDOMETHACIN

Administration Guidelines

• Give with a full glass of water.

• Give with food or immediately after meals to avoid stomach upset.

• Shake the suspension well before measuring each dose.

• Do not crush or allow your child to chew the extended-release capsules.

• Give on a regular basis if your child is taking this drug for arthritis.

• Missed doses: Give it as soon as you remember if it is within 2 hours of the missed dose. Otherwise, skip the missed dose and give the next dose at the scheduled time. Do not give double doses.

Side Effects

Tell your child's doctor about any side effects that are persistent or particularly bothersome.

More Common. Heartburn, nausea, vomiting, stomach pain, dizziness, drowsiness, light-headedness, indigestion

Less Common. Bitter taste, constipation, decreased appetite, flushing. Contact the doctor if your child experiences bloody or black, tarry stools; changes in vision; spitting up or vomiting of blood; severe stomach upset; skin rash; hives; trouble breathing; wheezing; ringing in the ears; difficult or painful urination.

Possible Drug Interactions

• Other anti-inflammatory medications and aspirin can increase stomach upset when used with this drug.

• May increase the effect of digoxin, methotrexate, and lithium.

• May decrease the effect of diuretics.

• Blood thinners may increase bleeding complications when used with this drug.

Tell Your Child's Doctor If

• Your child has had allergic reactions to any medications, especially other nonsteroidal anti-inflammatory drugs or aspirin.

• Your child has any diseases, especially asthma, stomach problems, or liver or kidney disease.

• Your daughter is or becomes pregnant.

• Your daughter is breast-feeding her baby. This drug can pass into breast milk; however, the American Academy of Pediatrics

Brand Name: Indocin

Generic Available: Yes

Type of Drug: Nonsteroidal anti-inflammatory analgesic

Use: Relieves mild to moderate pain and inflammation (swelling and stiffness); helps manage arthritis.

Time Required for Drug to Take Effect: 1 to 2 hours for pain relief. Begins to relieve inflammation of arthritis in 1 to 2 weeks, with full effect in 4 weeks.

Dosage Forms and Strengths: Capsules (25 mg, 50 mg); Capsules, extended-release (75 mg); Suspension (25 mg per 5 mL); Rectal suppositories (50 mg)

Storage: Store at room temperature in tightly closed, light-resistant containers. Suppositories also may be stored in the refrigerator.

How This Drug Works: Decreases the production of the chemical prostaglandin.

considers it compatible with breast-feeding in most cases.

Special Instructions

• Before your child has any medical or dental surgery, tell the doctor performing the procedure your child is taking this drug.

Symptoms of Overdose: Fainting, fast or irregular breathing, confusion, ringing in the ears, convulsions, sweating, blurred vision

Measuring Up

Remember: Never use an ordinary tableware teaspoon to measure liquid doses. Instead, use a cylindrical dosing spoon, dosage cup, dropper, or syringe. These measuring devices can be found at your local drug store and sometimes at supermarkets, toy stores, and department stores.

INSULIN

Administration Guidelines

• Use disposable needles and syringes.

• Clean the injection site with an antiseptic alcohol swab before injecting.

• Change injection site every time.

• Always check the dose in the syringe at least twice before injecting it.

• Do not inject cold insulin.

• Gently roll vial before withdrawing insulin. Do not shake.

• Never use a vial of insulin if there are lumps in it.

• If giving 2 different types of insulin, draw the regular (clear) insulin into the syringe first.

• Missed doses: Contact your child's doctor.

Side Effects

Tell your child's doctor about any side effects that are persistent or particularly bothersome.

More Common. Redness and/or rash at the site of injection

Less Common. Tell the doctor if your child experiences palpitations, fainting, shortness of breath, skin rash, or sweating.

Possible Drug Interactions

• Oral contraceptives, adrenocorticosteroids, furosemide, thyroid replacement, thiazide diuretics, and phenytoin can increase insulin requirements.

• Monoamine oxidase (MAO) inhibitors, sulfinpyrazone, tetracycline, alcohol, or large doses of aspirin can increase the effects of this drug, leading to hypoglycemia.

• Beta blockers, atenolol, metoprolol, nadolol, propranolol, and timolol may prolong the effects of this drug and mask the signs of hypoglycemia such as rapid heartbeat.

Tell Your Child's Doctor If

• Your child is currently taking any medication.

• Your child is allergic to a particular type of insulin.

• Your child has high fevers; infections; kidney, liver, or thyroid disease; or severe nausea and vomiting.

• Your daughter is or becomes pregnant. Diabetes must be well

Brand Names: Humulin L, Humulin N, Humulin R, Iletin I, Iletin II, Insulatard NPH, Mixtard, Novolin, Velosulin

Generic Available: No

Type of Drug: Antidiabetic

Use: Treats diabetes mellitus.

Time Required for Drug to Take Effect: Varies by type: ½ hour for short-acting (regular) insulin, 1 hour for intermediate-acting (NPH) insulin, 36 hours for long-acting (leute) insulin

Dosage Forms and Stengths: Injectable, all types (100 units/mL); Injectable, regular (100 units/mL, 500 units/mL)

Storage: Refrigerate unopened vials. After opening, keep all forms (except 500 units/mL) at room temperature and use within 6 months.

How This Drug Works: Regulates blood-sugar levels when the pancreas does not produce enough of its own insulin.

controlled under a doctor's supervision during pregnancy.

Special Instructions

• Make sure friends and family are aware of the symptoms of too much or too little insulin and know what to do if they notice any of the symptoms in your child.

• Have your child carry a card or wear a bracelet as identification for a child with diabetes.

• Always have insulin and syringes available. When traveling, do not pack them in your luggage.

• Do not store insulin in a car's glove compartment or anywhere it might be subjected to extreme temperatures.

• Check with the doctor or pharmacist before giving any nonprescription products.

• The requirements of this drug may change if your child becomes ill. Consult the doctor.

Symptoms of Overdose: Too much insulin can cause hypoglycemia (low blood sugar), which can lead to anxiety, chills, cold sweats, drowsiness, fast heart rate, headache, loss of consciousness, nausea, nervousness, tremors, unusual hunger, or unusual weakness. A child experiencing these symptoms should eat a quick source of sugar (such as table sugar, orange juice, honey, or a nondiet cola). You should also be sure to tell the doctor that your child had this reaction.

Special Notes

• Too little insulin can cause symptoms of hyperglycemia (high blood sugar), such as confusion, drowsiness, dry skin, fatigue, flushing, frequent urination, fruitlike breath odor, loss of appetite, or rapid breathing. If your child experiences any of these symptoms, contact the doctor, who may want to modify your child's dosing schedule or insulin dosage.

IPRATROPIUM BROMIDE

Administration Guidelines

• Shake inhalation container well just before each use to distribute the ingredients and equalize doses.

• Wait 1 full minute between doses to receive the full benefit of the first dose if more than 1 inhalation is necessary.

• Do not exceed the recommended dosage of this drug. Excessive use may lead to an increase in side effects or a loss of effectiveness.

• Do not spray aerosol near the eyes.

• Do not puncture, break, or burn the aerosol container. The contents are under pressure and may explode.

Side Effects

Tell your child's doctor about any side effects that are persistent or particularly bothersome.

More Common. Nosebleed, nasal dryness, dry mouth and throat, nasal congestion, dry nasal discharge

Less Common. Fast heartbeat, flushing, low blood pressure, high blood pressure, dizziness, fatigue, drowsiness, insomnia, itching, loss of hair, nausea, constipation, thirst, urinary difficulty, blurred vision, hoarseness

Tell Your Child's Doctor If

• Your child has had unusual or allergic reactions to any medications.

• Your daughter is pregnant or breast-feeding her baby. No adequate and well-controlled studies have been conducted in pregnant women. Use during pregnancy only if clearly needed. Severe forms of asthma should be controlled by the doctor during pregnancy. Although it is unlikely that this drug would reach the infant to an important extent, it is not known whether this drug passes into breast milk.

Special Instructions

• Do not use for immediate relief of asthma symptoms.

Symptoms of Overdose: Acute overdosage by inhalation is unlikely.

Brand Name: Atrovent

Generic Available: No

Type of Drug: Bronchodilator

Use: Treats bronchospasms associated with asthma, COPD (chronic obstructive pulmonary disease), and bronchitis.

Time Required for Drug to Take Effect: 1 to 3 minutes

Dosage Forms and Strengths: Aerosol (18 mcg/actuation); Solution for inhalation, nebulizing (0.02%); Nasal spray (0.03%, 0.06%)

Storage: Store solution at room temperature in tightly closed, light-resistant containers. Keep inhalation aerosol away from excessive heat; the contents are pressurized and can explode if heated.

How This Drug Works: Blocks the action of neurotransmitter (a chemical substance released by nerve endings), causing bronchodilation.

Brand Names: Laniazid, Nydrazid

Generic Available: Yes

Type of Drug: Antitubercular antibiotic

Use: Treats and prevents tuberculosis.

Time Required for Drug to Take Effect: 6 months to 2 years

Dosage Forms and Strengths: Tablets (50 mg, 100 mg, 300 mg); Syrup (50 mg/mL); Injection (100 mg/mL). Also available in combination products.

Storage: Store at room temperature in tightly closed, light-resistant containers.

How This Drug Works: Destroys the tuberculosis bacteria.

ISONIAZID

Administration Guidelines

• Works best if given on an empty stomach 1 hour before or 2 hours after meals. Give with food if your child experiences stomach upset.

• Usually given once a day. May be given 2 or 3 times a week under special circumstances.

• Give this drug for the entire time prescribed by the doctor, even if your child feels better.

• Missed doses: Give as soon as possible. However, if it's within 6 to 8 hours of the next dose, skip the missed dose and give the next regular dose. Do not give double doses.

Side Effects

Tell your child's doctor about any side effects that are persistent or particularly bothersome.

More Common. Upset stomach, diarrhea. Contact the doctor if your child experiences weakness or tingling of the fingers or toes.

Less Common. Liver damage, low blood counts, fever, rashes, swollen lymph nodes, drunken appearance, ringing in the ears. Contact the doctor if your child experiences fatigue, blurred vision, convulsions, confusion, mouth sores, unusual bleeding or bruising, yellowing of the eyes or skin, or dark-colored urine.

Possible Drug Interactions

• Antacids may reduce the absorption of this drug.

• Regular alcohol consumption may increase the risk of liver damage.

• May increase the effect of oral anticoagulants, benzodiazepines, carbamazepine, phenytoin, and meperidine.

Tell Your Child's Doctor If

• Your child has had allergic reactions to any medications.

• Your child has any other diseases.

• Your child is taking any other medications.

• Your child has ever had epilepsy or liver or kidney disease.

• Your daughter is or becomes pregnant.

• Your daughter is breast-feeding her baby. This drug can pass into breast milk; however, the American Academy of Pediatrics considers it compatible with breast-feeding in most cases.

Symptoms of Overdose: Nausea, vomiting, dizziness, blurred vision, hallucinations, slurred speech

Special Notes

• It may be best to avoid foods such as cheese, tuna, sauerkraut, salami, broad beans, liver, and wine since they can cause headache, fainting, and excessive sweating when consumed during therapy with this drug.

• Your child may require pyridoxine (vitamin B$_6$) supplements while taking this drug.

• Your child will need eye exams, blood tests, and liver function tests while taking this drug.

• The risk of liver disease caused by this drug is much less in children than in adults.

• This drug may be used in combination with other antitubercular medications.

• A variety of dosing schedules exist. It is very important that you adhere to the regimen prescribed for your child.

Teach Your Children Well

Let's face it. Kids can be pretty stubborn when it comes to accepting medication. When appropriate, try giving your child information about his or her condition and how the medicine works. In a nonthreatening voice, talk about the consequences of not taking the medication, perhaps reminding the child of how uncomfortable he or she was before beginning the medication. Use reasoning when possible, but don't scare the child. Children who understand the importance of antibiotics for infection, insulin for diabetes, or inhalants for asthma are more likely to take the medication without objection.

Brand Name: Accutane

Generic Available: No

Type of Drug: Acne preparation

Use: Treats severe cystic acne.

Time Required for Drug to Take Effect: It may take 1 to 2 months to achieve maximum effect.

Dosage Form and Strengths: Capsules (10 mg, 20 mg, 40 mg)

Storage: Store at room temperature in tightly closed, light-resistant containers.

How This Drug Works: The exact mechanism of action is unknown.

ISOTRETINOIN

Administration Guidelines

• Give with meals for maximum benefit.

• Capsules may be chewed before swallowing.

• Open the capsule with a large needle and sprinkle the contents on apple sauce or ice cream if your child is unable to swallow the capsule.

• Missed doses: Give as soon as possible. However, if it is time for the next dose, double it, and then return to your regular dosing schedule.

Side Effects

Tell your child's doctor about any side effects that are persistent or particularly bothersome.

More Common. It is especially important to tell the doctor if your child experiences bruising; burning or tingling sensation of the skin; depression; dizziness; hives; muscle pain; peeling of the palms and soles; rash; visual disturbances; or weight loss.

Less Common. Changes in skin color, drowsiness, dry lips or mouth, fatigue, fluid retention, headache, indigestion, inflammation of the eyelids or the lips, irritation of the eyes, thinning of the hair, nosebleeds, decreased night vision. These side effects may disappear as your child's body adjusts to this drug. May also cause increased sensitivity to sunlight.

Possible Drug Interactions

• Concurrent use of alcohol and this drug can lead to an increase in blood-lipid (fat) level, which can be dangerous.

• Taking vitamin supplements containing vitamin A can result in increased toxic effects.

• May decrease effectiveness of carbamazapine.

Tell Your Child's Doctor If

• Your child has had unusual or allergic reactions to any medications, especially to this drug, vitamin A, or the preservative parabens.

• Your child is taking any other medications.

• Your child has or ever had diabetes mellitus or hyperlipidemia (high-lipid levels).

• Your child's mouth remains dry after 2 weeks.

• Your daughter is or becomes pregnant. This drug has been shown to cause birth defects in humans. An effective form of birth control should be used while taking this drug and for at least 1 month before and after your child stops taking it.

• Your daughter is breast-feeding her baby. It is not known whether this drug passes into breast milk.

Special Instructions

• Your child should avoid prolonged exposure to sunlight and sunlamps. Have your child wear an effective sunscreen, protective clothing, and sunglasses when out-of-doors.

Symptoms of Overdose: Transient headache; vomiting; facial flushing (red face); swollen, cracked, bright-red lips; abdominal pain; headache; dizziness; and shaky movement and unsteady walk

Special Notes

• Your child's acne may become worse for the first few days of treatment.

• Your child should not participate in any activity that requires alertness, such as riding a bicycle, if this drug causes drowsiness.

Be Accurate

If you don't give medication correctly, it may be ineffective or even cause side effects. An estimated 10 to 30 percent of medications aren't effective because they have been given incorrectly. To do it right, you have to give the exact amount of medicine prescribed at the scheduled time, for the specified duration, and in the appropriate manner. Always read the label, follow the directions carefully, and use the appropriate equipment for measuring and administering the medication. Also, be sure to wash your hands before you give any medication to your child.

Brand Name: Kapectolin

Generic Available: Yes

Type of Drug: Antidiarrheal

Use: Treats uncomplicated diarrhea.

Time Required for Drug to Take Effect: Response is highly variable.

Dosage Form and Strengths: Liquid (90 gm kaolin and 2 gm pectin/ 30 mL, 5.2 gm kaolin and 260 mg pectin/30 mL, 3.9 gm kaolin and 194 mg pectin/ 30 mL)

Storage: Store at room temperature in tightly closed containers. Do not freeze.

How This Drug Works: Adsorbs bacteria and toxins and reduces water loss.

KAOLIN AND PECTIN
Administration Guidelines
• Shake well before measuring each dose.

• Do not give within 2 to 3 hours of other medications.

• Do not give to children younger than 3 years of age unless prescribed by the doctor because of the increased risk of dehydration.

Side Effects
Tell your child's doctor about any side effects that are persistent or particularly bothersome.

More Common. Constipation

Possible Drug Interactions
• Decreases the absorption of other medications.

Tell Your Child's Doctor If
• Your child has had an allergic reaction to any medication.

• Your child is taking any other prescription or nonprescription medicine or has recently taken antibiotics.

• Your child has a fever, dysentery, severe diarrhea, or any other medical condition.

• Your child's diarrhea does not stop after 1 or 2 days.

• Your child develops symptoms of dehydration such as decreased urination, dizziness, light-headedness, dry mouth, increased thirst, no tears with crying, or wrinkled skin.

• Your daughter becomes pregnant or is breast-feeding her baby.

Special Instructions
• Do not give if your child has fever, abdominal pain, appendicitis, intestinal blockage, or blood or mucus in the stools.

• Keep your child well hydrated. It is very important to replace the water lost because of the diarrhea. Even if the stools look better, your child will continue to lose water into the intestine.

Symptoms of Overdose: Severe constipation

Special Notes
• This drug is not recommended for the treatment of sudden onset diarrhea in children of any age according to the American Academy of Pediatrics 1996 guidelines.

• Attapulgite has replaced this drug in many products such as Kaopectate, Parepectolin, Donnagel, and Diasorb.

KETOCONAZOLE

Administration Guidelines

- May be given on an empty stomach or with food to decrease nausea and vomiting.

- Tablets are generally given 1 or 2 times a day.

- Works best when blood concentrations are kept within a safe and effective range. Give at evenly spaced intervals around the clock. If you are to give 2 doses a day, space the doses 12 hours apart.

- Missed doses: Give immediately. However, if you do not remember until it is time for the next dose, give the missed dose and space the next dose about halfway through the regular interval between doses; then return to the regular schedule. Do not skip any doses.

- Apply the shampoo 2 times a week, at least 3 days apart. Massage over the entire scalp for 1 minute; rinse hair thoroughly and reapply for 3 minutes. Then wash it off.

- Apply the cream 1 or 2 times a day. Rub it into the affected area gently as instructed by your child's doctor.

- Give for the entire time prescribed by the doctor (usually until the infection has cleared and sometime thereafter as determined by the doctor). If the drug is stopped too soon, resistant yeast can continue growing, and the infection could recur.

Side Effects

Tell your child's doctor about any side effects that are persistent or particularly bothersome.

More Common. Fever, chills, headache, dizziness, lethargy, nervousness, itching, rash, dry skin, nausea, vomiting, abdominal discomfort, diarrhea, local irritation, and stinging with topical preparations

Less Common. It is especially important to tell the doctor if your child experiences bloody or prolonged diarrhea, fever, chills, fatigue, weakness, any other unusual bleeding or bruising, increased itching, yellow skin or eyes, dark urine, or enlarged breasts.

Possible Drug Interactions

- Antacids, ranitidine, cimetidine, famotidine, and sodium bicarbonate can decrease the amount of this drug absorbed from the stomach and, therefore, decrease its effectiveness.

- Rifampin and isoniazid can decrease blood concentrations of this drug and, therefore, decrease its effectiveness.

Brand Name: Nizoral

Generic Available: No

Type of Drug: Antifungal

Use: Treats yeast infections of the mouth, skin, and bloodstream.

Time Required for Drug to Take Effect: It may take a few days for this drug to be effective.

Dosage Forms and Strengths: Cream (2%); Shampoo (2%); Tablets (200 mg)

Storage: Store at room temperature in tightly closed containers; tablet containers also must be light-resistant.

How This Drug Works: Inhibits the manufacture of nutrients in the yeast cell wall, preventing further growth.

- Can increase blood concentrations of phenytoin, cyclosporine, astemizole, corticosteroids, terfenadine, and warfarin.

- Can cause serious heart complications when used with terfenadine or astemizole.

- A disulfiram-type reaction (severe nausea, vomiting, and discomfort) can result from the use of alcohol with this drug.

Tell Your Child's Doctor If
- Your child is taking any prescription or non-prescription medications, especially those listed above.

- Your child has had unusual or allergic reactions to any medications, especially to this drug.

- Your child has had liver, kidney, or blood diseases.

- Symptoms of infection seem to be getting worse rather than improving.

- Your daughter is or becomes pregnant.

- Your daughter is breast-feeding her baby. It is unknown whether this drug passes into breast milk.

Special Instructions
- Keep cream away from the eyes.

- Do not give antacids, famotidine, ranitidine, or cimetidine within 2 hours of a dose of this drug.

Symptoms of Overdose: Severe forms of side effects listed above.

Special Notes
- Cream contains sodium sulfite, an ingredient to which many people are allergic.

Just Call

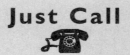

If you have any concerns about any side effects, even minor ones, you should be sure to discuss them with your child's doctor. The doctor may be able to minimize or eliminate the side effects by prescribing a different medication or changing your child's dosage, dosing schedule, or the way the drug is given. (Do not make adjustments on your own without discussing them with your doctor.) At the very least, the doctor can assure you that the medication's benefits far outweigh its side effects.

KETOPROFEN

Administration Guidelines

• Give with a full glass of water.

• Give with food or immediately after meals to avoid stomach upset.

• Do not crush or allow your child to chew extended-release capsules.

• Give on a regular basis if your child is taking this drug for arthritis.

• Missed doses: Give as soon as you remember if it is within 2 hours of the missed dose. Otherwise, skip the missed dose and give the next dose at the scheduled time. Do not give double doses.

Side Effects

Tell your child's doctor about any side effects that are persistent or particularly bothersome.

More Common. Heartburn, nausea, vomiting, stomach pain, dizziness, drowsiness, light-headedness, indigestion

Less Common. Bitter taste, constipation, decreased appetite, flushing. Contact the doctor if your child experiences bloody or black, tarry stools; changes in vision; spitting up or vomiting of blood; severe stomach upset; skin rash; hives; trouble breathing; wheezing; ringing in the ears; difficult or painful urination.

Possible Drug Interactions

• Other anti-inflammatory medications (ibuprofen) and aspirin can increase stomach upset.

• May decrease the effect of diuretics.

• Blood thinners may increase bleeding complications when used with this drug.

Tell Your Child's Doctor If

• Your child has had allergic reactions to any medications, especially other nonsteroidal anti-inflammatory drugs or aspirin.

• Your child has any diseases, especially asthma, stomach problems, or liver or kidney disease.

• Your daughter is or becomes pregnant.

• Your daughter is breast-feeding her baby.

Special Instructions

• Before your child has any medical or dental surgery, tell the doctor performing the procedure your child is taking this drug.

Brand Names: Orudis, Oruvail, Orudis KT

Generic Available: No

Type of Drug: Nonsteroidal anti-inflammatory analgesic

Use: Relieves mild to moderate pain and inflammation (swelling and stiffness) of arthritis.

Time Required for Drug to Take Effect: Relieves pain in 1 to 2 hours. Begins to relieve inflammation of arthritis in 1 to 2 weeks, with full effect in 4 weeks.

Dosage Forms and Strengths: Capsules (25 mg, 50 mg, 75 mg); Capsules, extended-release (200 mg)

Storage: Store at room temperature in tightly closed, light resistant containers.

How This Drug Works: Decreases the production of the chemical prostaglandin.

Symptoms of Overdose: Fainting, fast or irregular breathing, confusion, ringing in the ears, convulsions, sweating, blurred vision

Special Notes
• Available over the counter

• Not recommended for use in children younger than 16 years of age for fever without the supervision of the doctor. Its use in young children (between 2 and 16 years of age) is primarily for treating juvenile rheumatoid arthritis.

🗎 Keep a Lid on It

Pharmacists are required to put drugs in bottles that have child-resistant caps. Don't switch to a bottle that's easier for you to open—children may also find it easier to open. Remember, too, that child-resistant does not mean childproof. Children older than five years of age may be able to open most medicine bottles. That's why it's essential for you to teach them that drugs can be harmful if not taken correctly and that they need supervision before taking anything. And, just to be on the safe side, keep all medicines out of your child's reach.

LABETALOL

Administration Guidelines

- Usually given 2 times a day. Try to give it at the same times each day.

- May be given on an empty stomach or with food, but be consistent.

- Missed doses: Give as soon as possible and space remaining doses for the day at equal intervals. However, if it's within 6 hours of the next dose, skip the missed dose and give the next regular dose. Do not give double doses.

- Do not stop giving this drug without first speaking with your child's doctor.

Side Effects

Tell your child's doctor about any side effects that are persistent or particularly bothersome.

More Common. Fatigue, dizziness, headache, diarrhea, nausea, vomiting, vivid dreams

Less Common. Fainting, muscle cramps, tingling of fingers and toes, skin rash, stuffy nose, dry eyes, low blood counts, palpitations. Contact the doctor if your child experiences wheezing, swollen feet or ankles, yellowing of the eyes or skin, difficulty urinating, fainting, or confusion.

Possible Drug Interactions

- Can decrease the effectiveness of asthma medications.

- Cimetidine can increase the effectiveness of this drug, possibly leading to toxicity.

- Nonsteroidal anti-inflammatory agents (ibuprofen) may decrease the effectiveness of this drug.

- Clonidine, furosemide, and phenothiazine-type drugs such as prochlorperazine (Compazine), promethazine (Phenergan), and chlorpromazine (Thorazine) may increase the effectiveness of this drug.

Tell Your Child's Doctor If

- Your child has had allergic reactions to any medications.

- Your child has any other diseases.

- Your child is taking any other medications.

- Your child has ever had asthma, bronchitis, diabetes, or heart disease.

- Your daughter is or becomes pregnant.

Brand Names: Normodyne, Trandate

Generic Available: No

Type of Drug: Alpha- and beta-blocker

Use: Treats high blood pressure.

Time Required for Drug to Take Effect: Several days to weeks

Dosage Forms and Strengths: Tablets (100 mg, 200 mg, 300 mg); Injection (5 mg/mL)

Storage: Store at room temperature in tightly closed, light-resistant containers.

How This Drug Works: Slows the heart rate and dilates blood vessels.

- Your daughter is breast-feeding her baby. This drug can pass into breast milk; however, the American Academy of Pediatrics considers it compatible with breast-feeding in most cases.

Special Instructions
- Do not give medications for asthma, cough, cold, allergy, sinus problems, or weight control without first checking with the doctor or pharmacist.

Symptoms of Overdose: Excessively low blood pressure and heart rate, fainting, dizziness, convulsions, wheezing

Special Notes
- Can hide the signs and symptoms of low blood sugar in children with diabetes.

- Do not abruptly stop giving this drug.

Outdated Doses

Safe and proper medication disposal is essential, especially when you have children in the house. Do not keep medication—whether prescription or nonprescription—past the expiration date, even if it appears normal. Expired medication may be ineffective and can even be dangerous. Make a habit of regularly checking the expiration date on all medicines in your home. Flush leftover medication down the toilet or pour it down the sink. Rinse the container before throwing it out. If your medication does not display an expiration date, throw it out after one year.

LACTULOSE

Administration Guidelines

• Can be diluted in water, fruit juice, or milk, or added to food.

• Give a full glass of water or other liquid with this drug unless it's been diluted in 8 oz. of liquid.

• Increase your child's intake of water or other fluids.

• Discard syrup if it is cloudy or very dark in color. Some darkening of color is normal.

• Usually given once a day for constipation and 3 to 4 times a day for hepatic encephalopathy.

• Do not give regularly for more than 1 week or to children younger than 6 years of age unless prescribed by your child's doctor.

Side Effects

Tell your child's doctor about any side effects that are persistent or particularly bothersome.

More Common. Intestinal gas, abdominal discomfort, diarrhea, vomiting, nausea, cramping, increased thirst

Less Common. Contact the doctor if your child experiences confusion, dizziness, light-headedness, unusual fatigue or weakness, irregular heartbeat, or muscle cramps.

Tell Your Child's Doctor If

• Your child is taking any other medications.

• Your child has had an allergic reaction to this drug, any other medication, foods, preservatives, or dyes.

• Your child experiences a sudden change in bowel movements that either lasts longer than 2 weeks or returns intermittently.

• Your child has diabetes mellitus, a galactose-restricted diet, appendicitis, intestinal obstruction, rectal bleeding, or any other medical condition.

• Your daughter is or becomes pregnant.

Special Instructions

• Do not use if your child has abdominal pain, appendicitis, intestinal blockage, nausea, vomiting, or rectal bleeding.

Symptoms of Overdose: Diarrhea, abdominal pain, dehydration, low blood pressure, or changes in electrolytes

Special Notes

• Some sugar is absorbed from this drug and may cause problems with blood sugar control in children with diabetes.

Brand Names: Cephulac, Chronulac, Duphalac, Lactulose PSE, Cholac, Constulose, Constilac

Generic Available: Yes

Type of Drug: Laxative, hyperosmotic

Use: Treats chronic constipation; lowers high ammonia levels in the blood due to liver disease (hepatic encephalopathy)

Time Required for Drug to Take Effect: 24 to 48 hours for the laxative effect; 12 to 48 hours for lowering blood ammonia levels

Dosage Form and Strength: Syrup (10 gm/15 mL)

Storage: Store at room temperature in tightly closed, light-resistant containers. Do not freeze.

How This Drug Works: Produces an osmotic effect, pulling water into the colon to soften the stool and increase its movement through the colon.

Brand Name: Lamictal

Generic Available: No

Type of Drug: Anticonvulsant

Use: Adjunct treatment of convulsions or seizures.

Time Required for Drug to Take Effect: It may take several weeks to achieve complete effectiveness.

Dosage Form and Strengths: Tablets (25 mg, 50 mg, 100 mg, 200 mg)

Storage: Store at room temperature in tightly closed, light-resistant containers.

How This Drug Works: How it works in the central nervous system to reduce the number and severity of seizures is not completely understood.

LAMOTRIGINE

Administration Guidelines

• May be given with food to avoid stomach upset.

• Give at evenly spaced intervals around the clock to maintain a constant concentration of this drug in your child's bloodstream. If it is to be given 2 times a day, space the doses 12 hours apart.

• Missed doses: Give as soon as you remember, then stagger subsequent doses evenly for the rest of the day. Do not give double doses. If you miss 2 or more doses, contact your child's doctor.

• Do not increase the dose or give more frequently than the doctor prescribed.

Side Effects

Tell your child's doctor about any side effects that are persistent or particularly bothersome.

More Common. Dizziness, drowsiness, stomach upset, headache

Less Common. Agitation, increased skin sensitivity to the sun, vomiting. Contact the doctor if your child has a skin rash, flulike symptoms, itching, difficulty breathing, clumsiness, seizures, abnormal eye movements, or rapid or irregular heartbeat.

Possible Drug Interactions

• Acetaminophen may decrease the effectiveness of this drug if given at the same time. Do not give this drug within 2 to 3 hours of giving acetaminophen.

• Carbamazepine may increase some side effects of this drug if given at the same time. Do not give this drug within 2 hours of giving carbamazepine.

• Alcohol, antidepressants, antihistamines, pain relievers, or tranquilizers may increase drowsiness caused by this drug.

Tell Your Child's Doctor If

• Your child has had allergic reactions to any medications.

• Your child has any diseases.

• Your child is taking any medications.

• Your daughter is or becomes pregnant. Seizure disorders should be controlled by the doctor during pregnancy.

• Your daughter is breast-feeding her baby.

• Phenobarbital and phenytoin can decrease the effectiveness of this drug.

• Valproic acid may increase the effect of this drug. If your child is taking valproic acid and this drug, check carefully for rash, which is more common when these two drugs are taken together.

Special Instructions

• Before your child has surgery or any medical or dental treatment, tell the doctor performing the treatment that your child is taking this drug.

• Do not suddenly stop giving this drug. Abruptly stopping this drug could cause seizures.

• Check your child frequently for rash, especially during the first 1 to 2 months of therapy. Tell the doctor about any signs of rash.

Symptoms of Overdose: Severe dizziness or clumsiness, severe drowsiness, blurred or double vision, seizures or abnormal twitching, severe vomiting, abnormal eye movements, staggered walk, slurred speech

Special Notes

• This drug is usually given in addition to another seizure medication.

• Initially, the doctor will gradually increase the dose to ascertain the proper amount for your child.

• The doctor will want to follow your child's progress with regular office visits.

• Your child's dose will be determined, in part, by other medications your child is taking.

Teach Your Children Well

Let's face it. Kids can be pretty stubborn when it comes to accepting medication. When appropriate, try giving your child information about his or her condition and how the medicine works. In a nonthreatening voice, talk about the consequences of not taking the medication, perhaps reminding the child of how uncomfortable he or she was before beginning the medication. Use reasoning when possible, but don't scare the child. Children who understand the importance of antibiotics for infection, insulin for diabetes, or inhalants for asthma are more likely to take the medication without objection.

Brand Names: Synthroid, Levothroid

Generic Available: Yes

Type of Drug: Thyroid hormone

Use: Treats low thyroid hormone levels and other thyroid problems.

Time Required for Drug to Take Effect: Onset within 3 to 5 days; full effect in 3 to 4 weeks

Dosage Forms and Strengths: Tablets (0.025 mg, 0.05 mg, 0.075 mg, 0.088 mg, 0.1 mg, 0.112 mg, 0.125 mg, 0.137 mg, 0.15 mg, 0.175 mg, 0.2 mg, 0.3 mg)

Storage: Store at room temperature in tightly closed, light-resistant containers.

How This Drug Works: Replaces the thyroid hormone.

LEVOTHYROXINE

Administration Guidelines

• Give on an empty stomach.

• Usually given once a day.

• Missed doses: If a once-a-day dose is missed, give it as soon as you remember on the day missed. Otherwise, skip the missed dose and go back to the regular dosing schedule. Do not give double doses.

• Doses may be gradually increased in children to decrease the behavioral side effects.

Side Effects
Tell your child's doctor about any side effects that are persistent or particularly bothersome.

More Common. Temporary decrease in school performance due to short attention, hyperactivity, insomnia, irritability, and behavior difficulties

Less Common. Contact the doctor if your child develops headache, hives, skin rash, chest pain, rapid or irregular heartbeat, or shortness of breath.

Possible Drug Interactions

• Increases the effect of warfarin.

• Cholestyramine and colestipol decrease the absorption of this drug.

Tell Your Child's Doctor If

• Your child has thyroid, heart, lung, or adrenal gland disease; high blood pressure; diabetes mellitus; diabetes insipidus; asthma; or any other medical condition.

• Your child has taken or is taking any other prescription or nonprescription medication.

• Your child has had an allergic reaction to this drug, any other medications, foods, preservatives, or dyes.

• Your child experiences changes in appetite, diarrhea, fever, hand tremors, headache, irritability, leg cramps, an increase or decrease in weight, nervousness, sweating, trouble sleeping, vomiting, or changes in menstrual periods. A change in dosage may be necessary.

• Your child develops a new medical problem.

• Your child is taking this drug before having any medical tests, surgery, or dental work.

• Your daughter is or becomes pregnant.

Special Instructions
• Do not interchange brands without checking with the doctor.

• Do not suddenly stop giving this drug before speaking to the doctor.

• Give only as directed by the doctor.

• Take your child to the doctor regularly to monitor progress.

Symptoms of Overdose: Fever, low blood sugar, or heart failure in an acute overdose; weight loss, nervousness, sweating, fast heart rate, insomnia, heat intolerance, fever, or psychosis in a chronic overdose

Special Notes
• Children with long-standing, severe thyroid underactivity will experience temporary behavioral changes if thyroid hormone is replaced too fast. These children need to start at a low dose, increasing it slowly to decrease these side effects.

• Some products contain tartrazine dye. If your child is allergic to this dye, ask the pharmacist for a tartrazine-free product.

• Your child may have to take this drug for the rest of his or her life.

Keep It Out of Reach

Do not rely on a child-resistant cap to deter your child from opening a bottle of medication. Child-resistant does not mean childproof. Legally, a cap can be called child-resistant if 80 percent of all five-year-olds need more than five minutes to open it. That means the other 20 percent could get into it in even less time. Put the bottle in a hard-to-reach cabinet with a childproof lock. Do not keep it on the countertop, kitchen table, or nightstand.

Brand Name: EMLA

Generic Available: No

Type of Drug: Topical anesthetic

Use: Prevents pain prior to insertion of intravenous needles, harvesting of skin grafts, or other superficial skin surgery.

Time Required for Drug to Take Effect: At least 60 to 90 minutes

Dosage Form and Strength: Cream (5-g or 3-g tube with occlusive dressing)

Storage: Store at room temperature in tightly closed containers. Do not freeze.

How This Drug Works: Blocks the pain receptors in the skin, preventing the conduction of pain impulses.

LIDOCAINE 2.5% AND PRILOCAINE 2.5%

Administration Guidelines
• Wash your hands thoroughly before and after applying this drug.

• Apply a thick layer on the skin surface. If you are to apply an occlusive dressing, be sure you understand the instructions. Occlusive dressings are usually provided in the package with the cream.

• Be sure to apply the cream at the time your child's doctor tells you to, as it takes 60 to 90 minutes to take effect.

• Be careful not to touch your child's eyes with this drug, either directly from the tube or accidentally from cream that remains on your hands. This drug can cause severe eye irritation.

Side Effects
Tell your child's doctor about any side effects that are persistent or particularly bothersome.

More Common. Paleness or blanching (loss of color) of the skin, irritation, swelling, itching, alterations in temperature sensation, and rash

Less Common. It is especially important to tell the doctor if your child experiences any blueness of the lips, headache, weakness, difficulty in breathing, changes in blood pressure, or severe rash.

Possible Drug Interactions
• This drug generally does not interact with any other medications when used according to instructions.

Tell Your Child's Doctor If
• Your child has had unusual or allergic reactions to any medications, especially to lidocaine, prilocaine, or other local anesthetic agents.

• Your child has or ever had liver or kidney disease, anemia, or G6PD enzyme deficiency.

Special Instructions
• Do not give this drug to your child longer than is recommended by the doctor.

Special Notes
• Some children with congenital enzyme deficiency and infants younger than 3 months of age are at increased risk of side effects from this drug.

LINDANE

Administration Guidelines

- Wear plastic or rubber gloves when applying this drug to avoid absorbing it through the skin.

- Shake the lotion well before measuring each dose to distribute the ingredients evenly and equalize the doses.

- Your child should bathe and wash off lotion or cream 6 to 8 hours after application. (For infants, wash off 6 hours after application.)

- Apply shampoo and lather for 4 to 5 minutes. Rinse hair thoroughly and comb with a fine-tooth comb to remove nits (eggs).

- Be sure to rinse off this product completely according to the directions or too much of this drug will be absorbed.

- Do not use this drug more than once unless you are certain that lice are still present. Repeated use increases the risk of side effects. Speak to your child's doctor before applying a second time.

- When hair is dry, remove nits with a nit comb (fine-toothed comb) or fingernails. Wash combs and brushes, including the nit comb, with lice shampoo to prevent the spread of lice.

- Do not use on the face. If your child gets this drug in the eyes, flush them out immediately.

- Avoid using on any open wounds, cuts, or sores to minimize absorption through the skin.

- Do not give orally.

- When applying on young children, cover their hands to prevent accidental ingestion from finger or thumb sucking.

Side Effects

Tell your child's doctor about any side effects that are persistent or particularly bothersome.

More Common. The serious side effects associated with this drug, such as clumsiness, convulsions, irritability, muscle cramps, awareness of one's heartbeat, restlessness, unsteadiness, unusual nervousness, or vomiting, are due to absorption through the skin. This should not happen if the product is used according to directions. Contact the doctor if your child experiences any of these symptoms.

Less Common. Rash or skin irritation when product is applied incorrectly or repeatedly.

Brand Names: G-well, Kwell, Lindane (various manufacturers), Scabene

Generic Available: Yes

Type of Drug: Pediculicide and scabicide

Use: Eliminates crab lice, head lice, and scabies.

Time Required for Drug to Take Effect: One application is usually curative.

Dosage Forms and Strengths: Cream (1%); Lotion (1%); Shampoo (1%)

Storage: Store at room temperature in tightly closed containers. Do not freeze.

How This Drug Works: Stimulates the nervous system of the parasites, causing seizures and death.

Possible Drug Interactions
• Do not use other skin preparations (lotions, ointments, or oils) because they increase the absorption of this drug through the skin, which can lead to serious side effects.

Tell Your Child's Doctor If
• Your child has had unusual or allergic reactions to any medications, especially to this drug.

• Your daughter is or becomes pregnant. This drug is absorbed through the skin and may cause central nervous system side effects in the mother and fetus.

• Your daughter is breast-feeding her baby. This drug probably passes into breast milk and may cause central nervous system side effects in nursing infants.

Special Instructions
• After using the shampoo for head lice, you must remove the dead nits. Use a fine-tooth comb to remove them from the hair, or mix a solution of equal parts of water and vinegar and apply to the affected area. Rub the solution in well. After several minutes, shampoo with your regular shampoo and then brush your child's hair. This process should remove all the nits.

• Use with caution on infants, small children, and patients with preexisting seizure disorders as it has potential for neurologic toxicity.

Symptoms of Overdose: Central
nervous system excitation (restlessness, awareness of one's heartbeat, unusual nervousness) and, if used in sufficient quantities, seizures

Special Notes
• Itching can occur for several weeks after lice treatment. Itching by itself is not a sign of lice. Do not reuse lice treatments just because of itching.

• Cream and lotion are used only to treat scabies infections. Shampoo is used only to treat lice infestations.

LITHIUM
Administration Guidelines
• Give with meals to decrease stomach upset.

• Tablets are usually given 3 to 4 times a day; long-acting tablets are usually given 2 times a day.

• Dilute the syrup with juice or other beverages.

• Do not mix the syrup with other medications.

• Must be given every day at the prescribed times to keep blood concentrations constant.

• Doses are started low and adjusted weekly based on serum concentrations and response.

• Do not crush or allow your child to chew long-acting tablets; they must be swallowed whole.

• Missed doses: For tablets, capsules, and syrup, give as soon as possible. However, if it's within 2 hours of the next dose, skip the missed dose and go back to the regular schedule. For long-acting capsules, give as soon as possible. However, if it's within 6 hours of the next dose, skip the missed dose and go back to the regular schedule. For all forms: Do not give double doses.

Side Effects
Tell your child's doctor about any side effects that are persistent or particularly bothersome.

More Common. Increased urination, increased thirst, mild nausea, impaired taste, slight trembling of hands, weakness, fatigue, skin rash

Less Common. Contact the doctor if your child experiences diarrhea; drowsiness; loss of appetite; muscle weakness; slurred speech; trembling; blurred vision; clumsiness; unsteadiness; confusion; fainting; fast, slow, or irregular heartbeat; trouble breathing; unusual fatigue or weakness; weight gain; dry, rough skin; hair loss; hoarseness; mental depression; sensitivity to cold; swelling of feet or legs; swelling of neck; or unusual excitement.

Possible Drug Interactions
• Thiazide diuretics such as hydrochlorothiazide and nonsteroidal anti-inflammatory agents such as aspirin, ibuprofen, and naproxen may increase serum levels of this drug. This can lead to toxicity.

• Chlorpromazine, haloperidol, and molindone need to be dosed carefully when used with this drug. Concurrent use of any of these medications with this drug can lead to increased side effects.

Brand Names: Eskalith, Lithane, Lithonate, Lithotabs, Cibalith-S

Generic Available: Yes

Type of Drug: Antimanic agent

Use: Manages acute manic episodes, bipolar disorders, and depression.

Time Required for Drug to Take Effect: Full benefit may take 1 to several weeks.

Dosage Forms and Strengths: Capsules (150 mg, 300 mg, 600 mg); Tablets (300 mg); Tablets, long-acting (300 mg, 450 mg); Syrup (300 mg/5 mL)

Storage: Store at room temperature in tightly closed containers. Do not freeze syrup.

How This Drug Works: Changes the transport of cations across cell membranes in nerve and muscle cells, and changes the reuptake of serotonin and norepinephrine.

Tell Your Child's Doctor If

• Your child has taken or is taking any other prescription or nonprescription medicine.

• Your child has had an allergic reaction to this drug or any other medications, foods, preservatives, or dyes.

• Your child is dehydrated or has heart, kidney, or thyroid disease; seizures; leukemia; problems with urination; or any other medical condition.

• Your child develops a new medical problem.

• Your child has an illness that causes sweating, vomiting, or diarrhea.

• Your daughter is or becomes pregnant.

• Your daughter is breast-feeding her baby. This drug can pass into breast milk, and the American Academy of Pediatrics considers it incompatible with breast-feeding.

Special Instructions

• Keep your child's salt intake from food and table salt consistent from day to day. Changing the amount of salt in the body will change the amount of this drug removed by the kidneys.

• Give this drug only as directed by the doctor.

• Take your child to the doctor regularly to monitor progress.

• Do not stop giving this drug even if symptoms improve.

• Keep your child well hydrated. Your child should avoid heavy sweating, saunas, hot baths, or hot weather. It is dangerous for your child to lose too much water and salt.

• Limit your child's caffeine intake.

• Your child should not drink alcohol while taking this drug.

• Ask the pharmacist or the doctor before giving any other medication with this drug.

Symptoms of Overdose: Sedation, confusion, tremors, joint pain, trouble seeing, seizures, or coma

Special Notes

• Make sure you know how your child is reacting to this drug before allowing participation in activities that require alertness and coordination, such as riding a bicycle. This drug may make your child dizzy, drowsy, or less alert.

• Toxicity can occur at or near therapeutic serum levels of this drug.

• Some products contain tartrazine dye. If your child is allergic to it, ask the pharmacist for a tartrazine-free product.

• Long-acting tablet products are not interchangeable. Do not switch products without speaking with the doctor.

• Measurements of blood concentrations of this drug are used by the doctor to determine the correct dosage and to prevent toxicities. Early in therapy, blood concentrations may need to be measured 2 times a week. Later, blood concentrations may be measured every 1 to 2 months.

• Various laboratory tests will be needed to monitor your child.

LOPERAMIDE

Administration Guidelines
• Give with food or milk.

• Missed Doses: Give as soon as possible. However, if it's within 4 hours of the next dose, skip the missed dose. Do not give double doses.

• Have your child drink plenty of fluids.

• Do not give this drug for more than 10 days at a time unless your child's doctor specifically tells you to.

Side Effects
Tell your child's doctor about any side effects that are persistent or particularly bothersome.

More Common. Constipation, dizziness, drowsiness, dry mouth, fatigue, loss of appetite, nausea or vomiting, stomach upset

Less Common. Tell the doctor if your child experiences abdominal bloating or pain, fever, rash, or sore throat.

Tell Your Child's Doctor If
• Your child is allergic to this drug.

• Your child has had colitis, diarrhea caused by infectious organisms, drug-induced diarrhea, liver disease, dehydration, or conditions in which constipation must be avoided such as hemorrhoids, diverticulitis, heart or blood vessel disorders, or blood clotting disorders.

• Your child's diarrhea does not subside within 3 days.

• Your daughter is or becomes pregnant.

• Your daughter is breast-feeding her baby. This drug can pass into breast milk and cause side effects in the infant.

Special Instructions
• Do not give to children who have diarrhea caused by an infecting organism. Consult the doctor.

• Make sure you know how your child is reacting to this drug before allowing participation in activities that require alertness, such as riding a bicycle.

Symptoms of Overdose: Severe nausea, dizziness, fatigue, drowsiness

Special Notes
• Available over the counter.

• Not recommended for short-term bouts (1-2 days) of diarrhea when stools are produced frequently.

Brand Name: Imodium

Generic Available: Yes

Type of Drug: Antidiarrheal

Use: Treats acute and chronic diarrhea.

Time Required for Drug to Take Effect: 30 to 60 minutes

Dosage Forms and Strengths: Capsules (2 mg); Liquid (1 mg per 5 mL); Caplet (2 mg). Liquid and caplets are available over the counter.

Storage: Store at room temperature in tightly closed containers.

How This Drug Works: Slows the movement of the gastrointestinal tract, and decreases the passage of water and other substances into the bowel.

Brand Name: Claritin

Generic Available: No

Type of Drug: Antihistamine

Use: Provides symptomatic relief of seasonal allergic rhinitis such as hay fever.

Time Required for Drug to Take Effect: 1 to 3 hours

Dosage Form and Strength: Tablets (10 mg)

Storage: Store at room temperature in tightly closed, light-resistant containers.

How This Drug Works: Blocks the action of histamine, a chemical released from the body during an allergic reaction.

LORATADINE

Administration Guidelines
• Give on an empty stomach to achieve effective blood concentrations.

• Give once a day.

• Try to give at the same time each day, preferably in the morning.

• Missed doses: Give as soon as possible if it is during the day. Otherwise skip the missed dose and return to your regular dosing schedule. Do not give double doses.

Side Effects
Tell your child's doctor about any side effects that are persistent or particularly bothersome.

More Common. Blurred vision; confusion; constipation, diarrhea; difficult or painful urination; dizziness; dry mouth, throat, or nose; dry skin or hair; headache; increased or decreased appetite; irritability; itching; nausea; restlessness; stomach upset; migraines; palpitations; rash; shortness of breath; sleeping disorders; sore throat or fever; tightness in the chest or back; trouble breathing; unusual bleeding or bruising; unusual fatigue or weakness; urine discoloration; or yellowing of the eyes or skin. These effects should disappear as the body adjusts to this drug. This drug can cause increased sensitivity to sunlight.

Less Common. It is especially important to tell the doctor if your child experiences anxiety, clumsiness, feeling faint, or flushing of the face.

Possible Drug Interactions
• Can cause extreme drowsiness when used with central nervous system depressants such as alcohol, barbiturates, benzodiazepine tranquilizers, muscle relaxants, narcotics, pain medications, and phenothiazine tranquilizers, or with tricyclic antidepressants.

• Monoamine oxidase (MAO) inhibitors such as isocarboxazid, pargyline, phenelzine, and tranylcypromine can increase the side effects of this drug.

Tell Your Child's Doctor If
• Your child is taking any other medications.

• Your child has had unusual or allergic reactions to any medications, especially to this drug, cyproheptadine, azatadine, or any other antihistamine such as astemizole, brompheniramine, carbinoxamine, chlorpheniramine, clemastine, dimenhydrinate, dimethindene, diphenhydramine, diphenylpyraline, doxylamine, hydroxyzine, and terfenadine.

- Your child has or ever had asthma, blood vessel disease, high blood pressure, kidney disease, liver disease, peptic ulcers, or thyroid disease.

- Your daughter is or becomes pregnant. The effects of this drug during pregnancy have not been thoroughly studied in humans.

- Your daughter is breast-feeding her baby. This drug should not be used by nursing mothers.

Special Instructions
- Make sure your child avoids prolonged exposure to sunlight and sunlamps. When out-of-doors, your child should wear an effective sunscreen and protective clothing.

Symptoms of Overdose: Intensified symptoms of side effects listed above.

Special Notes
- Your child should not participate in any activity that requires alertness, such as riding a bicycle, if this drug causes drowsiness.

- Because this drug is metabolized primarily by the liver, patients with liver disease may require a lower dosage.

Just Call

If you have any concerns about any side effects, even minor ones, you should be sure to discuss them with your child's doctor. The doctor may be able to minimize or eliminate the side effects by prescribing a different medication or changing your child's dosage, dosing schedule, or the way the drug is given. (Do not make adjustments on your own without discussing them with your doctor.) At the very least, the doctor can assure you that the medication's benefits far outweigh its side effects.

Brand Names: Ativan, Alzapam

Generic Available: Yes

Type of Drug: Benzodiazepine

Use: Treats general anxiety or panic disorders and some types of seizures disorders. Provides sedation and/or amnesia for test procedures. Relaxes skeletal muscles.

Time Required for Drug to Take Effect: Within 60 minutes for sedation. Full benefit may not be achieved for a few weeks when used for anxiety or seizure disorders or for muscle relaxation.

Dosage Forms and Strengths: Tablets (0.5 mg, 1 mg, 2 mg); Solution (2 mg/mL); Injection (2 mg/mL, 4 mg/mL)

Storage: Store tablets at room temperature in tightly closed, light-resistant containers. Refrigerate the solution and injection; do not freeze.

How This Drug Works: Depresses the central nervous system by enhancing the action of GABA; suppresses the spread of seizure activity in the brain.

LORAZEPAM

Administration Guidelines

- May be given with food or water to decrease stomach upset.

- Usually given 2 to 4 times a day.

- Doses may be increased slowly.

- Solution should be diluted with water, soda, juice, applesauce, pudding, or other liquids and semisolid foods.

- Missed doses: If you remember within 1 hour, give the missed dose. Otherwise skip the missed dose and go back to the regular schedule. Do not give double doses.

- Do not suddenly stop giving this drug before speaking to your child's doctor. Abruptly stopping this drug can lead to seizures.

Side Effects

Tell your child's doctor about any side effects that are persistent or particularly bothersome.

More Common. Clumsiness, unsteadiness, dizziness, light-headedness, drowsiness, slurred speech, headache, dry mouth, constipation, diarrhea, nausea, change in appetite

Less Common. Contact the doctor if your child experiences behavioral changes, difficulty concentrating, outbursts of anger, confusion, depression, seizures, hallucinations, impaired memory, muscle weakness, skin rash, itching, sore throat, fever, chills, sores in the mouth, uncontrolled movements of the body, unusual bleeding or bruising, unusual excitement or nervousness, irritability, unusual fatigue or weakness, or yellow skin.

Possible Drug Interactions

- Central nervous system depressants such as alcohol, antihistamines, cold preparations, muscle relaxants, tranquilizers, and some pain medications may cause extreme drowsiness when used with this drug.

Tell Your Child's Doctor If

- Your child has taken or is taking any other prescription or nonprescription medicine.

- Your child has had an allergic reaction to this drug, any other medications, foods, preservatives, or dyes.

- Your child has asthma, lung disease, seizures, glaucoma, liver disease, kidney disease, uncontrolled pain, or any other medical condition.

- Your daughter is or becomes pregnant.

• Your daughter is breast-feeding her baby. This drug can pass into breast milk, and the American Academy of Pediatrics is concerned about its effect on the baby.

Special Instructions
• Give this drug only as directed by the doctor.

• Do not allow your child to drink alcohol while taking this drug.

• Do not give other medicines that may make your child sleepy.

• Limit your child's intake of caffeine.

Symptoms of Overdose: Slurred
speech, confusion, severe drowsiness, severe weakness, shakiness, low blood pressure, trouble breathing, slow heartbeat, staggering, coma, or trouble walking

Special Notes
• Drowsiness is common. Make sure you know how your child is reacting to this drug before allowing participation in activities that require alertness and coordination, such as riding a bicycle.

• Children and patients with preexisting brain damage have more behavioral problems with this drug.

• It is important to have the doctor check your child's progress regularly.

• When this drug is stopped after long-term use, your child's body may take up to 3 weeks to adjust.

Be Accurate

If you don't give medication correctly, it may be ineffective or even cause side effects. An estimated 10 to 30 percent of medications aren't effective because they have been given incorrectly. To do it right, you have to give the exact amount of medicine prescribed at the scheduled time, for the specified duration, and in the appropriate manner. Always read the label, follow the directions carefully, and use the appropriate equipment for measuring and administering the medication. Also, be sure to wash your hands before you give any medication to your child.

Brand Name: Vermox

Generic Available: No

Type of Drug: Anthelmintic

Use: Treats pinworm, whipworm, roundworm, hookworm, and capillariasis infections.

Time Required for Drug to Take Effect: A few days to a few weeks, depending on the type of infection being treated.

Dosage Form and Strength: Tablets, chewable (100 mg)

Storage: Store at room temperature in tightly closed containers.

How This Drug Works: Deprives the infecting worms of nutrition, causing them to die.

MEBENDAZOLE

Administration Guidelines

• Give with food to decrease stomach irritation and to increase absorption.

• Can be crushed and mixed with food. May also be chewed or swallowed whole.

• Generally given 1 to 2 times a day.

• The duration of treatment varies with the type of infection. For pinworms, a single dose is sufficient. For whipworms, roundworms, and hookworms, give 2 times a day for 3 consecutive days. For capillariasis, give 2 times a day for 2 to 3 weeks.

• Works best when drug concentrations in the blood are kept constant. Give at evenly spaced intervals around the clock.

• Missed doses: Give immediately. However, if you do not remember until it is time for the next dose, give the missed dose and space the next dose about halfway through the regular interval between doses. Then return to the regular schedule. Do not skip any doses.

• Give this drug for the entire time prescribed by your child's doctor, even if the symptoms disappear before the end of that period. If the drug is stopped too soon, the infection could recur.

• Do not give to children younger than 2 years of age.

Side Effects

Tell your child's doctor about any side effects that are persistent or particularly bothersome.

More Common. Dizziness, fever, headache, rash, itching, hair loss, diarrhea, abdominal pain, nausea, vomiting, ringing in the ears

Less Common. It is especially important to tell the doctor about blood in the urine, persistent fever, or headache.

Possible Drug Interactions

• Anticonvulsants such as carbamazepine and phenytoin can increase the breakdown of this drug in the body, decreasing its effectiveness.

Tell Your Child's Doctor If

• Your child is taking any prescription or nonprescription medications, especially those listed above.

• Your child has or ever had unusual or allergic reactions to any medications, especially to this drug.

• Your child has any liver, kidney, or blood disease.

- Symptoms of infection are getting worse rather than improving.

- Your daughter is or becomes pregnant. This drug's safety in pregnancy has not been established in humans.

- Your daughter is breast-feeding her baby. This drug's safety during breast-feeding has not been established.

Symptoms of Overdose: Severe forms of side effects listed above.

Special Notes
- If your child is not cured within 3 to 4 weeks following treatment, the doctor may repeat the course of treatment.

- Strict hygiene (daily disinfection of toilets and daily laundering of undergarments, bed linens, towels, and night clothing) is essential to prevent reinfection.

Keep a Lid on It

Pharmacists are required to put drugs in bottles that have child-resistant caps. Don't switch to a bottle that's easier for you to open—children may also find it easier to open. Remember, too, that child-resistant does not mean childproof. Children older than five years of age may be able to open most medicine bottles. That's why it's essential for you to teach them that drugs can be harmful if not taken correctly and that they need supervision before taking anything. And, just to be on the safe side, keep all medicines out of your child's reach.

Brand Names: Amen, Curretab, Cycrin, Provera

Generic Available: Yes

Type of Drug: Progesterone

Use: Treats abnormal menstrual bleeding, difficult menstruation, and lack of menstruation.

Time Required for Drug to Take Effect: Menstrual bleeding usually occurs 3 to 7 days after stopping this drug.

Dosage Form and Strength: Tablets (2.5 mg, 5 mg, 10 mg)

Storage: Store at room temperature in tightly closed containers.

How This Drug Works: Mimics the body's natural female hormone that regulates the menstrual cycle.

MEDROXYPROGESTERONE

Administration Guidelines
• Give with food or immediately after a meal to avoid stomach upset.

• Missed doses: Give as soon as you remember. If you give more than 1 dose off schedule, call your child's doctor.

Side Effects
Tell your child's doctor about any side effects that are persistent or particularly bothersome.

More Common. Changes in appetite, changes in weight, fatigue, weakness, dizziness

Less Common. Acne, brown-colored skin spots, increase in body or facial hair, slight loss of scalp hair, fever, breast tenderness, nausea, trouble sleeping. Contact the doctor if your child experiences double vision, loss of vision, discharge from the breasts, depression, rash, yellow eyes or skin, sudden headache, sudden loss of coordination, chest pain, numbness or pain in the leg, slurred speech, shortness of breath, swelling of the feet or ankles, increased sensitivity to sunlight.

Tell Your Child's Doctor If
• Your child has had allergic reactions to any medications.

• Your child has any diseases or is taking any other medications.

• Your daughter is or becomes pregnant.

• Your daughter is breast-feeding her baby. This drug passes into breast milk; however, the American Academy of Pediatrics considers it compatible with breast-feeding in most cases.

Special Instructions
• Make sure your child wears an effective sunscreen and protective clothing when out-of-doors. This drug may cause increased sensitivity to sunlight.

• Make sure medical and laboratory personnel know your child is taking this drug since it may interfere with some laboratory tests.

Symptoms of Overdose: Nausea, vomiting

MEPERIDINE

Administration Guidelines
• Give with food or milk to avoid stomach upset.

• Do not increase the dose or give it more often than your child's doctor prescribed.

• Works best if given at the onset of your child's pain rather than waiting until the pain increases.

• Missed doses: Give as soon as you remember if it is within 2 hours of the missed dose. Otherwise, skip the missed dose and give the next dose at the scheduled time. Do not give double doses.

Side Effects
Tell your child's doctor about any side effects that are persistent or particularly bothersome.

More Common. Constipation, dizziness, drowsiness, dry mouth, flushing, light-headedness, loss of appetite, nausea, or sweating

Less Common. Blurred vision, nightmares or unusual dreams, trouble sleeping. Call the doctor immediately if your child has breathing difficulties, palpitations, tremors, excitation, rash, sore throat and fever, anxiety, severe weakness, or difficult or painful urination.

Possible Drug Interactions
• Other central nervous system depressants such as alcohol, antihistamines, cold preparations, muscle relaxants, tranquilizers, and other pain medicines can cause extreme drowsiness.

Tell Your Child's Doctor If
• Your child has had allergic reactions to this drug or to other narcotic analgesics.

• Your child has any diseases, such as asthma.

• Your child is taking any other medications.

• Your daughter is or becomes pregnant.

• Your daughter is breast-feeding her baby.

Special Instructions
• Increase the amount of fluid and fiber in your child's diet to avoid constipation.

• If you have been giving this drug to your child for several weeks, do not suddenly stop giving it without first talking with the doctor. The doctor may want to decrease the dose gradually to avoid withdrawal side effects.

Brand Name: Demerol

Generic Available: Yes

Type of Drug: Narcotic analgesic

Use: Relieves moderate to severe pain.

Time Required for Drug to Take Effect: 30 to 60 minutes

Dosage Forms and Strengths: Tablets (50 mg, 100 mg); Syrup (50 mg per 5 mL)

Storage: Store at room temperature in tightly closed, light-resistant containers.

How This Drug Works: Acts directly on the central nervous system (brain and spinal cord) to relieve pain.

Symptoms of Overdose: Convulsions (tremors), confusion, severe nervousness or restlessness, severe dizziness, severe drowsiness, slow or difficult breathing, severe weakness, pinpoint pupils of the eyes

Special Notes

• Tolerance (decreased effectiveness) may be seen with long-term use.

• This drug can cause drowsiness. Make sure you know how your child is reacting to this drug before allowing participation in activities that require alertness, such as riding a bicycle.

Measuring Up

Remember: Never use an ordinary tableware teaspoon to measure liquid doses. Instead, use a cylindrical dosing spoon, dosage cup, dropper, or syringe. These measuring devices can be found at your local drug store and sometimes at supermarkets, toy stores, and department stores.

MESALAMINE

Administration Guidelines

• Give with food to avoid stomach irritation.

• Tablets and capsules should be swallowed whole without breaking the outer coating.

• Tablets and capsules are generally given 3 to 4 times a day.

• The rectal suspension is given once at nighttime. Shake the enema well to redistribute the active ingredient. Lay your child on the back or side, and gently insert the enema's nozzle high into the rectum; gently squeeze the container. Ask your child to try and retain it for 8 hours or as long as practical. Enema treatment is usually given for 3 to 6 weeks.

• The rectal suppository is generally administered 2 times a day. Your child should try to retain the suppository for 1 to 3 hours. Treatment with rectal suppositories usually lasts 3 to 6 weeks.

• Do not stop giving this drug without first consulting your child's doctor.

Side Effects

Tell your child's doctor about any side effects that are persistent or particularly bothersome.

More Common. Chills, dizziness, fever, headache, anxiety, dry skin, itching, stomach pain, flatulence, bloody diarrhea, anal irritation, vomiting, constipation, hemorrhoids, altered taste, breathing difficulty

Less Common. It is especially important to tell the doctor about chest pain; bloody, prolonged diarrhea; itching; insomnia; yellow skin; abdominal pain; and breathing difficulty.

Possible Drug Interactions

• Can reduce the absorption of digoxin.

Tell Your Child's Doctor If

• Your child is currently taking any prescription or nonprescription medications, especially those listed above.

• Your child has or ever had unusual or allergic reactions to any medications, including this drug, aspirin, or sulfa drugs.

• Your child has or ever had liver or kidney disease.

• Your child's symptoms are getting worse rather than improving.

• Your daughter is or becomes pregnant. This drug has been shown to be safe during pregnancy in animal and human studies.

Brand Names: Asacol Oral, Pentasa Oral, Rowasa Rectal

Generic Available: No

Type of Drug: Anti-inflammatory agent

Use: Treats inflammation in the intestine, colon, and rectum (ulcerative colitis, proctitis, and procto-sigmoiditis).

Time Required for Drug to Take Effect: It may take 1 to 2 weeks to achieve maximum effect.

Dosage Forms and Strengths: Tablets, enteric-coated (400 mg); Capsules, controlled-release (250 mg); Suppository, rectal (500 mg); Suspension, rectal (4 Gm/60 mL)

Storage: Store tablets, capsules, and rectal enema in light-resistant containers at room temperature in a dry place. After removing the suspension's outer foil wrapper, use within 1 year.

How This Drug Works: Thought to reduce the number of substances that cause inflammation.

- Your daughter is breast-feeding her baby. This drug should be used with caution during breast-feeding. It passes into breast milk and may produce adverse effects such as profuse diarrhea in the nursing infant.

Symptoms of Overdose: Severe forms of side effects listed above.

Special Notes
- May cause urine to turn yellow-brown.

- This drug contains 5-Aminosalicylic acid derivative (aspirin derivative).

Teach Your Children Well

Let's face it. Kids can be pretty stubborn when it comes to accepting medication. When appropriate, try giving your child information about his or her condition and how the medicine works. In a nonthreatening voice, talk about the consequences of not taking the medication, perhaps reminding the child of how uncomfortable he or she was before beginning the medication. Use reasoning when possible, but don't scare the child. Children who understand the importance of antibiotics for infection, insulin for diabetes, or inhalants for asthma are more likely to take the medication without objection.

METAPROTERENOL

Administration Guidelines

- Give tablets or syrup with food to decrease stomach upset.

- Shake the inhalation aerosol well just before each use to distribute the ingredients evenly and equalize the doses.

- If more than 1 inhalation is necessary, wait at least 1 full minute between doses to receive the full therapeutic benefit of the first dose.

- Do not spray the aerosol in or near the eyes.

- Do not use the syrup or solution if it contains particles or if it turns brown or darker than slightly yellow.

- Missed doses: Give if you remember within 1 hour; then follow the regular dosing schedule. However, if you miss the dose by more than 1 hour, skip the missed dose and wait for the next scheduled dose. Do not give double doses.

- If you also are giving an aerosol corticosteroid such as beclomethasone, dexamethasone, or triamcinolone, use this drug first and wait about 5 minutes before using the corticosteroid inhalation. This allows the corticosteroid inhalation to better reach your child's lungs.

Side Effects

Tell your child's doctor about any side effects that are persistent or particularly bothersome.

More Common. It is especially important to tell the doctor about chest pain, difficulty breathing, difficult or painful urination, palpitations, rash, or tremors.

Less Common. Anxiety, dizziness, headache, flushing, irritability, insomnia, loss of appetite, muscle cramps, nausea, nervousness, restlessness, sweating, vomiting, weakness, or dryness or irritation of the mouth or throat (from the inhalation aerosol). These side effects should disappear as your child's body adjusts to this drug.

Possible Drug Interactions

- Beta blockers (acebutolol, atenolol, betaxolol, carteolol, esmolol, labetalol, metoprolol, nadolol, penbutolol, pindolol, propranolol, timolol) decrease the effectiveness of this drug.

- Monoamine oxidase (MAO) inhibitors; tricyclic antidepressants; antihistamines; levothyroxine; and nonprescription cough, cold, allergy, asthma, diet, and sinus medications may increase the side effects of this drug. At least 14 days should separate the use of this drug and an MAO inhibitor.

Brand Name: Alupent, Arm-a-Med Metaproterenol, Dey-Dose, Metaprel, Prometa

Generic Available: No

Type of Drug: Bronchodilator

Use: Relieves wheezing and shortness of breath caused by lung diseases such as asthma and bronchitis.

Time Required for Drug to Take Effect: Oral: within 30 minutes; Inhalation: 1 to 2 minutes

Dosage Forms and Strengths: Aerosol, oral (0.65 mg/dose); Aerosol, micronized powder in inert propellant (0.65 mg/inhalation); Solution for nebulization (4 mg/mL, 6 mg/mL, 50 mg/mL); Syrup (10 mg/5mL); Tablets (10 mg, 20 mg)

Storage: Store tablets and syrup at room temperature in tightly closed, light-resistant containers. Store the inhalation aerosol at room temperature away from excessive heat; the container can explode if heated. Refrigerate the solution for nebulization.

How This Drug Works: Relaxes the smooth muscle on the bronchial tree and the blood vessels located outside the central part of the body.

- May increase the blood-pressure-lowering effects of guanethidine.

- Other bronchodilator drugs (either oral or inhaled) can make side effects more severe when used with this drug. Discuss this with the doctor.

Tell Your Child's Doctor If

- Your child is taking any other medications, especially any of those listed above.

- Your child has had unusual or allergic reactions to any medications, especially to this drug or any related drugs such as albuterol, amphetamines, ephedrine, epinephrine, isoproterenol, norepinephrine, phenylephrine, phenylpropanolamine, pseudoephedrine, or terbutaline.

- Your child has or ever had diabetes, high blood pressure, epilepsy, heart disease, or thyroid disease.

- Your child is taking this drug before having surgery or any other medical or dental treatment.

- Your child does not respond to the usual dose of this drug. It may be a sign of worsening asthma, which may require additional therapy.

- Your daughter is or becomes pregnant. The effects of this drug during pregnancy have not been thoroughly studied in humans.

- Your daughter is breast-feeding her baby. It is not known whether this drug passes into breast milk.

Special Instructions

- Do not allow your child to perform tasks that require alertness, such as riding a bicycle, if this drug causes dizziness.

- If you notice a decrease in the effects produced during continuous use or constantly repeated administration of the inhalant, do not increase the dosage or the frequency of administration. Contact the doctor if your child does not respond to the usual dose of this drug.

- Do not puncture, break, or burn the aerosol container. The contents are under pressure and may explode.

Symptoms of Overdose: Chest pain, heart flutters, tremors, dry mouth, insomnia

Special Notes

- Deaths have been reported from the excessive use of inhalants. Monitor your child's use of the inhaler.

- The dosage requirements for insulin or oral antidiabetic medications may need to be changed when this drug is started.

METHENAMINE

Administration Guidelines
• Give with food; do not give with milk.

• Shake suspension well before measuring each dose.

• Enteric-coated tablets should be swallowed whole. Do not break, crush, or allow your child to chew them.

• Dissolve the oral granules in at least 2 to 4 ounces of water just before giving.

• Missed doses: Give as soon as possible. However, if it's within 4 hours of the next dose, skip the missed dose. Do not give double doses.

Side Effects
Tell your child's doctor about any side effects that are persistent or particularly bothersome.

More Common. Abdominal cramps, diarrhea, headache, loss of appetite, nausea, vomiting

Less Common. Tell the doctor about difficulty in breathing, difficult or painful urination, itching, mouth sores, rapid weight gain (3 to 5 pounds in a week), shortness of breath, skin rash.

Possible Drug Interactions
• Sodium bicarbonate, antacids, and diuretics can decrease the effectiveness of this drug.

• Sulfonamide antibiotics may cause an insoluble precipitate to form in acidic urine, decreasing the effectiveness of this drug.

Tell Your Child's Doctor If
• Your child is allergic to this drug, to the color additive FD&C Yellow No. 5 (tartrazine), or is sensitive to aspirin.

• Your child is taking any other medication.

• Your child has kidney or liver disease.

• Your daughter is or becomes pregnant.

• Your daughter is breast-feeding her baby. This drug can pass into breast milk and cause side effects in the infant.

Special Instructions
• This drug works best when the urine is acidic. Give your child vitamin C or cranberry juice and avoid giving milk products.

Symptoms of Overdose: Severe headache, nausea, vomiting, ringing in the ears

Brand Names: Hiprex, Mandameth, Mandelamine, Methenamine Hippurate (various manufacturers), Methenamine Mandelate (various manufacturers), Urex

Generic Available: Yes

Type of Drug: Antibiotic

Use: Prevents bacterial infections of the urinary tract.

Time Required for Drug to Take Effect: 2 to 3 days

Dosage Forms and Strengths: Tablets (500 mg, 1 g); Tablets, enteric-coated (500 mg, 1 g); Suspension (250 and 500 mg per 5 mL); Granules (1-g packets)

Storage: Store at room temperature in tightly closed containers.

How This Drug Works: Destroys susceptible bacteria.

Brand Names: Methylphenidate Hydrochloride (various manufacturers), Ritalin, Ritalin-SR

Generic Available: Yes

Type of Drug: Adrenergic, psychotherapeutic agent

Use: Treats hyperkinetic syndrome and Attention Deficit Hyperactivity Disorder (ADHD).

Time Required for Drug to Take Effect: Immediate-release tablets: Within 2 hours; Sustained-release tablets: 4 to 7 hours. Full benefit may take 4 to 6 weeks.

Dosage Forms and Strengths: Tablets (5 mg, 10 mg, 20 mg); Tablets, sustained-release (20 mg)

Storage: Store at room temperature in tightly closed, light-resistant containers.

How This Drug Works: The way this drug works in abnormal behavioral syndrome in children is not clearly understood.

METHYLPHENIDATE

Administration Guidelines

- Give with food, milk, or a full glass of water.

- Give the first dose soon after your child awakens.

- Give the last dose of the regular tablets 4 to 6 hours before bedtime.

- Give the sustained-release tablets at least 8 hours before bedtime.

- Sustained-release tablets should be swallowed whole; do not crush, break, or allow your child to chew them.

- Missed doses: Skip the missed dose and give the next dose at its scheduled time. Do not give double doses.

Side Effects

Tell your child's doctor about any side effects that are persistent or particularly bothersome.

More Common. Abdominal pain, dizziness, drowsiness, dry mouth, headache, insomnia, loss of appetite, nausea, nervousness, vomiting, weakness

Less Common. Tell the doctor if your child experiences chest pain, fever, rash, hallucinations, hives, joint pain, mood changes, palpitations, seizures, or bleeding or bruising.

Possible Drug Interactions

- Decreases the blood-pressure-lowering effects of antihypertensive medications.

- Increases the side effects of blood thinners; tricyclic antidepressants such as amitriptyline, desipramine, imipramine, and nortriptyline; and anticonvulsants such as phenytoin, phenobarbital, and primidone.

Tell Your Child's Doctor If

- Your child is allergic to this drug.

- Your child has ever had epilepsy, high blood pressure, Tourette syndrome, anxiety, agitation, depression, or tension.

- Your daughter is or becomes pregnant.

Special Instructions

- Make sure your child uses caution while participating in physical activity.

- Limit your child's caffeine intake. Caffeine is found in colas, coffee, tea, and chocolate.

Symptoms of Overdose: Severe nausea, chest pain, vomiting, headache

Special Notes
• This drug is related to amphetamines and may be habit-forming when taken for long periods of time. Both physical and psychological dependence can occur.

• May slow growth in children. The doctor may recommend drug-free periods during school holidays and summer vacations. Growth spurts often occur during these drug-free periods.

Keep It Out of Reach

Do not rely on a child-resistant cap to deter your child from opening a bottle of medication. Child-resistant does not mean childproof. Legally, a cap can be called child-resistant if 80 percent of all five-year-olds need more than five minutes to open it. That means the other 20 percent could get into it in even less time. Put the bottle in a hard-to-reach cabinet with a childproof lock. Do not keep it on the countertop, kitchen table, or nightstand.

Brand Name: Medrol

Generic Available: Yes

Type of Drug: Adreno-corticosteroid hormone

Use: Treats a variety of disorders, including endocrine and rheumatic disorders; asthma; blood diseases; certain cancers; eye disorders; gastrointestinal disturbances such as ulcerative colitis; respiratory diseases; and inflammatory diseases such as arthritis, dermatitis, and poison ivy.

Time Required for Drug to Take Effect: Varies based on the illness being treated. It may be several days before an effect is achieved.

Dosage Form and Strengths: Tablets (2 mg, 4 mg, 8 mg, 16 mg, 24 mg, 32 mg)

Storage: Store at room temperature in tightly closed containers.

How This Drug Works: Not completely understood. This drug is similar to the cortisonelike chemicals naturally produced by the adrenal gland. These chemicals are involved in various regulatory processes in the body such as fluid balance, temperature, and reaction to inflammation.

METHYLPREDNISOLONE (SYSTEMIC)

Administration Guidelines
• Give with food or milk to prevent stomach irritation.

• If your child is taking only 1 dose of this drug a day, try to give it before 9:00 A.M. This will mimic the body's normal production of this chemical.

• Missed doses: It is important not to miss a dose of this drug. Follow these guidelines if you do miss giving a dose:

   1. If given more than once a day, give the missed dose as soon as possible, and return to the regular schedule. If it is already time for the next dose, double the dose given.

   2. If given once a day, give the missed dose as soon as possible. If you do not remember until the next day, do not give the missed dose at all, just follow the regular dosing schedule. Do not double the next dose.

   3. If given every other day, give the missed dose as soon as you remember. If you miss the scheduled time by a whole day, give it when you remember, then skip a day before you give the next dose. Do not double the next dose. If you miss more than one dose, contact your child's doctor.

Side Effects
Tell your child's doctor about any side effects that are persistent or particularly bothersome.

More Common. Dizziness, false sense of well-being, fatigue, increased appetite, increased sweating, indigestion, leg cramps, menstrual irregularities, muscle weakness, nausea, swelling of the skin on the face, restlessness, sleep disorders, or weight gain

Less Common. Tell the doctor if your child experiences abdominal enlargement or pain; acne; back or rib pain; bloody or black, tarry stools; blurred vision; convulsions; eye pain; fever and sore throat; headaches; slow healing of wounds; increased thirst and urination; depression; mood changes; muscle wasting; nightmares; peptic ulcers; rapid weight gain (3 to 5 pounds in a week); rash; shortness of breath; unusual bleeding or bruising; or unusual weakness.

Possible Drug Interactions
• Aspirin and anti-inflammatory medications such as ibuprofen, indomethacin, and ketoprofen may increase stomach problems.

• Cholestyramine and colestipol can prevent the absorption of this drug.

Tell Your Child's Doctor If

• Your child has had allergic reactions to this drug or other adrenocorticosteroids such as betamethasone, cortisone, dexamethasone, fluocinolone, hydrocortisone, prednisolone, prednisone, and triamcinolone.

• Your child is taking any other medications.

• Your child has recently been exposed to or currently has chicken pox or measles.

• Your child has any medical problems, especially diabetes; glaucoma; fungal infections; heart disease; high blood pressure; peptic ulcers; thyroid, kidney, or liver disease; tuberculosis; or ulcerative colitis.

• Your daughter is or becomes pregnant. This drug can have adverse effects on the fetus.

• Your daughter is breast-feeding her baby.

Special Instructions

• With long-term use, the doctor may need to increase your child's dose during times of stress such as serious infection, injury, or surgery.

• Do not have your child vaccinated or immunized while giving this drug. This drug decreases the effectiveness of vaccines and can lead to infection if a live virus vaccine is given.

• Do not suddenly stop giving this drug before speaking with the doctor.

Symptoms of Overdose: Severe restlessness

Special Notes

• If your child is taking this drug for a long time, the doctor may want your child to be on a low-salt and potassium-rich diet. The doctor may also want your child's eyes examined periodically during treatment to detect glaucoma and cataracts.

Brand Names:
Metoclopramide, Maxolon, Octamide, Reglan, Clopra

Generic Available: Yes

Type of Drug: Antiemetic

Use: Relieves symptoms of gastric reflux; prevents nausea and vomiting.

Time Required for Drug to Take Effect: 30 to 60 minutes

Dosage Forms and Strengths: Tablets (5 mg, 10 mg); Solution (10 mg/mL); Syrup (5 mg per 5 mL)

Storage: Store at room temperature in tightly closed containers.

How This Drug Works: Acts directly on the vomiting center in the brain to prevent nausea and vomiting. It also accelerates gastric emptying and intestinal transit time.

METOCLOPRAMIDE

Administration Guidelines

• Give 30 minutes before each meal.

• Missed doses: Give as soon as possible. However, if it's within 4 to 6 hours of the next dose, skip the missed dose. Do not give double doses.

Side Effects

Tell your child's doctor about any side effects that are persistent or particularly bothersome.

MORE COMMON. Diarrhea, dizziness, drowsiness, dry mouth, fatigue, headache, insomnia, nausea, restlessness, weakness

LESS COMMON. Tell the doctor if your child experiences anxiety; confusion; depression; disorientation; involuntary movements of the eyes, face, or limbs; muscle spasms; rash; or trembling of the hands.

Possible Drug Interactions

• Can cause extreme drowsiness when used with other central nervous system depressants such as alcohol, antihistamines, barbiturates, muscle relaxants, narcotics, pain medications, and sleeping medications or with tricyclic antidepressants.

• Narcotic analgesics may block the effectiveness of this drug.

• Decreases the effectiveness of cimetidine and digoxin.

• Increases the absorption of acetaminophen, tetracycline, and alcohol.

• May alter the insulin requirements for children with diabetes.

Tell Your Child's Doctor If

• Your child is taking any other medication.

• Your child is allergic to this drug, procaine, or procainamide.

• Your child has ever had epilepsy, kidney or liver disease; intestinal bleeding or blockage; or pheochromocytoma.

• Your daughter is or becomes pregnant.

• Your daughter is breast-feeding her baby. This drug can pass into breast milk and cause side effects in the infant.

Special Instructions

• Make sure you know how your child is reacting to this drug before allowing participation in activities that require alertness, such as riding a bicycle.

Symptoms of Overdose: Drowsiness, disorientation, extrapyramidal reactions (see below), irritability, and agitation

Special Notes
• Extrapyramidal reactions may occur in children and young adults, usually within 24 to 48 hours of starting therapy. Be sure to contact the doctor immediately if your child exhibits any of these symptoms: involuntary movements of the limbs; facial grimacing; rhythmic protrusion of the tongue; unusual speech; tremor; or any unusual movement of the tongue, face, mouth or jaw, trunk, or extremities.

Just Call

If you have any concerns about any side effects, even minor ones, you should be sure to discuss them with your child's doctor. The doctor may be able to minimize or eliminate the side effects by prescribing a different medication or changing your child's dosage, dosing schedule, or the way the drug is given. (Do not make adjustments on your own without discussing them with your doctor.) At the very least, the doctor can assure you that the medication's benefits far outweigh its side effects.

Brand Names: Zaroxolyn, Mykrox, Diulo

Generic Available: No

Type of Drug: Diuretic

Use: Treats edema due to congestive heart failure, liver disease, and nephrotic syndrome. Also treats hypertension.

Time Required for Drug to Take Effect: Several days to several weeks

Dosage Form and Strengths: Tablets (0.5 mg, 2.5 mg, 5 mg, 10 mg)

Storage: Store at room temperature in tightly closed, light-resistant containers.

How This Drug Works: Increases the elimination of salt and water through the kidneys.

METOLAZONE

Administration Guidelines

- Usually given 1 or 2 times a day. Try to give it at the same time(s) each day.

- Give with food or milk.

- Do not give doses late in the evening or your child may have to get up at night to urinate.

- Missed doses: Give as soon as possible. However, if it's less than 6 hours (if given 2 times a day) or less than 12 hours (if given 1 time a day) of the next dose, skip the missed dose. Do not give double doses.

Side Effects

Tell your child's doctor about any side effects that are persistent or particularly bothersome.

More Common. Constipation, diarrhea, upset stomach, increased sensitivity to sunlight, headache. Contact the doctor if your child experiences muscle cramps.

Less Common. Dizziness, fatigue. Contact the doctor if your child experiences blurred vision, confusion, difficulty breathing, dry mouth or excessive thirst, excessive weakness, fever, itching, joint pain, palpitations, tingling fingers or toes, yellowing of the eyes or skin, or unusual bleeding or bruising.

Possible Drug Interactions

- Can decrease the effectiveness of oral anticoagulants, insulin, oral antidiabetic medications, and methenamine.

- Nonsteroidal anti-inflammatory medications such as ibuprofen can decrease the effectiveness of this drug.

- Can increase the side effects of calcium supplements, digoxin, and lithium.

- Some diuretics (such as furosemide) may increase the effects of this drug.

Tell Your Child's Doctor If

- Your child is taking any other medications.

- Your child has had allergic reactions to any medications, especially to sulfa drugs.

- Your child has any other diseases, particularly kidney, liver, or pancreatic disease; diabetes mellitus; asthma; or lupus.

- Your daughter is or becomes pregnant. High blood pressure should be controlled by a physician during pregnancy.

• Your daughter is breast-feeding her baby. This drug can pass into breast milk, and it is not known if side effects can occur in the infant.

Special Instructions
• Make sure the pharmacist always dispenses the same brand of this drug. Some brands are not interchangeable.

Symptoms of Overdose: Excessive urination, dehydration, lethargy, and severe dizziness or fainting

Special Notes
• This drug can increase potassium loss, leading to muscle cramps and weakness. The doctor will do blood tests to check the levels of electrolytes, including potassium, in your child's blood.

• Blood glucose levels may be increased in children with diabetes.

Be Accurate

If you don't give medication correctly, it may be ineffective or even cause side effects. An estimated 10 to 30 percent of medications aren't effective because they have been given incorrectly. To do it right, you have to give the exact amount of medicine prescribed at the scheduled time, for the specified duration, and in the appropriate manner. Always read the label, follow the directions carefully, and use the appropriate equipment for measuring and administering the medication. Also, be sure to wash your hands before you give any medication to your child.

Brand Names: Lopressor, Toprol XL

Generic Available: No

Type of Drug: Beta-adrenergic blocking agent

Use: Treats high blood pressure and chest pain. Has also been used to treat abnormally fast heart rhythms, tremors, and some emotional disturbances. May be given after heart attacks to prevent further heart attacks. Also may be used to prevent migraine headaches.

Time Required for Drug to Take Effect: Several days to several weeks

Storage: Store at room temperature in tightly closed, light-resistant containers.

Dosage Forms and Strengths: Tablets (50 mg, 100 mg); Tablets, extended-release (50 mg, 100 mg, 200 mg); Injection (1 mg/mL)

How This Drug Works: Blocks nerve receptors in the heart and controls nerve impulses that excite the heart, causing it to beat more slowly.

METOPROLOL

Administration Guidelines

- Usually given 1 or 2 times a day. Extended-release tablets are given once a day. Give the dose at approximately the same time(s) each day.

- May be given on an empty stomach or with meals, but be consistent.

- Do not stop giving this drug without first speaking with your child's doctor. Stopping this drug abruptly may cause high blood pressure.

- Missed doses: Give as soon as possible. However, if it's within 8 hours of the next dose, skip the missed dose. Do not give double doses.

Side Effects

Tell your child's doctor about any side effects that are persistent or particularly bothersome.

More Common. Cold hands or feet, constipation or diarrhea, upset stomach, difficulty sleeping, fatigue, weakness. Some side effects may improve with time as your child gets used to this drug. Contact the doctor if your child experiences nightmares or difficulty breathing.

Less Common. Allergic reactions, dry eyes and mouth. Contact the doctor if your child experiences swelling of the feet or legs, hallucinations, confusion, unusual bleeding or bruising, or tingling of the fingers or toes.

Possible Drug Interactions

- Decongestants in cough, cold, allergy, asthma, weight control, and sinus medications can increase blood pressure when taken with this drug.

- Alcohol, barbiturate sedatives, nonsteroidal anti-inflammatory drugs, and rifampin can decrease the effectiveness of this drug.

- Can offset the therapeutic effect of asthma medications such as theophylline, albuterol, terbutaline, and metaproterenol.

- Oral contraceptives, haloperidol, cimetidine, hydralazine, and monoamine oxidase (MAO) inhibitors can increase the effects of this drug.

Tell Your Child's Doctor If

- Your child has had allergic reactions to any medications.

- Your child is taking any other medications.

- Your child has allergies; asthma; wheezing; slow heartbeat; diabetes mellitus; heart or blood vessel disease; liver, thyroid, or kidney disease; or any other diseases.

- Your daughter is or becomes pregnant. High blood pressure should be controlled by a physician during pregnancy.

- Your daughter is breast-feeding her baby. This drug can pass into breast milk; however, the American Academy of pediatrics considers it compatible with breast-feeding in most cases.

Symptoms of Overdose: Excessively slow heartbeat and low blood pressure, difficulty breathing, unconsciousness

Special Notes
- May cause fewer side effects in children with respiratory illnesses and diabetes than other beta blockers.

- Can affect blood sugar levels in children with diabetes and mask the signs and symptoms of low blood sugar.

Keep a Lid on It

Pharmacists are required to put drugs in bottles that have child-resistant caps. Don't switch to a bottle that's easier for you to open—children may also find it easier to open. Remember, too, that child-resistant does not mean childproof. Children older than five years of age may be able to open most medicine bottles. That's why it's essential for you to teach them that drugs can be harmful if not taken correctly and that children need supervision before taking anything. And, just to be on the safe side, keep all medicines out of your child's reach.

Brand Names: Flagyl, Protostat, MetroGel

Generic Available: Yes

Type of Drug: Antibiotic, antiparasitic

Use: Treats a wide variety of infections, including those of the vagina, urinary tract, lower respiratory tract, bones, joints, intestinal tract, and skin. Also used topically to treat acne rosacea.

Time Required for Drug to Take Effect: It may take a few days to affect the infection.

Dosage Forms and Strengths: Tablets (250 mg, 500 mg); Gel (0.75%)

Storage: Store at room temperature in a tightly closed, light-resistant container. Do not freeze the gel.

How This Drug Works: Kills bacteria or parasites.

METRONIDAZOLE

Administration Guidelines

- Give with food or a full glass of water or milk to avoid stomach irritation, unless your child's doctor directs you to do otherwise.

- Generally given 3 times a day.

- Works best when drug concentrations are kept constant. Give doses at evenly spaced intervals around the clock. If you are to give 3 doses a day, space them approximately 8 hours apart.

- Missed doses: Give immediately. However, if you don't remember the missed dose until it is time for the next dose, give the missed dose and space the next dose about halfway through the regular interval between doses; then return to the regular dosing schedule. Do not give double doses, and do not skip any doses.

- Shake the suspension well just before measuring each dose to distribute the ingredients evenly and equalize the doses.

- Give this drug for the entire time prescribed by the doctor (usually 7 to 14 days), even if symptoms disappear. If the drug is stopped too soon, resistant bacteria and parasites may continue to grow, and the infection could recur.

Side Effects

Tell your child's doctor about any side effects that are persistent or particularly bothersome.

More Common. Abdominal cramps, constipation, diarrhea, dizziness, dry mouth, headache, insomnia, irritability, loss of appetite, metallic taste in the mouth, nasal congestion, nausea, restlessness, or vomiting. These side effects should disappear as your child's body adjusts to this drug.

Less Common. It is especially important to tell the doctor if your child experiences confusion, convulsions, flushing, hives, itching, joint pain, loss of bladder control, mouth sores, numbness or tingling in the fingers or toes, rash, a sense of pressure inside the abdomen, unexplained sore throat and fever, or unusual weakness.

Possible Drug Interactions

- Concurrent use of alcohol and this drug can lead to a severe reaction including abdominal cramps, nausea, vomiting, headache, and flushing, the severity of which is dependent upon the amount of alcohol ingested.

- Disulfiram can lead to confusion when used with this drug.

- May increase the effects of oral anticoagulants (blood thinners such as warfarin), which can lead to bleeding complications.

- May increase the risk of lithium toxicity.

- Barbiturates can decrease the effectiveness of this drug.

- Cimetidine can increase the chance of side effects from this drug.

Tell Your Child's Doctor If

- Your child is currently taking any prescription or nonprescription medications, especially any of those listed above.

- Your child has had unusual or allergic reactions to any medications.

- Your child has or ever had blood disorders, a central nervous system (brain or spinal cord) disease, or liver disease.

- Your child is taking this drug before having surgery or any other medical or dental treatment.

- Your child's symptoms seem to be getting worse rather than improving.

- Your daughter is or becomes pregnant.

- Your daughter is breast-feeding her baby. This drug passes into breast milk.

Special Instructions

- When used to treat a vaginal infection, sexual partners should receive concurrent therapy in order to prevent reinfection. In addition, sexual intercourse should be avoided or condoms should be used until treatment is completed.

- Your child should avoid alcohol for at least 48 hours after discontinuing this drug.

- This drug may cause the urine to darken or turn reddish-brown.

Outdated Doses

Safe and proper medication disposal is essential, especially when you have children in the house. Do not keep medication—whether prescription or nonprescription—past the expiration date, even if it appears normal. Expired medication may be ineffective and can even be dangerous. Make a habit of regularly checking the expiration date on all medicines in your home. Flush leftover medication down the toilet or pour it down the sink. Rinse the container before throwing it out. If your medication does not display an expiration date, throw it out after one year.

Brand Name: Phillips Milk of Magnesia

Generic Available: Yes

Type of Drug: Laxative, saline hyperosmotic, antacid

Use: Treats occasional constipation, heartburn, and acid ingestion; cleans out the large bowel prior to surgery or medical tests. Also used for magnesium replacement.

Time Required for Drug to Take Effect: Within minutes for heartburn relief; 30 minutes to 6 hours to produce a bowel movement. Larger doses given on an empty stomach produce a bowel movement more rapidly.

Dosage Forms and Strengths: Liquid (400 mg/ 5 mL, 800 mg/5 mL); Tablets, chewable (311 mg)

Storage: Store at room temperature in tightly closed containers. Do not freeze the liquid.

How This Drug Works: Draws water into the small intestine, producing distention and increased movement of stool through the intestine. Neutralizes the acid in the stomach.

MILK OF MAGNESIA (MOM)

Administration Guidelines

• Shake well before measuring each dose.

• Liquid may be mixed in water or juice.

• Chewable tablets must be chewed completely.

• Give each dose with a large amount (4 to 8 ounces) of water or juice.

• Increase your child's intake of water or other fluids.

• Do not give within 2 hours of other medications.

• Do not give late in the day unless given with food at bedtime.

• Do not give to children younger than 6 years of age unless prescribed by your child's doctor.

• Do not give regularly for more than 1 week unless prescribed by the doctor.

Side Effects

Tell your child's doctor about any side effects that are persistent or particularly bothersome.

More Common. Cramping, diarrhea, gas, or increased thirst

Less Common. Whitish speckling or color of stools. Contact the doctor if your child experiences confusion, dizziness, lightheadedness, irregular heartbeat, muscle cramps, unusual fatigue, or weakness.

Possible Drug Interactions

• Decreases tetracycline absorption. Do not give the medications within 2 hours of each other.

• Decreases the absorption of warfarin, digoxin, and etidronate.

• Decreases the absorption of ciprofloxacin, norfloxacin, or ofloxacin. If possible, stop giving this drug while giving these medications. Otherwise, do not give these medications within less than 2 hours of each other.

Tell Your Child's Doctor If

• Your child has had an allergic reaction to this drug or to any other medication.

• Your child has taken or is taking any other prescription or nonprescription medicine.

• Your child has kidney or liver disease, swelling of the legs or feet, intestinal blockage, other intestinal problems, diabetes mellitus, high blood pressure, rectal bleeding, or any other medical condition.

- Your child has a sudden change in bowel movements that lasts longer than 2 weeks or returns intermittently.

- Your daughter is or becomes pregnant.

- Your daughter is breast-feeding her baby. The American Academy of Pediatrics considers this drug compatible with breast-feeding in most cases.

Special Instructions
- Do not use this drug if your child has abdominal pain, appendicitis, intestinal blockage, nausea, vomiting, or rectal bleeding.

Symptoms of Overdose: Diarrhea, low blood pressure, trouble breathing, lethargy, weakness, feeling hot, flushing, central nervous system depression, seizures, or cessation of heartbeat

Over-the-Counter Wisdom

Keep in mind that even a medication that is available without a doctor's prescription may still be harmful and should be given appropriately and only when necessary. Talk to your pediatrician about what to do if your child gets sick. Some illnesses can be treated at home, some require a call to the pediatrician's office, and some will require a visit to the doctor. In addition, ask the doctor what situations constitute an emergency. If you're not sure if it's safe or appropriate to give your child a particular over-the-counter medication, be sure to talk to the doctor first.

Brand Names: Dynacin, Minocin

Generic Available: No

Type of Drug: Antibiotic

Use: Treats a wide range of bacterial infections, and prevents meningococcal meningitis. Also used to treat acne.

Time Required for Drug to take Effect: It may take a few days to affect the infection.

Dosage Forms and Strengths: Capsules (50 mg, 100 mg); Tablets (50 mg, 100 mg); Suspension (50 mg per 5 mL, with 5% alcohol)

Storage: Store at room temperature in tightly closed, light-resistant containers. Do not refrigerate.

How This Drug Works: Kills susceptible bacteria, but it is not effective against viruses or fungi.

MINOCYCLINE
Administration Guidelines
• Give with food to avoid stomach upset unless your child's doctor directs you to do otherwise.

• Give with a full glass of water.

• Generally administered 2 times a day.

• Works best when drug concentrations in the blood are kept constant. Give doses at evenly spaced intervals around the clock. For example, if you are to give 2 doses a day, the doses should be spaced 12 hours apart.

• Missed doses: Give immediately. However, if you do not remember until it is time for the next dose, give the missed dose and space the following dose about halfway through the regular interval between doses; then return to the regular dosing schedule. Try not to skip any doses.

• Shake suspension well just before measuring each dose to distribute ingredients and equalize doses. The contents tend to settle on the bottom of the bottle.

• Give this drug for the entire time prescribed by the doctor, even if symptoms disappear. If you stop giving the drug too soon, resistant bacteria are given a chance to continue growing, and the infection could recur.

• Do not give to infants or children younger than 8 years of age. This drug can cause permanent discoloration of the teeth and can inhibit tooth and bone growth if used during their development.

Side Effects
Tell your child's doctor about any side effects that are persistent or particularly bothersome.

More Common. Diarrhea, dizziness, headache, light-headedness, loss of appetite, nausea, stomach cramps and stomach upset, vomiting, or discoloration of the nails. These side effects should disappear as the body adjusts to this drug.

Less Common. It is especially important to tell the doctor if your child experiences darkened tongue, difficulty in breathing, joint pain, mouth irritation, rash, rectal or vaginal itching, sore throat and fever, unusual bleeding or bruising, or yellowing of the eyes or skin.

Possible Drug Interactions
• Increases the absorption of digoxin, which may lead to digoxin toxicity.

- Can increase the gastrointestinal side effects (nausea, vomiting, and stomach upset) of theophylline.

- Antacids, calcium channel blockers, and iron may decrease the effects of this drug if they are taken at the same time. Doses of these medications and this drug should be separated by 2 to 3 hours.

- Decreases the intestinal bacteria that produce vitamin K, which is important for blood thinning. Therefore, the dosage of oral anticoagulants (blood thinners, such as warfarin) may need to be adjusted when this drug is started.

- May decrease the effectiveness of birth control pills. Your child should use a different or additional form of birth control while taking this drug.

Tell Your Child's Doctor If

- Your child is currently taking any prescription or nonprescription medications.

- Your child has had unusual or allergic reactions to any medications, especially to this drug or to oxytetracycline, doxycycline, or tetracycline.

- Your child has or ever had kidney or liver disease.

- Your child's symptoms of infection seem to be getting worse rather than improving.

- Your daughter is or becomes pregnant.

- Your daughter is breast-feeding her baby. This drug can pass into breast milk and cause side effects in the infant.

- Your child has syphilis. This drug can affect tests for the disease.

Special Instructions

- Your child should avoid prolonged exposure to direct sunlight. When out-of-doors, have your child wear protective clothing, an effective sunscreen, and sunglasses as this drug can increase the body's sensitivity to sunlight.

- Make sure your child is cautious when performing tasks that require alertness, such as riding a bicycle. This drug can cause dizziness or light-headedness.

Brand Names: MS Contin, MSIR, Oramorph SR, RMS, Roxanol, Roxanol SR

Generic Available: Yes

Type of Drug: Narcotic analgesic

Use: Relieves moderate to severe pain.

Time Required for Drug to Take Effect: 30 to 60 minutes

Dosage Forms and Strengths: Capsules (15 mg, 30 mg); Tablets (15 mg, 30 mg); Tablets, sustained-release (15 mg, 30 mg, 60 mg, 100 mg); Solution (10 mg and 20 mg per 5 mL with 10% alcohol, 20 mg per mL, 100 mg per 5 mL); Rectal suppositories (5 mg, 10 mg, 20 mg, 30 mg)

Storage: Store tablets and solution at room temperature in tightly closed, light-resistant containers. Keep rectal suppositories in the refrigerator.

How This Drug Works: Acts directly on the central nervous system (brain and spinal cord) to relieve pain.

MORPHINE

Administration Guidelines

• Give with food or milk to avoid stomach upset.

• Works best if given at the onset of your child's pain rather than waiting until the pain increases.

• The solution may be mixed with fruit juice after measuring to improve the taste.

• Your child should not crush or chew the sustained-release tablets.

• Do not increase the dose or give it more often than your child's doctor prescribed.

• Missed doses: Give as soon as you remember if it is within 2 hours of the missed dose. Otherwise, skip the missed dose and give the next dose at the scheduled time. Do not give double doses.

Side Effects

Tell your child's doctor about any side effects that are persistent or particularly bothersome.

More Common. Constipation, dizziness, drowsiness, dry mouth, flushing, light-headedness, loss of appetite, nausea, or sweating

Less Common. Blurred vision, nightmares or unusual dreams, trouble sleeping. Call the doctor immediately if your child experiences breathing difficulties, palpitations, tremors, excitation, rash, sore throat and fever, anxiety, severe weakness, or difficult or painful urination.

Possible Drug Interactions

• Other central nervous system depressants such as alcohol, antihistamines, cold preparations, muscle relaxants, tranquilizers, and other pain medicines can cause extreme drowsiness.

Tell Your Child's Doctor If

• Your child has had allergic reactions to this drug or other narcotic analgesics.

• Your child has any diseases such as asthma.

• Your child is taking any other medications.

• Your daughter is or becomes pregnant.

• Your daughter is breast-feeding her baby. This drug can pass into breast milk; however, the American Academy of Pediatrics considers it compatible with breast-feeding in most cases.

Special Instructions

• Increase the fluid and fiber in your child's diet to avoid constipation.

• If you have been giving this drug for several weeks, do not suddenly stop giving it without first talking with the doctor. The doctor may want to decrease the dose gradually to avoid withdrawal side effects.

Symptoms of Overdose: Convulsions (tremors), confusion, severe nervousness or restlessness, severe dizziness, severe drowsiness, slow or difficult breathing, severe weakness, pinpoint pupils of the eyes

Special Notes

• Tolerance (decreased effectiveness) may be seen with long-term use of this drug.

• This drug can cause drowsiness. Make sure you know how your child is reacting to this drug before allowing participation in activities that require alertness, such as riding a bicycle.

Measuring Up

Remember: Never use an ordinary tableware teaspoon to measure liquid doses. Instead, use a cylindrical dosing spoon, dosage cup, dropper, or syringe. These measuring devices can be found at your local drug store and sometimes at supermarkets, toy stores, and department stores.

Brand Names: Aleve, Anaprox, Naprosyn, Anaprox DS, E-C Naprosyn

Generic Available: No

Type of Drug: Nonsteroidal anti-inflammatory analgesic

Use: Relieves mild to moderate pain and inflammation (swelling and stiffness) of arthritis.

Time Required for Drug to Take Effect: 1 to 2 hours for pain relief. Begins to relieve inflammation of arthritis in 1 to 2 weeks, with full effect in 4 weeks.

Dosage Forms and Strengths: Tablets (200 mg, 250 mg, 375 mg, 500 mg); Tablets, enteric-coated (375 mg, 500 mg) Suspension (125 mg per 5 mL)

Storage: Store at room temperature in tightly closed, light-resistant containers.

How This Drug Works: Decreases the production of the chemical prostaglandin.

NAPROXEN

Administration Guidelines

• Give with a full glass of water.

• Give with food or immediately after meals to avoid stomach upset.

• Shake the suspension well before measuring each dose.

• Give this drug on a regular basis if your child has arthritis.

• Missed doses: Give as soon as you remember if it is within 2 hours of the missed dose. Otherwise, skip the missed dose and give the next dose at the scheduled time. Do not give double doses.

• Do not give to children younger than 2 years of age without first consulting the doctor.

Side Effects

Tell your child's doctor about any side effects that are persistent or particularly bothersome.

More Common. Heartburn, nausea, vomiting, stomach pain, dizziness, drowsiness, light-headedness, indigestion

Less Common. Bitter taste, constipation, decreased appetite, flushing. Contact the doctor if your child experiences bloody or black, tarry stools; changes in vision; spitting up or vomiting of blood, severe stomach upset; skin rash, hives; trouble breathing; wheezing; ringing in the ears; or difficult or painful urination.

Possible Drug Interactions

• Other anti-inflammatory medications and aspirin can increase stomach upset when given with this drug.

• May decrease the effect of diuretics.

• Blood thinners may increase bleeding complications when used with this drug.

Tell Your Child's Doctor If

• Your child has had allergic reactions to any medications, especially other nonsteroidal anti-inflammatory drugs or aspirin.

• Your child has any diseases, especially asthma, stomach problems, or liver or kidney disease.

• Your daughter is or becomes pregnant.

• Your daughter is breast-feeding her baby. This drug can pass into breast milk; however, the American Academy of Pediatrics considers it compatible with breast-feeding in most cases.

Special Instructions

• Before your child has any medical or dental surgery, tell the doctor performing the procedure that your child is taking this drug.

• Make sure you know how your child is reacting to this drug before allowing participation in activities that require alertness, such as riding a bicycle.

Symptoms of Overdose: Fainting, fast or irregular breathing, confusion, ringing in the ears, convulsions, sweating, blurred vision

Special Notes

• Available over the counter.

Keep It Out of Reach

Do not rely on a child-resistant cap to deter your child from opening a bottle of medication. Child-resistant does not mean childproof. Legally, a cap can be called child-resistant if 80 percent of all five-year-olds need more than five minutes to open it. That means the other 20 percent could get into it in even less time. Put the bottle in a hard-to-reach cabinet with a childproof lock. Do not keep it on the countertop, kitchen table, or nightstand.

Brand Name: Tilade

Generic Available: No

Type of Drug: Anti-inflammatory

Use: Maintenance therapy in the management of patients with mild to moderate bronchial asthma.

Time Required for Drug to Take Effect: After being added to a bronchodilator regimen, a beneficial effect should be detected within 2 weeks.

Dosage Form and Strength: Aerosol (1.75 mg/activation)

Storage: Store away from excessive heat; the contents are pressurized and can explode if heated. Do not freeze.

How This Drug Works: The principal effect following oral inhalation of nedocromil is bronchodilation resulting from relaxation of smooth muscles of the bronchial tree (breathing pipes).

NEDOCROMIL SODIUM

Administration Guidelines

• Give exactly as prescribed by your child's doctor.

• Shake the container just before each use to distribute the ingredients evenly and equalize the doses.

• Wait at least 1 full minute between inhalations to receive the full benefit of the first dose.

• Missed doses: Give immediately if you remember within 1 hour; then follow your regular dosing schedule for the next dose. If you miss the dose by more than 1 hour, wait until the next scheduled dose. Do not give double doses.

• This drug must be used regularly, even during symptom-free periods, to be beneficial.

Side Effects

Tell your child's doctor about any side effects that are persistent or particularly bothersome.

More Common. Headache, nausea, cough, unpleasant taste upon inhalation

Less Common. Chest pain, fatigue, dizziness, rash, nausea, vomiting, diarrhea, abdominal pain, dry mouth, tremor, cough, inflammation of the throat, inflammation of the mucous membrane of the nose, bronchitis, upper respiratory infection, bronchospasm, increased sputum production

Tell Your Child's Doctor If

• Your child has had unusual or allergic reactions to any drugs.

• Your daughter is pregnant or is breast-feeding her baby. Extensive safety studies in humans have not been conducted. It is not known whether this drug passes into breast milk.

Special Notes

• This is not the drug of choice for rapid onset episodes of bronchospasm.

NEOMYCIN (TOPICAL)

Administration Guidelines
• Use externally only.

• Cleanse affected area before applying unless directed otherwise.

• Cover with sterile bandage if needed.

Side Effects
Tell your child's doctor about any side effects that are persistent or particularly bothersome.

More Common. Side effects are not common with topical use.

Less Common. Inflammation of the skin, flushing of the skin, rash, urticaria (allergic reaction in which red, round wheals develop on the skin)

Tell Your Child's Doctor If
• Your child's condition worsens.

• Your child develops a rash or skin irritation.

Special Instructions
• Do not use in the eyes.

• Dosage should be carefully controlled in children with bad skin burns (those who have burns on more than 20% of the body surface), especially if the patient has impaired renal function or is receiving other aminoglycoside antibiotics such as amikacin, gentamicin, kanamycin, netilmicin, streptomycin, or tobramycin.

Brand Names: Neomycin (various manufacturers), Myciguent

Generic Available: Yes

Type of Drug: Topical antibiotic

Use: Protects against infection in minor cuts, wounds, burns, and skin abrasions.

Time Required for Drug to Take Effect: 4 to 7 days

Dosage Forms and Strengths: Cream (0.5%); Ointment (0.5%)

Storage: Store at room temperature in tightly closed containers. Do not freeze.

How This Drug Works: Interferes with bacterial protein synthesis, killing off the offending bacteria.

Brand Names: Procardia, Procardia XL, Adalat, Adalat CC

Generic Available: Yes

Type of Drug: Calcium channel blocker

Use: Treats high blood pressure and chest pain. May also be used to treat congestive heart failure, swallowing difficulties, and to prevent migraines.

Time Required for Drug to Take Effect: Several minutes to several hours. Full effect is achieved in several days with regular dosing.

Dosage Forms and Strengths: Capsules (10 mg, 20 mg); Tablets, sustained-release (30 mg, 60 mg, 90 mg)

Storage: Store at room temperature in tightly closed, light-resistant containers.

How This Medication Works: Relaxes blood vessels, lowering blood pressure.

NIFEDIPINE

Administration Guidelines

- May be given on an empty stomach or with meals, but be consistent.

- Do not crush or allow your child to chew the sustained-release tablets.

- Do not stop giving this drug without first checking with your child's doctor.

- Missed doses: Give as soon as possible. However, if it's almost time for the next dose, skip the missed dose and give the next regular dose. Do not give double doses. Call the doctor or pharmacist for more specific instructions.

Side Effects

Tell your child's doctor about any side effects that are persistent or particularly bothersome.

More Common. Dizziness, headache, flushing, nervousness, weakness, nausea, diarrhea or constipation, upset stomach, dry mouth, skin rash, stuffy nose, cough. Call the doctor if your child experiences swelling of the feet or ankles, palpitations, wheezing, or difficulty breathing.

Less Common. Fainting, difficulty sleeping, tingling fingers and toes, low blood counts. Contact the doctor if your child experiences unusual bleeding or bruising, chest pain, or yellowing of the eyes or skin.

Possible Drug Interactions

- Cimetidine or ranitidine may increase the effects of this drug.

- Quinidine and beta blockers may increase the side effects of this drug.

- May increase the effects of warfarin, theophylline, digoxin, and phenytoin. Dosing adjustment of these drugs may be necessary.

Tell Your Child's Doctor If

- Your child has had allergic reactions to any medications or is taking any other medications.

- Your child has liver, kidney, or heart disease.

- Your daughter is pregnant.

• Your daughter is breast-feeding her baby. This drug can pass into breast milk; however, the American Academy of Pediatrics considers it safe to use while breast-feeding.

Symptoms of Overdose: Nausea, dizziness, weakness, drowsiness, confusion, fainting, excessively low heart rate and blood pressure

Special Notes
• If your child is taking sustained-release tablets, it is normal to see empty tablets in the stool.

Just Call

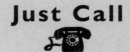

If you have any concerns about any side effects, even minor ones, you should be sure to discuss them with your child's doctor. The doctor may be able to minimize or eliminate the side effects by prescribing a different medication or changing your child's dosage, dosing schedule, or the way the drug is given. (Do not make adjustments on your own without discussing them with your doctor.) At the very least, the doctor can assure you that the medication's benefits far outweigh its side effects.

Brand Names: Furadantin, Macrobid, Macrodantin, Nitrofurantoin (various manufacturers)

Generic Available: Yes

Type of Drug: Antibiotic

Use: Treats bacterial infections of the urinary tract.

Time Required for Drug to Take Effect: It may take 1 to 2 days to achieve maximum effect.

Dosage Forms and Strengths: Capsules (25 mg, 50 mg, 100 mg); Capsules, dual-release (equivalent to 100 mg); Suspension (25 mg per 5 mL)

Storage: Store all forms at room temperature in tightly closed, light-resistant containers. Do not freeze.

How This Drug Works: Kills susceptible bacteria by breaking down their cell membranes and interfering with their production of vital nutrients.

NITROFURANTOIN

Administration Guidelines

• Give with meals or a glass of water or milk to increase the effectiveness of this drug and to avoid stomach irritation.

• Tablets and capsules should be swallowed whole for maximum benefit.

• Generally given 4 times a day.

• Works best when the level of this drug in the urine is kept constant. Give doses at evenly spaced intervals around the clock. For example, if you are to give 3 doses a day, the doses should be spaced 8 hours apart.

• Missed doses: Give immediately. However, if you do not remember until it is time for the next dose, give the missed dose and space the following dose halfway through the regular interval between doses; then return to the regular dosing schedule. Try not to skip any doses.

• Shake the suspension well just before measuring each dose to distribute the ingredients evenly and equalize the doses. You can then dilute the dose with water, milk, fruit juice, or infant's formula to mask the unpleasant taste.

• Give this drug for the entire time prescribed by your child's doctor (usually 7 to 14 days), even if symptoms disappear. If this drug is stopped too soon, resistant bacteria can continue growing, and the infection could recur.

Side Effects

Tell your child's doctor about any side effects that are persistent or particularly bothersome.

More Common. Abdominal cramps, diarrhea, dizziness, drowsiness, loss of appetite, nausea, or vomiting. These side effects should disappear as your child's body adjusts to this drug.

Less Common. It is especially important to tell the doctor if your child experiences chest pain, chills, cough, difficulty in breathing, fainting, fever, hair loss, irritation of the mouth, muscle aches, numbness or tingling, rash, rectal or vaginal itching, unusual bleeding or bruising, weakness, or yellowing of the eyes or skin.

Possible Drug Interactions

• Probenecid and sulfinpyrazone can decrease the effectiveness and increase the side effects of this drug.

• Certain antacids such as magnesium trisilicate can decrease the absorption of this drug.

Tell Your Child's Doctor If

• Your child is taking any prescription or non-prescription medications, especially any of those listed above.

• Your child has had unusual or allergic reactions to any medications, especially to this drug, nitrofurazone, or furazolidone.

• Your child has or ever had anemia, diabetes mellitus, electrolyte abnormalities, G6PD deficiency, kidney or lung disease, nerve damage, or vitamin B deficiencies.

• Your child is taking this drug before having surgery or undergoing other medical or dental treatment.

• Your child's symptoms of infection seem to be getting worse rather than improving.

• Your daughter is or becomes pregnant. This drug is contraindicated in pregnant women at term.

• Your daughter is breast-feeding her baby. Small amounts of this drug may pass into breast milk and temporarily alter the bacterial balance in the intestine of the nursing infant, causing diarrhea. Breast-feeding infants younger than 1 month of age is not recommended, especially if G6PD deficiency is present since it can have an adverse effect on the baby's red blood cells.

Special Instructions

• Do not permit participation in activities that require alertness if this drug makes your child dizzy or drowsy.

• Children with diabetes may have a false-positive sugar reaction with a Clinitest urine glucose test. To avoid this problem, switch to Clinistix or Tes-Tape during treatment. Be sure to check with the doctor before adjusting your insulin dose.

Symptoms of Overdose: Severe forms of side effects listed above.

Special Notes

• Can cause urine to change color (to rust, yellow, or brown). This is harmless, but it may stain underclothing. The color change will disappear after your child stops taking this drug.

• Not recommended for children younger than 1 month of age.

Brand Names: Aventyl, Pamelor

Generic Available: No

Type of Drug: Antidepressant, tricyclic

Use: Treats depression, bed-wetting, panic disorders, and some types of chronic pain.

Time Required for Drug to Take Effect: 7 to 21 days. It may take 3 to 6 weeks to achieve full antidepressant benefit.

Dosage Forms and Strengths: Capsules (10 mg, 25 mg, 50 mg, 75 mg); Liquid (10 mg/5 mL)

Storage: Store at room temperature in tightly closed containers. Protect the liquid from light and do not freeze.

How This Drug Works: Increases the concentration of serotonin and nor-epinephrine in the central nervous system.

NORTRIPTYLINE

Administration Guidelines

• Give with food to decrease stomach upset.

• Usually given 3 or 4 times a day or as a single daily dose at bedtime.

• Give 30 minutes before bedtime if used for bed-wetting.

• Mix the liquid with ½ cup water, milk, or juice (not grape juice or carbonated beverages) just before giving each dose.

• Missed doses: Give as soon as possible. However, if it's within 2 hours of the next dose, skip the missed dose. Do not give double doses. If you miss a once-a-day bedtime dose, do not give the missed dose the next day.

• Do not suddenly stop giving this drug before speaking to your child's doctor.

• Do not give to children younger than 6 years of age for treatment of bed-wetting.

Side Effects

Tell your child's doctor about any side effects that are persistent or particularly bothersome.

More Common. Drowsiness, mouth dryness, dizziness, light-headedness, headache, nausea, increased appetite, weight gain, unpleasant taste, constipation, weakness

Less Common. Contact the doctor if your child experiences blurred vision, confusion, difficulty in speaking or swallowing, eye pain, fainting, fast or irregular heartbeat, hallucinations, loss of balance, masklike face, nervousness or restlessness, problems urinating, shakiness, or slow movements.

Possible Drug Interactions

• Clonidine (Catapres) may lead to very high blood pressure when used with this drug.

• Monoamine oxidase (MAO) inhibitors such as isocarboxazid (Marplan), phenelzine (Nardil), and tranylcypromine (Parnate) can cause very serious reactions and death when used with this drug.

• Central nervous system depressants such as alcohol, antihistamines, cold preparations, muscle relaxants, tranquilizers, and some pain medications may cause extreme drowsiness when used with this drug.

• Cimetidine (Tagamet and Tagamet HB) and methylphenidate (Ritalin) may increase the effect and side effects of this drug.

- Phenobarbital may decease the effectiveness of this drug.

- Eyedrops and nasal sprays or drops that contain naphazoline, oxymetazoline, epinephrine, phenylephrine, or xylometazoline may cause an increase in heart rate and blood pressure.

- Antithyroid drugs can cause an increase in rare blood disorders when used with this drug.

Tell Your Child's Doctor If

- Your child has had an allergic reaction to this drug or any other medication.

- Your child has heart disease, seizures, glaucoma, thyroid disease, urinary retention, liver or kidney disease, or any other medical condition.

- Your child is or has been taking MAO inhibitors such as isocarboxazid (Marplan), phenelzine (Nardil), or tranylcypromine (Parnate).

- Your child has been or is taking any other prescription or nonprescription medicine.

- Your daughter is or becomes pregnant.

- Your daughter is breast-feeding her baby. This drug can pass into breast milk, and the American Academy of Pediatrics is concerned about its effect on the baby.

Special Instructions

- Do not allow your child to drink alcohol while taking this drug.

- Do not give other medicines that may make your child sleepy.

- Have your child stand up slowly to prevent dizziness or light-headedness.

- Limit your child's caffeine intake.

- This drug may cause a skin rash or severe sunburn when your child is exposed to direct sunlight or ultraviolet light. Your child should avoid exposure to sunlight and sunlamps and wear an effective sunscreen and protective clothing when out-of-doors.

Symptoms of Overdose: Agitation; dry mouth; confusion; hallucinations; severe drowsiness; enlarged pupils; fever; vomiting; trouble breathing; urinary retention; low blood pressure; seizures; or fast, slow, or irregular heartbeat

Special Notes

- Drowsiness is common. Make sure you know how your child is reacting to this drug before allowing participation in activities that require alertness and coordination, such as riding a bicycle.

- Doses may be increased slowly to decrease the side effects.

- The effects of this drug may last for 1 or 2 weeks after you stop giving it.

- May cause urine to turn blue-green.

- Your child's progress should be checked by the doctor regularly.

Brand Names: Mycostatin, Nilstat, Nystat-Rx, O-V Staticin

Generic Available: Yes

Type of Drug: Antifungal

Use: Treats fungal infections of the throat, gastro-intestinal tract, skin, and vagina.

Time Required for Drug to Take Effect: 24 to 72 hours

Dosage Forms and Strengths: Cream (100,000 units/g); Ointment (100,000 units/g); Powder (100,000 units/g); Suspension (100,000 units/mL); Tablet (500,000 units); Vaginal (100,000 units); Troche (lozenge) (200,000 units)

Storage: Keep vaginal inserts in the refrigerator. Store all other forms at room temperature in tightly closed, light-resistant containers. Do not freeze.

How This Drug Works: Binds chemically to the cell membranes of fungal organisms, causing the cell contents to leak out, killing the fungi.

NYSTATIN

Administration Guidelines

- Tablets may be given on an empty stomach or with food or milk, as directed by your child's doctor.

- Shake the suspension well just before giving each dose to distribute the ingredients evenly and equalize the doses. Place half the dose in each side of your child's mouth. The child should try to hold the suspension in the mouth or swish it through the mouth for as long as possible before swallowing it.

- Your child should let the lozenge slowly dissolve in the mouth.

- Vaginal tablets occasionally are prescribed to be taken orally to treat mouth or throat infections. Your child should suck on the tablets to increase contact time with the mouth and throat.

- Wash and pat dry the affected area before applying the cream, ointment, or powder. Then apply a sufficient amount to cover the area without any excess after rubbing it in. Do not cover with an occlusive dressing (such as kitchen plastic wrap) unless the doctor directs you to do so.

- Sprinkle the powder liberally into your child's shoes and socks when using it to treat a foot infection.

- Missed Doses: Try not to miss any doses. If you do miss a dose, give it as soon as possible. However, if it is within 1 to 2 hours of the next dose, skip the missed dose and return to your regular dosing schedule. Do not give double doses.

- Give for the entire time prescribed by the doctor (usually 7 to 14 days), even if symptoms disappear before the end of that time. If your child stops taking this drug too soon, resistant fungi may continue growing, and your child's infection could recur.

Side Effects

Tell your child's doctor about any side effects that are persistent or particularly bothersome.

More Common. It is especially important to tell the doctor about a rash.

Less Common. Oral forms: diarrhea, nausea, or vomiting. Topical and vaginal forms: itching. These side effects should disappear as your child's body adjusts to this drug.

Tell Your Child's Doctor If

- Your child has had unusual or allergic reactions to any medications, especially this drug.

• The symptoms of infection do not begin to improve within 2 or 3 days after your child begins this drug. This drug may not be effective against the organism that is causing your child's infection.

• The symptoms seem to be getting worse rather than improving.

• Your daughter is or becomes pregnant. Although this drug appears to be safe during pregnancy, extensive and conclusive studies in humans have not been conducted.

• Your daughter is breast-feeding her baby. It is not known whether this drug passes into breast milk.

Special Instructions

• When being treated for a vaginal infection, your daughter should use the vaginal tablets continuously, even during her menstrual period. She should wear cotton underpants, rather than those made of nylon or other nonporous materials. Wearing a sanitary napkin or panty liner will help protect her under-clothes from vaginal drainage.

• If your daughter is sexually active, she should avoid sexual intercourse or ask her partner to wear a condom until treatment for a vaginal infection has been completed. This will help prevent reinfection.

Outdated Doses

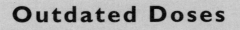

Safe and proper medication disposal is essential, especially when you have children in the house. Do not keep medication—whether prescription or nonprescription—past the expiration date, even if it appears normal. Expired medication may be ineffective and can even be dangerous. Make a habit of regularly checking the expiration date on all medicines in your home. Flush leftover medication down the toilet or pour it down the sink. Rinse the container before throwing it out. If your medication does not display an expiration date, throw it out after one year.

Brand Name: Prilosec

Generic Available: No

Type of Drug: Gastric-acid-secretion inhibitor

Use: Treats peptic ulcer disease, gastroesophageal reflux, and hypersecretory syndromes.

Time Required for Drug to Take Effect: 1 hour

Dosage Form and Strengths: Capsules, delayed-release (10 mg, 20 mg)

Storage: Store at room temperature in tightly closed containers.

How This Drug Works: Suppresses stomach-acid secretion.

OMEPRAZOLE

Administration Guidelines

• Capsules should not be opened, chewed, or crushed.

• Give on an empty stomach with a full glass of water.

• Missed doses: Give as soon as possible. However, if it's within 8 to 12 hours of the next dose, skip the missed dose. Do not give double doses.

Side Effects

Tell your child's doctor about any side effects that are particularly bothersome.

MORE COMMON. Stomach ache, burning sensation in the mouth, constipation, diarrhea, dizziness, dry mouth, fatigue, headache, palpitations

LESS COMMON. Tell the doctor if your child experiences itching, rash, joint pain, chest pain, numbness or tingling of fingers or toes, or yellowing of the eyes and skin.

Possible Drug Interactions

• Increases the effects of diazepam, warfarin, and phenytoin.

Tell Your Child's Doctor If

• Your child is taking any other medication.

• Your child is allergic to this drug.

• Your child has ever had thyroid disease, liver disease, Addison disease, or Cushing disease.

• Your daughter is or becomes pregnant.

• Your daughter is breast-feeding her baby. This drug can pass into breast milk and cause side effects in the infant.

Special Instructions

• Make sure your child uses caution when participating in activities that require alertness as this drug causes dizziness and light-headedness.

Symptoms of Overdose: Sedation, convulsions, decreased respiratory rate

ONDANSETRON

Administration Guidelines
• Use for prevention of symptoms only.

Side Effects
Tell your child's doctor about any side effects that are persistent or particularly bothersome.

More Common. Constipation, diarrhea, dizziness, drowsiness, dryness of the mouth, fever or chills, headache, light-headedness, skin rash

Less Common. Tell the doctor if your child experiences shortness of breath, tightness of the chest, troubled breathing, or wheezing.

Tell Your Child's Doctor If
• Your child is allergic to this drug.

• Your child has had liver or kidney disease.

• Your daughter is or becomes pregnant.

• Your daughter is breast-feeding her baby. This drug can pass into breast milk and cause side effects in the infant.

Special Instructions
• Make sure you know how your child is reacting to this drug before allowing participation in activities that require alertness, such as riding a bicycle.

Symptoms of Overdose:
Sudden blindness, severe constipation, heart problems

Brand Name: Zofran

Generic Available: No

Type of Drug: Antiemetic

Use: Prevents (does not treat) nausea, vomiting, and retching associated with cancer chemotherapy or surgery.

Time Required for Drug to Take Effect: 1 to 2 hours

Dosage Form and Strengths: Tablets (4 mg, 8 mg)

Storage: Store in tightly closed containers at room temperature, away from heat and direct sunlight.

How This Drug Works: Blocks the release of certain chemicals that stimulate the impulse to vomit.

Brand Names: Bactocill, Prostaphlin, Oxacillin (various manufacturers)

Generic Available: Yes

Type of Drug: Penicillin antibiotic

Use: Treats a wide variety of bacterial infections, especially those involving *Staphylococcus* bacteria.

Time Required for Drug to Take Effect: It may be a few days before this drug affects the infection.

Dosage Forms and Strengths: Capsules (250 mg, 500 mg); Solution (250 mg per 5 mL)

Storage: Store capsules at room temperature in tightly closed containers. Keep solution in the refrigerator in tightly closed containers; do not freeze. Discard any unused portion of the solution after 14 days.

How This Drug Works: Kills susceptible bacteria, but is not effective against viruses, parasites, or fungi.

OXACILLIN

Administration Guidelines

• Give on an empty stomach or with a glass of water 1 hour before or 2 hours after a meal. Do not give with fruit juices or carbonated beverages because the acidity of these drinks destroys the drug in the stomach.

• Generally given 4 times a day.

• Works best when blood concentrations are kept within a safe and effective range. Give doses at evenly spaced intervals around the clock. If you are to give 4 doses a day, space them 6 hours apart.

• Missed doses: Give immediately. However, if you do not remember until it is time for the next dose, give the missed dose and space the following dose about halfway through the regular interval between doses. Then return to a regular dosing schedule. Try not to skip any doses.

• Give this drug for the entire time prescribed by your child's doctor (usually 7 to 14 days), even if symptoms disappear. If you stop the drug too soon, resistant bacteria may continue to grow, and the infection could recur.

Side Effects

Tell your child's doctor about any side effects that are persistent or particularly bothersome.

More Common. Diarrhea, heartburn, nausea, or vomiting. These side effects should disappear as your child's body adjusts to this drug.

Less Common. It is especially important to tell the doctor if your child experiences bloating, chills, cough, darkened tongue, difficulty in breathing, difficult or painful urination, fever, irritation of the mouth, muscle aches, rash, rectal or vaginal itching, severe diarrhea, sore throat, or yellowing of the eyes or skin.

Possible Drug Interactions

• Probenecid can increase the blood concentrations of this drug.

• May decrease the effectiveness of birth control pills. Your daughter should use another form of birth control while taking this drug.

Tell Your Child's Doctor If

• Your child is taking any prescription or nonprescription medications, especially any listed above.

• Your child has had unusual or allergic reactions to any medications, especially to this drug or other penicillins such as amoxicillin, cephalosporin antibiotics, penicillamine, or griseofulvin.

- Your child has or ever had kidney disease, asthma, or allergies.
- Your child's symptoms seem to be getting worse rather than improving.
- Your daughter is or becomes pregnant.
- Your daughter is breast-feeding her baby. Small amounts of this drug pass into breast milk and may temporarily alter the bacterial balance in the intestinal tract of the nursing infant, causing diarrhea.

Special Instructions
- Children with diabetes may have a false-positive sugar reaction with a Clinitest urine glucose test. To avoid this problem, switch to Clinistix or Tes-tape urine glucose tests during treatment with this drug.

To Each His Own

If one of your children has been prescribed an antibiotic and your other child gets sick, it is not safe to give the antibiotic to the child for whom it was not prescribed. The medication may not be the appropriate one for another child—even if the children's symptoms are similar. Treating an infection with the wrong drug may make the condition worse instead of better. What's more, children respond to the same drug differently and may need different dosages. The child who became ill first needs the drug in the amount prescribed for the time advised; otherwise, it may not be effective. If you think another child needs medication, consult the doctor.

Brand Names: Ditropan, Oxybutynin (various manufacturers)

Generic Available: Yes

Type of Drug: Antispasmodic

Use: Relieves the symptoms associated with urinary incontinence or urinary frequency.

Time Required for Drug to Take Effect: 30 to 60 minutes

Dosage Forms and Strengths: Tablets (5 mg); Syrup (5 mg per 5 mL)

Storage: Store at room temperature in tightly closed containers.

How This Drug Works: Stops spasms of the smooth muscles.

OXYBUTYNIN

Administration Guidelines

• Give with food or milk.

• Missed doses: Give as soon as possible. However, if it's within 3 to 4 hours of the next dose, skip the missed dose. Do not give double doses.

Side Effects

Tell your child's doctor about any side effects that are persistent or particularly bothersome.

More Common. Bloating, blurred vision, constipation, decreased sweating, dizziness, drowsiness, dry mouth, insomnia, nausea, vomiting, weakness.

Less Common. Tell your doctor if your child experiences difficult or painful urination, eye pain, itching, fever, diarrhea, palpitations, or skin rash.

Possible Drug Interactions

• May increase sedation if given with central nervous system depressants, antihistamines or anticholinergics.

• Increases digoxin blood levels.

Tell Your Child's Doctor If

• Your child is allergic to this drug.

• Your child has ever had bleeding disorders; glaucoma; hiatal hernia; high blood pressure; intestinal blockage; kidney, liver, thyroid, or heart disease; ulcerative colitis; or urinary retention.

• Your child is taking any other medications.

• Your daughter is or becomes pregnant or is breast-feeding her baby. This drug can pass into breast milk and cause side effects in the infant.

Special Instructions

• Make sure you know how your child is reacting to this drug before allowing participation in activities that require alertness.

• This drug can decrease sweating and heat release. Make sure your child avoids strenuous exercise in hot weather and use caution with hot baths, showers, and saunas. Have your child drink plenty of fluids.

• Give your child sunglasses to help relieve discomfort caused by bright lights as this drug increases eye sensitivity to sunlight.

Symptoms of Overdose: Central nervous system excitation, restlessness, tremors, irritability, convulsions, nausea, vomiting, rapid heart rate

OXYCODONE

Administration Guidelines
- May be given with food or milk to avoid stomach upset.

- Do not increase the dose or give it more often than your child's doctor prescribed.

- Works best if given at the onset of your child's pain rather than when the pain increases.

- Missed doses: Give as soon as you remember if it's within 2 hours of the missed dose. Otherwise, skip the missed dose and give the next dose at the scheduled time. Do not give double doses.

Side Effects
Tell your child's doctor about any side effects that are persistent or particularly bothersome.

More Common. Constipation, dizziness, drowsiness, dry mouth, flushing, light-headedness, loss of appetite, nausea, or sweating

Less Common. Blurred vision, nightmares or unusual dreams, trouble sleeping. Call the doctor immediately if your child experiences breathing difficulties, palpitations, tremors, excitation, rash, sore throat and fever, anxiety, severe weakness, or difficult or painful urination.

Possible Drug Interactions
- Other central nervous system depressants such as alcohol, antihistamines, cold preparations, muscle relaxants, tranquilizers, and other pain medicines can cause extreme drowsiness when used with this drug.

Tell Your Child's Doctor If
- Your child has had allergic reactions to this drug or to other narcotic analgesics.

- Your child has any diseases, such as asthma.

- Your child is taking any other medications.

- Your daughter becomes pregnant.

- Your daughter is breast-feeding her baby.

Special Instructions
- Increase the fluid and fiber in your child's diet to avoid constipation.

- Do not suddenly stop giving this drug without first talking with the doctor if you have been giving it for several weeks. The doctor may want to decrease the dose gradually to avoid withdrawal side effects.

Brand Names: Roxicodone (in combination with acetaminophen: Percocet, Tylox, Roxilox; in combination with aspirin: Percodan and Roxiprin)

Generic Available: No

Type of Drug: Narcotic analgesic

Use: Relieves moderate to moderately severe pain.

Time Required for Drug to Take Effect: 10 to 15 minutes

Dosage Forms and Strengths: Tablets with acctamenophen (5 mg); Tablets with aspirin (2.25 mg, 4.5 mg); Solution (5 mg per 5 mL)

Storage: Store at room temperature in tightly closed, light-resistant containers.

How This Drug Works: Acts directly on the opiate receptors of the central nervous system to relieve pain.

- Tylox contains metabisulfite. Avoid this product if your child is allergic to sulfites.

- Do not give an oxycodone-aspirin combination product if your child has signs of a fever or chicken pox.

- Make sure you know how your child is reacting to this drug before allowing participation in activities that require alertness, such as riding a bicycle.

Symptoms of Overdose: Convulsions (tremors), confusion, severe nervousness or restlessness, severe dizziness, severe drowsiness, slow or difficult breathing, severe weakness, pinpoint pupils of the eyes

Special Notes

- Tolerance (decreased effectiveness) may be seen with long-term use of this drug.

Measuring Up

Remember: Never use an ordinary tableware teaspoon to measure liquid doses. Instead, use a cylindrical dosing spoon, dosage cup, dropper, or syringe. These measuring devices can be found at your local drug store and sometimes at supermarkets, toy stores, and department stores.

OXYMETAZOLINE

Administration Guidelines
• For intranasal use only.

• Usually applied 2 times daily. Do not exceed recommended dosage.

• Use the 0.05% solution for children 6 years of age and older. Use the 0.025% solution for children between 2 and 6 years of age. Do not give to children younger than 2 years of age unless directed to do so by your child's doctor.

Side Effects
Tell your child's doctor about any side effects that are persistent or particularly bothersome.

More Common. Burning, stinging, dryness of the nose, sneezing

Less Common. Nausea, dizziness, headache, nervousness, palpitations, difficulty sleeping

Tell Your Child's Doctor If
• Your child has had allergic reactions to any medications.

• Your child has any other diseases.

• Your child is taking any other medications.

• Your child has heart or blood vessel disease or high blood pressure.

• Your daughter becomes pregnant.

Symptoms of Overdose: Drinking the nasal solution can cause drowsiness, low blood pressure, and unconsciousness.

Special Notes
• Prolonged use (longer than 3 days) can cause rebound congestion in which nasal congestion may persist and worsen rather than improve.

• Available over the counter.

Brand Names: Afrin, Afrin Children's, Allerest 12 Hour, Dristan Long-Acting, Duramist Plus 12 Hour, Duration 12 Hour, 4-Way Long Acting, Genasal, Neo-Synephrine 12 Hour, Nostrilla Long Acting, NTZ, Oxymeta-12, Sinarest 12 Hour, Vicks Sinex Long-Acting

Generic Available: Yes

Type of Drug: Topical nasal decongestant

Use: Relieves nasal congestion caused by the common cold, sinusitis, hay fever, and allergies.

Time Required for Drug to Take Effect: 5 to 10 minutes

Dosage Forms and Strengths: Nasal drops and spray (0.025% and 0.05%)

Storage: Store at room temperature in tightly closed, light-resistant containers.

How This Drug Works: Causes blood vessels in the nose to constrict, which relieves nasal congestion.

Brand Names: Cotazym, Cotazym-S, Ilozyme, Ku-Zyme HP, Pancrease, Pancrease MT, Protilase, Ultrase MT, Viokase, Zymase

Generic Available: No

Type of Drug: Pancreatic enzymes

Use: Replaces pancreatic enzymes for those with malabsorption syndrome due to insufficient functioning of the pancreas.

Time Required for Drug to Take Effect: It may take a week or more before maximum effect is achieved.

Dosage Forms: Capsules; Spheres, enteric-coated; Beads, microencapsulated; Powder; Tablets, sustained-release. (Each product contains different amounts of the various enzymes.)

Storage: Store all products in tightly closed containers in a cool, dry place.

How This Drug Works: Replaces the endogenous pancreatic enzymes, assisting in the absorption of protein, starch, and fat.

PANCRELIPASE

Administration Guidelines
• Give with food to enhance the absorption of fats.

• Tablets and capsules should be swallowed whole. The microencapsulated beads and the powder may be mixed with food. Open the microencapsulated beads and sprinkle the contents on soft food. Your child should swallow the food without chewing on the beads.

• Generally given with each main meal. Your child's doctor may instruct you to give additional doses with snacks between meals.

Side Effects
Tell your child's doctor about any side effects that are persistent or particularly bothersome.

More Common. Nausea, stomach pain, sneezing, wheezing, and rash

Less Common. It is especially important to tell the doctor if your child experiences difficulty breathing.

Possible Drug Interactions
• Calcium carbonate and magnesium hydroxide, present in some nonprescription antacid preparations, may decrease the effectiveness of this drug.

• May decrease the amount of iron absorbed from the stomach if iron supplements are taken at the same time as this drug.

Tell Your Child's Doctor If
• Your child is taking any other prescription or nonprescription medications, especially those listed above.

• Your child has had unusual or allergic reactions to any medications.

Special Instructions
• Do not spill the powder on your hands as it is a skin irritant and may also produce an asthmatic attack if inhaled.

Symptoms of Overdose:
Severe forms of side effects listed above, especially nausea and vomiting with severe dehydration.

Special Notes
• The various products listed are not equivalent; each contains a variety of enzymes in different amounts. These products are not interchangable and should not be substituted without first consulting the doctor or pharmacist.

• This product is made from hog pancreas enzymes. Use with caution in children with hypersensitivity to hog protein.

PAROXETINE

Administration Guidelines

- May be given with or without food. Food will help to decrease stomach upset.

- Usually given as a single dose in the morning.

- Missed doses: Give as soon as possible on the same day as the missed dose. Do not give double doses.

- Do not suddenly stop giving this drug before speaking to the doctor. The doctor may first want to gradually reduce the dose.

Side Effects

Tell your child's doctor about any side effects that are persistent or particularly bothersome.

More Common. Constipation, dizziness, drowsiness, dry mouth, diarrhea, increased sweating, decreased appetite, headache, nausea, difficulty urinating, tremor, trouble sleeping, unusual fatigue or weakness, vomiting, increased intestinal gas. Contact the doctor if your child experiences agitation, light-headedness, fainting, muscle pain or weakness, or skin rash.

Less Common. Anxiety, nervousness, blurred vision, tingling or prickly sensations, change in sense of taste, increased appetite, fast or irregular heartbeat, change in weight. Contact the doctor if your child experiences difficulty speaking; fever; inability to move the eyes; loss of or decrease in body movements; mood or behavior changes; fast heartbeat; restlessness; shivering or shaking; sudden or unusual body or face movements; talking, feeling, or acting with excitement; or activity that your child cannot control.

Possible Drug Interactions

- Monoamine oxidase (MAO) inhibitors such as isocarboxazid (Marplan), phenelzine (Nardil) or tranylcypromine (Parnate) can lead to very serious reactions and death when used with this drug.

- Central nervous system depressants such as alcohol, antihistamines, cold preparations, muscle relaxants, tranquilizers, sleeping medicine, sedatives, narcotics, and some pain medications may cause extreme drowsiness when used with this drug.

- The side effects of tricyclic antidepressants such as amitriptyline, imipramine, desipramine, and doxepin may increase when these medications are used with this drug.

- The risk of bleeding from warfarin is increased.

Brand Name: Paxil

Generic Available: No

Type of Drug: Antidepressant

Use: Treats depression.

Time Required for Drug to Take Effect: It may takes 4 weeks or more to achieve full benefit.

Dosage Form and Strengths: Tablets (20 mg, 30 mg)

Storage: Store at room temperature in tightly closed containers.

How This Drug Works: Increases the concentration of serotonin in the central nervous system.

Tell Your Child's Doctor If

• Your child has had an allergic reaction to this drug, any other medication, foods, preservatives, or dyes.

• Your child has seizures; cardiac, liver, or kidney disease; mania; suicidal tendencies; drug abuse problems; or any other medical condition.

• Your child is or has been taking MAO inhibitors such as isocarboxazid (Marplan), phenelzine (Nardil), or tranylcypromine (Parnate).

• Your child is or has been taking other antidepressants.

• Your child is taking any other prescription or nonprescription medicine.

• Your child has a dry mouth after taking this drug for 2 weeks.

• Your child develops side effects after this drug has been stopped.

• Your daughter is or becomes pregnant.

• Your daughter is breast-feeding her baby. This medicine can pass into breast milk and may affect the infant.

Special Instructions

• Give only as directed by the doctor.

• Do not give tryptophan supplements to your child. They can cause dangerous side effects.

• Do not allow your child to drink alcohol while taking this drug.

• Do not give other medicines that may make your child sleepy.

• Have your child stand up slowly to prevent light-headedness or dizziness.

• Do not give any other medications without first talking to the pharmacist or doctor.

Symptoms of Overdose: Severe drowsiness, severe mouth dryness, irritability, large pupils, severe nausea and vomiting, racing heartbeat, severe tremor

Special Notes

• This drug may cause your child to be dizzy, drowsy, less alert, or to have blurred vision. Make sure you know how your child is reacting to this drug before allowing participation in any activity that requires alertness and coordination, such as riding a bicycle.

• The safety and efficacy of this drug have not been established for children younger than 12 years of age.

• Doses generally are increased every 7 days to decrease the side effects.

• It is important to have the doctor check your child's progress regularly.

• The effects of this drug may last for 1 to 2 weeks after you stop giving it.

PEMOLINE

Administration Guidelines
• Give in the morning.

• Chewable tablets must be chewed before swallowing.

• Do not increase the dose or give it more often than your child's doctor prescribed.

• Missed doses: Skip the missed dose and give the next dose at the scheduled time. Do not give double doses.

Side Effects
Tell your child's doctor about any side effects that are persistent or particularly bothersome.

More Common. Loss of appetite, trouble sleeping, weight loss

Less Common. Dizziness, drowsiness, increased irritability, depression, nausea, skin rash, stomach ache. Contact the doctor if your child has yellow eyes or skin, seizures, hallucinations, or severe headache

Possible Drug Interactions
• Central nervous system depressants such as alcohol, antihistamines, muscle relaxants, tranquilizers, and pain relievers may increase drowsiness when used with this drug.

Tell Your Child's Doctor If
• Your child has had allergic reactions to any medications.

• Your child has any diseases or is taking any other prescription or nonprescription medications.

• Your daughter becomes pregnant.

• Your daughter is breast-feeding her baby.

Special Instructions
• Your child should avoid caffeine and alcohol while taking this drug.

• If you have been giving this drug to your child for several weeks, do not suddenly stop giving it without first talking with your child's doctor. The doctor may want to decrease the dose gradually to avoid withdrawal side effects.

• Make sure you know how your child is reacting to this drug before allowing participation in activities that require alertness, such as riding a bicycle.

Symptoms of Overdose: Agitation, confusion, seizures, false sense of well-being, fast heartbeat, hallucinations, severe headache, high fever with sweating, large pupils, muscle tremors or twitches,

Brand Name: Cylert

Generic Available: No

Type of Drug: Central nervous system stimulant

Use: Treats attention deficit disorder with hyperactivity (ADHD). Also used to treat narcolepsy.

Time Required for Drug to Take Effect: Full effect may not be achieved for 3 to 4 weeks.

Dosage Forms and Strengths: Tablets (18.75 mg, 37.5 mg, 75 mg); Tablets, chewable (37.5 mg)

Storage: Store at room temperature in tightly closed, light-resistant containers.

How This Drug Works: It is not completely understood how this drug works in the central nervous system to increase attention and decrease restlessness in children who are hyperactive and cannot concentrate very long.

uncontrolled movement of the eyes or other parts of the body, nervousness, restlessness, vomiting

Special Notes

• The doctor will check your child's progress at regular visits to make sure this drug does not cause unwanted side effects.

• The doctor will ask you periodically to stop giving this drug to assess your child's continued need for it and to avoid the development of tolerance to its effect.

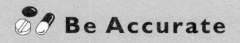 **Be Accurate**

If you don't give medication correctly, it may be ineffective or even cause side effects. An estimated 10 to 30 percent of medications aren't effective because they have been given incorrectly. To do it right, you have to give the exact amount of medicine prescribed at the scheduled time, for the specified duration, and in the appropriate manner. Always read the label, follow the directions carefully, and use the appropriate equipment for measuring and administering the medication. Also, be sure to wash your hands before you give any medication to your child.

PENICILLAMINE

Administration Guidelines

• Give on an empty stomach 1 hour before or 2 hours after a meal for maximum benefit.

• Separate each dose from doses of other medications by at least 1 hour for maximum absorption.

• Missed doses: Give as soon as possible. However, if it's time for the next dose, skip the missed dose and return to the regular dosing schedule. Do not give double doses.

Side Effects

Tell your child's doctor about any side effects that are persistent or particularly bothersome.

More Common. Altered taste sensations, diarrhea, loss of appetite, nausea, stomach upset, vomiting. These side effects should disappear as the body adjusts to this drug.

Less Common. It is especially important to tell the doctor if your child experiences breast enlargement (in both sexes), difficult or painful urination, difficulty in breathing, joint pain, loss of hair, mouth sores, ringing in the ears, skin rash, sore throat, tingling sensations in the fingers or toes, unusual bleeding or bruising, or wheezing.

Possible Drug Interactions

• Iron or antacids can decrease the absorption of this drug.

• Can decrease blood concentrations and beneficial effects of digoxin.

• Causes increased side effects to the blood and kidneys when used with gold salts, hydroxychloroquine, phenylbutazone, oxyphenbutazone, or anticancer drugs.

Tell Your Child's Doctor If

• Your child is taking any prescription or nonprescription medications, especially any of those listed above.

• Your child has had unusual or allergic reactions to any medications, especially to this drug or to penicillin or cephalosporin antibiotics.

• Your child has or ever had blood disorders or kidney disease.

• Your child is taking this drug before having surgery or any other medical or dental treatment.

• Your daughter is or becomes pregnant. This drug has been found to cause birth defects in both animals and humans. Its use during pregnancy is contraindicated.

Brand Names: Cuprimine, Depen Titratable Tablets

Generic Available: No

Type of Drug: Copper chelator and antirheumatic

Use: Treats Wilson disease (high blood-copper levels), severe rheumatoid arthritis, and cystinuria (high urine levels of cystine).

Time Required for Drug to Take Effect: The full benefits of this drug may not become apparent for as long as 3 months after therapy.

Dosage Forms and Strengths: Tablets (250 mg); Capsules (125 mg, 250 mg)

Storage: Store at room temperature in tightly closed containers.

How This Drug Works: Binds to copper and cystine, preventing their harmful effects on the body. It is not clearly understood how this drug relieves rheumatoid arthritis.

- Your daughter is breast-feeding her baby. Breast-feeding must be discontinued during treatment with this drug

Special Instructions

- Do not stop giving this drug unless you first check with the doctor.

Special Notes

- Can decrease the body's ability to repair wounds. Every attempt should be made to avoid injury while your child is taking this drug.

This warning is especially important for children with diabetes.

- The doctor may want your child to take pyridoxine (vitamin B) to prevent some of this drug's side effects, such as tingling sensations.

- Children with high levels of cystine in the urine should drink large amounts of water.

- The doctor may want to see your child often to monitor progress and prevent side effects.

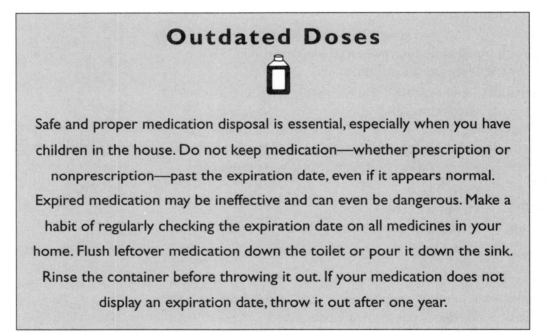

Outdated Doses

Safe and proper medication disposal is essential, especially when you have children in the house. Do not keep medication—whether prescription or nonprescription—past the expiration date, even if it appears normal. Expired medication may be ineffective and can even be dangerous. Make a habit of regularly checking the expiration date on all medicines in your home. Flush leftover medication down the toilet or pour it down the sink. Rinse the container before throwing it out. If your medication does not display an expiration date, throw it out after one year.

PENICILLIN VK

Administration Guidelines

• Give on an empty stomach or with a glass of water 1 hour before or 2 hours after a meal. Do not give with fruit juices or carbonated beverages because the acidity of these drinks destroys the drug in the stomach.

• Usually given 4 times a day.

• Works best when blood concentrations are kept within a safe and effective range. Give doses at evenly spaced intervals around the clock. If you are to give 4 doses a day, space them 6 hours apart.

• Missed doses: Give immediately. However, if it is time for the next dose, give the missed dose and space the next dose halfway through the regular interval between doses; then return to the regular dosing schedule. Try not to skip any doses.

• Give for the entire time prescribed by your child's doctor (usually 7 to 14 days), even if symptoms disappear. If the drug is stopped too soon, resistant bacteria can continue growing, and the infection could recur.

Side Effects

Tell your child's doctor about any side effects that are persistent or particularly bothersome.

More Common. Diarrhea, heartburn, nausea, or vomiting. These side effects should disappear as the body adjusts to this drug.

Less Common. It is especially important to tell the doctor if your child experiences bloating, chills, cough, darkened tongue, difficulty in breathing, fever, irritation of the mouth, muscle aches, rash, rectal or vaginal itching, severe diarrhea, or sore throat.

Possible Drug Interactions

• Probenecid can increase the blood concentrations of this drug.

• Oral neomycin may decrease the absorption of this drug.

• May decrease the effectiveness of oral contraceptives. Your daughter should use a different or additional form of birth control while taking this drug.

Tell Your Child's Doctor If

• Your child is taking any prescription or nonprescription medications, especially any of those listed above.

• Your child has had unusual or allergic reactions to any medications, especially to this drug or to other penicillin antibiotics such as ampicillin and amoxicillin, cephalosporin antibiotics, penicillamine, or griseofulvin.

Brand Names: Beepen-VK, Betapen-VK, Ledercillin VK, Robicillin VK, Uticillin VK, V-Cillin K, Veetids, Pen-Vee K, Penicillin VK (various manufacturers)

Generic available: Yes

Type of Drug: Penicillin antibiotic

Use: Treats a wide variety of bacterial infections, including those of the middle ear, the respiratory tract, and the urinary tract. It is not effective against viral or fungal infections.

Time Required for Drug to Take Effect: It may take a few days for this drug to affect the infection.

Dosage Forms and Strengths: Tablets (125 mg, 250 mg, 500 mg); Solution (125 mg and 250 mg per 5 mL)

Storage: Store tablets at room temperature in a tightly closed container. Refrigerate the solution in tightly closed containers; do not freeze. Discard any unused portion of the solution after 14 days.

How This Drug Works: Severely injures the cell membranes of infecting bacteria. Kills susceptible bacteria, but is not effective against viruses, parasites, or fungi.

- Your child has or ever had kidney disease, asthma, or allergies.

- Your child's infection seems to be getting worse rather than improving.

- Your daughter is or becomes pregnant.

- Your daughter is breast-feeding her baby. Small amounts of this drug pass into breast milk and may temporarily cause diarrhea in the nursing infant.

Special Instructions

- Children with diabetes may have a false-positive sugar reaction with a Clinitest urine glucose test. To avoid this problem, switch to Clinistix or Tes-tape urine glucose tests during treatment with this drug.

To Each His Own

If one of your children has been prescribed an antibiotic and another child gets sick, it is not safe to give the antibiotic to the child for whom it was not prescribed. The medication may not be the appropriate one for the other child—even if the children's symptoms are similar. Treating an infection with the wrong drug may make the condition worse instead of better. What's more, children respond to the same drug differently and may need different dosages. The child who became ill first needs the drug in the amount prescribed for the time advised; otherwise, it may not be effective. If you think another child needs medication, consult the doctor.

PERMETHRIN

Administration Guidelines

- Avoid contact with eyes, nose, and mouth. Flush eyes with water immediately if they come in contact with this drug.

- Shake well before using.

- For head lice, apply a sufficient volume of liquid to saturate the hair and scalp. Leave on hair for 10 minutes before rinsing off with water. Remove remaining nits. May be repeated in 1 week if lice and nits are still present.

- For scabies, apply cream head to toe; leave on for 8 to 14 hours. Wash off with water. For infants, apply on the hairline, neck, scalp, temple, and forehead.

- Do not exceed the prescribed dosage.

Side Effects

Tell your child's doctor about any side effects that are persistent or particularly bothersome.

More Common. Itching, reddening of the skin, rash of the scalp, burning, pain, stinging, tingling, numbness, scalp discomfort, swelling.

Tell Your Child's Doctor If

- Your child is hypersensitive to chrysanthemums or to any component of the product, including formaldehyde.

- Your daughter is pregnant. Use during pregnancy only if clearly needed.

- Your daughter is breast-feeding. It is not known whether this drug passes into breast milk. Consider discontinuing breast-feeding temporarily or withholding the drug while the mother is breast-feeding.

Special Instructions

- Use externally only.

- Discontinue use if your child develops hypersensitivity (extreme itching, swelling, or rash) to this drug.

Symptoms of Overdose: From oral ingestion of this drug: dizziness, vertigo, anorexia, nausea, vomiting, headache, weakness, coma, seizures

Special Notes

- Treatment with this drug may temporarily exacerbate the itching, red skin, and swelling that often accompany scabies and head lice infestation.

Brand Names: Elimite, Nix

Generic Available: No

Type of Drug: Antiparasitic agent, pediculicide (kills the head louse) and its nits (eggs); scabicidal agent (kills scabies).

Use: Treats scabies, head lice, and crab lice.

Time Required for Drug to Take Effect: Liquid, topical: 10 minutes (for head lice); Cream: 8 to 14 hours (for scabies)

Dosage Forms and Strengths: Cream (5%); Liquid (1%)

Storage: Store at room temperature in tightly closed containers. Do not freeze.

How This Drug Works: Paralyzes the infecting organisms.

- To remove nits, comb with a fine-toothed nit comb and apply a damp towel to the scalp for 30 to 60 minutes.

- For infestation of eyelashes, apply petrolatum ointment 3 to 4 times a day for 8 to10 days; remove nits from the eyelashes with a pair of tweezers.

- These products contain formaldehyde, which is a contact allergen.

- Wash clothing and bedding in hot water or dry clean to kill scabies.

Keep It Out of Reach

Do not rely on a child-resistant cap to deter your child from opening a bottle of medication. Child-resistant does not mean childproof. Legally, a cap can be called child-resistant if 80 percent of all five-year-olds need more than five minutes to open it. That means the other 20 percent could get into it in even less time. Put the bottle in a hard-to-reach cabinet with a childproof lock. Do not keep it on the countertop, kitchen table, or nightstand.

PHENOBARBITAL

Administration Guidelines

• Give with food or a full glass of water or milk to avoid stomach upset.

• The liquid may be mixed with water, milk, or juice.

• Give 30 to 60 minutes before bedtime if given as a sleep aid.

• If being given to control seizures, give at evenly spaced intervals around the clock to maintain a constant concentration of this drug in your child's bloodstream. If it is to be given 3 times a day, space the doses 8 hours apart.

• Missed doses: Give as soon as you remember, then stagger subsequent doses evenly for the rest of the day. Do not give double doses. For seizure disorders, contact the doctor if your child misses 2 or more doses.

• Do not use the liquid if it becomes cloudy.

Side Effects

Tell your child's doctor about any side effects that are persistent or particularly bothersome.

More Common. Constipation, dizziness, drowsiness, nausea

Less Common. Contact the doctor immediately if your child experiences difficulty breathing, confusion, depression, unusual excitement or fatigue, hives or itching, unusual clumsiness, muscle or joint pain, skin rash, slurred speech, sore throat, unusual bleeding or bruising, unusual weakness, or yellowing of the eyes or skin.

Possible Drug Interactions

• Alcohol, antidepressants, and tranquilizers will greatly increase the drowsiness from this drug.

• Birth control pills may not work properly while your child is taking this drug. Your daughter should use an additional form of birth control if she is sexually active.

Tell Your Child's Doctor If

• Your child is taking any other medications.

• Your child has any diseases.

• Your child has had allergic reactions to any medications.

• Your daughter is or becomes pregnant. Seizure disorders should be controlled by a doctor during pregnancy.

• Your daughter is breast-feeding her baby. This drug can pass into breast milk and cause significant effects in some nursing infants. It

Brand Names: Barbita, Solfoton

Generic Available: Yes

Type of Drug: Anticonvulsant and sedative

Use: Treats convulsions including febrile seizures; relieves anxiety or tension; promotes sleep.

Time Required for Drug to Take Effect: 20 to 60 minutes when used to promote sleep. It may take about 1 week for the complete control of seizures.

Dosage Forms and Strengths: Capsules (16 mg); Tablets (15 mg, 16 mg, 30 mg, 32 mg, 60 mg, 65 mg, 100 mg); Liquid (15 mg and 20 mg per 5 mL with 13.5% alcohol)

Storage: Store at room temperature in tightly closed, light-resistant containers.

How This Drug Works: Depresses the central nervous system (brain and spinal cord).

should be given to nursing mothers with caution, according to the American Academy of Pediatrics.

Special Instructions

• Before your child has surgery or any medical or dental treatment, tell the doctor performing the treatment that your child is taking this drug.

• Make sure you know how your child is reacting to this drug before allowing participation in activities that require alertness, such as riding a bicycle.

• If giving for seizures, do not suddenly stop giving this drug. Abruptly stopping this drug could cause seizures.

Symptoms of Overdose: Severe dizziness or clumsiness, severe drowsiness, blurred or double vision, seizures or abnormal twitching, severe vomiting, abnormal eye movements, staggered walk, slurred speech

Teach Your Children Well

Let's face it. Kids can be pretty stubborn when it comes to accepting medication. When appropriate, try giving your child information about his or her condition and how the medicine works. In a nonthreatening voice, talk about the consequences of not taking the medication, perhaps reminding the child of how uncomfortable he or she was before beginning the medication. Use reasoning when possible, but don't scare the child. Children who understand the importance of antibiotics for infection, insulin for diabetes, or inhalants for asthma are more likely to take the medication without objection.

PHENYLEPHRINE

Administration Guidelines
- Avoid contamination of the dropper or spray. Rinse with hot water following each use.

- For children 6 to 12 years of age, use the .025% nasal spray or drops.

- For children younger than 6 months of age, use the 0.16% nasal spray or drops.

- Do not use nasal products longer than 3 to 5 days.

Side Effects
Tell your child's doctor about any side effects that are persistent or particularly bothersome.

More Common. Insomnia, dizziness, weakness, or tremor

Less Common. High blood pressure, chest pain, slowing of the heart, restlessness, excitability, headache, anxiety, nervousness, dizziness, tremor, difficulty breathing, nasal stuffiness (when used as a decongestant too often)

Possible Drug Interactions
- Do not give if your child is taking a monoamine oxidase (MAO) inhibitor.

Tell Your Child's Doctor If
- Your child has had unusual or allergic reactions to any medications, especially to this drug, phenothiazine tranquilizers, or other adrenergic agents such as albuterol, amphetamines, ephedrine, epinephrine, isoproterenol, metaproterenol, norepinephrine, pseudoephedrine, phenylpropanolamine, and terbutaline.

- Your child has or ever had asthma, brain disease, blockage of the urinary or digestive tract, diabetes mellitus, colitis, heart or blood-vessel disease, high blood pressure, kidney disease, liver disease, lung disease, peptic ulcers, or thyroid disease.

- Your daughter is or becomes pregnant. The effects of this drug during the early stages of pregnancy have not been thoroughly studied in humans.

- Your daughter is breast-feeding her baby. Small amounts of this drug pass into breast milk and may cause unusual excitement or irritability in nursing infants.

Special Instructions
- Do not use if solution changes color, becomes cloudy, or contains particles.

Brand Names: AK-Nefrin Ophthalmic Solution, Alconefrin Nasal Solution,* Doktors Nasal Solution,* I-Phrine Ophthalmic Solution, Isopto Frin Ophthalmic Solution, Mydfrin Ophthalmic Solution, Neo-Synephrine Nasal Solution,* Neo-Synephrine Ophthalmic Solution, Nostril Nasal Solution,* Prefrin Ophthalmic Solution, Relief Ophthalmic Solution, Rhinall Nasal Solution,* Sinarest Nasal Solution,* St. Joseph Measured Dose Nasal Solution,* Vicks Sinex Nasal Solution (*available over the counter)

Generic Available: Yes

Type of Drug: Nasal decongestant, ophthalmic agent

Use: Treats nasal congestion; dilates pupils.

Time Required for Drug to Take Effect: Nasal: 5 to15 minutes; Oral: 15 to 30 minutes; Ophthalmic: 5 to 10 minutes

Dosage Forms and Strengths: Nasal, drops (0.125%, 0.16%, 0.25%, 0.5%, 1%); Nasal, spray (0.25%, 0.5%, 1%); Ophthalmic solution (0.12%, 2.5%, 10%)

Storage: Store in tightly closed, light-resistant containers.

How This Drug Works: Causes vasoconstriction.

Symptoms of Overdose: Sleepiness, sedation, or coma. Sedation may be accompanied by profuse sweating, low blood pressure, or shock.

Special Notes

• Children are less likely to swallow this drug when administered by spray rather than by drop. Sprays, therefore, may be preferable to avoid absorption of this drug in the stomach.

• Some combination products may contain sulfates. If your child is allergic to sulfites or sulfa drugs, choose a sulfite-free product.

Over-the-Counter Wisdom

Keep in mind that even a medication that is available without a doctor's prescription may still be harmful and should be given appropriately and only when necessary. Talk to your pediatrician about what to do if your child gets sick. Some illnesses can be treated at home, some require a call to the pediatrician's office, and some will require a visit to the doctor. In addition, ask the doctor what situations constitute an emergency. If you're not sure if it's safe or appropriate to give your child a particular over-the-counter medication, be sure to talk to the doctor first.

PHENYLPROPANOLAMINE

Administration Guidelines
- Give with food or a full glass of milk or water to avoid stomach upset.

- Do not break, crush, or allow your child to chew timed-release tablets. Your child should swallow them whole.

- Missed doses: Give as soon as possible. However, if it is almost time for the next dose, skip the missed dose and return to the regular dosing schedule. Do not give double doses.

- Your child should drink at least 8 glasses of water a day to loosen bronchial secretions while taking this drug.

Side Effects
Tell your child's doctor about any side effects that are persistent or particularly bothersome.

More Common. Nervousness, restlessness, insomnia, dizziness, headache, increase in blood pressure, nausea, awareness of one's heartbeat

Less Common. Headache, tightness in the chest area, greatly elevated blood pressure, rapid heart beat

Possible Drug Interactions
- Monoamine oxidase (MAO) inhibitors such as isocarboxazid, pargyline, phenelzine, and tranylcypromine can increase the side effects of this drug. At least 14 days should separate the use of this drug and a MAO inhibitor.

- May decrease the blood-pressure-lowering effects of guanethidine.

- Digoxin and nonprescription allergy, asthma, cough, cold, diet, or sinus preparations may increase the side effects of the decongestant component of this drug.

Tell Your Child's Doctor If
- Your child is taking any other medications, especially any of those listed above.

- Your child has had unusual or allergic reactions to any medications, especially to this drug or to similar agents such as albuterol, amphetamines, ephedrine, epinephrine, isoproterenol, metaproterenol, norepinephrine, pseudoephedrine, and terbutaline.

- Your child has or ever had diabetes mellitus, heart or blood-vessel disease, high blood pressure, or thyroid disease.

- Your daughter is pregnant or is breast-feeding her baby.

Brand Names:
Decongestant: Phenyl-Propanolamine HCl (various manufacturers),* Propagest, Rhindecon (dye free)*, Diet Aid: Acutrim 16 Hour,* Acutrim Late Day,* Acutrim II Maximum Strength,* Control,* Dexatrim Pre-Meal,* Maximum Strength Dex-A-Diet Caplets,* Maximum Strength Dexatrim,* Phenoxine,* Phenyldrine,* Prolamine* (*available over the counter)

Generic Available: Yes

Type of Drug: Nasal decongestant; non-prescription diet aid

Use: Relieves the symptoms of upper respiratory tract infections. Also used for weight reduction.

Time Required for Drug to Take Effect: 15 to 30 minutes

Dosage Forms and Strengths: Tablets (25 mg, 50 mg); Tablets, precision-release (75 mg); Tablets, timed-release (25 mg, 75 mg); Capsules, timed-release (75 mg)

Storage: Store at room temperature in tightly closed containers.

How This Drug Works: Constricts blood vessels in the nasal passages, reducing swelling and congestion.

Special Instructions

- Make sure you know how your child is reacting to this drug before allowing participation in activities that require alertness, such as riding a bicycle.

- Do not use decongestant products longer than 3 to 5 days.

Special Notes

- Available in combination with other ingredients.

Symptoms of Overdose: Vomiting, high blood pressure, increased body temperature, peripheral neuropathy/paresthesia

Keep a Lid on It

Pharmacists are required to put drugs in bottles that have child-resistant caps. Don't switch to a bottle that's easier for you to open—children may also find it easier to open. Remember, too, that child-resistant does not mean childproof. Children older than five years of age may be able to open most medicine bottles. That's why it's essential for you to teach them that drugs can be harmful if not taken correctly and that they need supervision before taking anything. And, just to be on the safe side, keep all medicines out of your child's reach.

PHENYTOIN

Administration Guidelines

• Give with food or a full glass of water to avoid stomach upset.

• The tablet form should be chewed before swallowing.

• Shake the suspension well just before measuring each dose.

• Give at evenly spaced intervals around the clock to maintain a constant concentration of this drug in your child's bloodstream. If it is to be given 3 times a day, the doses should be spaced 8 hours apart.

• Missed doses: Give as soon as you remember, then stagger subsequent doses evenly for the rest of the day. Do not give double doses. For seizure disorders, contact the doctor if your child misses 2 or more doses.

Side Effects

Tell your child's doctor about any side effects that are persistent or particularly bothersome.

More Common. Constipation, dizziness, drowsiness

Less Common. Trouble sleeping, unusual or excessive hair growth on the body and face. Contact the doctor immediately if your child experiences bleeding, tender, or enlarged gums; skin rash; clumsiness or unsteadiness; confusion; twitching of the eyes; enlarged glands in the neck or underarm; sore throat; blurred or double vision; unusual bleeding or bruising; yellow eyes or skin; behavioral changes; vomiting; increased number of seizures; difficulty speaking or slurred speech; dark urine; unusual fatigue, unusual weight loss; numbness or tingling in the hands or feet; joint pain; or muscle twitching.

Possible Drug Interactions

• Alcohol, antidepressants, and tranquilizers may decrease the effectiveness of this drug and your child may experience increased drowsiness.

• Antacids, sucralfate, calcium, and medications for diarrhea may decrease the absorption of this drug from the stomach. Do not give this drug within 2 to 3 hours of these medications.

• Birth control pills may not work properly while your daughter is taking this drug. She should use an additional form of birth control.

Tell Your Child's Doctor If

• Your child has had allergic reactions to any medications.

• Your child has any diseases.

Brand Names: Dilantin, Diphenylan, Dilantin Infatab

Generic Available: Yes

Type of Drug: Anticonvulsant

Use: Treats convulsions or seizures.

Time Required for Drug to Take Effect: It may take about 1 week to achieve complete effectiveness.

Dosage Forms and Strengths: Capsules (30 mg, 100 mg); Tablets, chewable (50 mg); Suspension (30 mg and 125 mg per 5 mL, with less than 0.6% alcohol)

Storage: Store tablets and suspension at room temperature in tightly closed, light-resistant containers.

How This Drug Works: It is not completely understood how this drug works in the central nervous system to reduce the number and severity of seizures. It may decrease the number of seizures by regulating the number of sodium ions crossing the cell membrane of the motor cortex in the brain.

- Your daughter is taking any other medications.

- Your daughter is or becomes pregnant. Seizures must be controlled by a doctor during pregnancy.

- Your daughter is breast-feeding her baby. This drug can pass into breast milk; however, the American Academy of Pediatrics considers it compatible with breast-feeding in most cases.

Special Instructions

- Do not switch from one brand of this drug to another; your child may respond differently to different brands.

- Before your child has surgery or any medical or dental treatment, tell the doctor performing the treatment that your child is taking this drug.

- Do not suddenly stop giving this drug. Abruptly stopping this drug could cause seizures.

- Do not give this drug at the same time as enteral nutritional therapy ("liquid food" such as Pediasure). Give this drug 2 hours before and 2 hours after the enteral feeding.

Symptoms of Overdose: Severe dizziness or clumsiness, severe drowsiness, blurred or double vision, seizures or abnormal twitching, severe vomiting, abnormal eye movements, staggered walk, slurred speech

Special Notes

- Frequent brushing and massaging of the gums with the rubber tip of a good toothbrush may minimize the gum enlargement caused by this drug.

- Make sure you know how your child is reacting to this drug before allowing participation in activities that require alertness, such as riding a bicycle.

- Your child will require blood tests to monitor the concentration of this drug in the body.

POTASSIUM CHLORIDE

Administration Guidelines

- Give with food or immediately after a meal to avoid stomach irritation.

- Give at the same time(s) each day.

- Dilute each dose of the liquid, powder, or effervescent tablet in at least 4 ounces (½ cup) of cold water or juice (not tomato juice). Be sure this drug is dissolved completely and is no longer fizzing before your child drinks it. Tell your child to sip it slowly.

- The sustained-release tablets and capsules should be swallowed whole. Chewing, crushing, or breaking them destroys their sustained-release activity and may increase the side effects.

- Missed doses: Give as soon as possible. However, if it is within 2 hours of the next scheduled dose skip the missed dose and return to the regular dosing schedule. Do not give double doses.

Side Effects

Tell your child's doctor about any side effects that are persistent or particularly bothersome.

More Common. Diarrhea, nausea, stomach pains, vomiting. These should disappear as the body adjusts to this drug.

Less Common. It is especially important to tell the doctor if your child experiences anxiety; bloody or black, tarry stools; confusion; difficulty in breathing; numbness or tingling in the arms, legs, or feet; palpitations; severe abdominal pain; or unusual weakness.

Possible Drug Interactions

- Amiloride, spironolactone, or triamterene can lead to hyperkalemia (high concentrations of potassium in the bloodstream).

- Digoxin can lead to heart problems when given with high doses of this drug.

Tell Your Child's Doctor If

- Your child is taking any prescription or nonprescription medications.

- Your child has had unusual or allergic reactions to any medications, especially to potassium.

- Your child has or had Addison disease, dehydration, heart disease, heat cramps, hyperkalemia, intestinal blockage, kidney disease, myotonia congenita, or peptic ulcers.

- Your daughter is or becomes pregnant.

Brand Names: Cena-K, Kaochlor, Kaon, Kato, Kay Ciel, K-Dur, K-Lor, Klorvess, Klotrix, K-Lyte/Cl, K-Tab, Micro-K, Micro-K Extencaps, Rum-K, Slow-K,

Generic Available: Yes

Type of Drug: Potassium replacement

Use: Prevents or treats potassium deficiency, especially when caused by diuretics.

Time Required for Drug to Take Effect: It may take a few days before the full effect is achieved.

Dosage Forms and Strengths: Tablets, effervescent (20 mEq, 25 mEq); Tablets, sustained-release (6.7 mEq, 8 mEq, 10 mEq, 20 mEq); Tablets, enteric-coated (2.5 mEq); Capsules, sustained-release (8 mEq, 10 mEq); Liquid (20 mEq, 30 mEq, and 40 mEq per 15 mL, with alcohol varying from 0% to 5%); Powder (15 mEq, 20 mEq, and 25 mEq per packet)

Storage: Store at room temperature in tightly closed containers. Do not refrigerate.

How This Drug Works: Provides normal amounts of potassium.

Special Instructions

- Ask the doctor about using a salt substitute instead of this drug. Salt substitutes are similar, but less expensive and more convenient. However, salt substitutes should only be used with the doctor's approval. Too much potassium can be dangerous.

Symptoms of Overdose: Severe nausea, vomiting, dehydration, gastrointestinal lesions and abdominal pain. These symptoms require immediate medical attention.

Special Notes

- It is normal to find what looks like a tablet in the stool if your child is taking the sustained-release tablets. This drug is contained in a wax core that is eliminated in the stool.

- Some of these products contain the color additive FD&C Yellow No. 5 (tartrazine), which can cause rash, shortness of breath, or fainting in susceptible individuals.

- Some products are sugar free and some contain varying amounts of alcohol (0 to 5%).

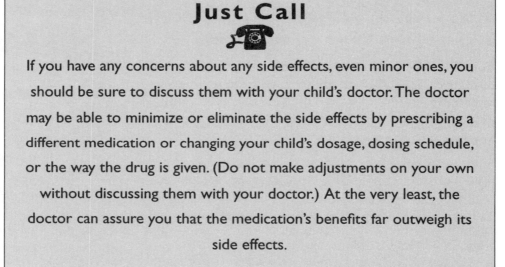

Just Call

If you have any concerns about any side effects, even minor ones, you should be sure to discuss them with your child's doctor. The doctor may be able to minimize or eliminate the side effects by prescribing a different medication or changing your child's dosage, dosing schedule, or the way the drug is given. (Do not make adjustments on your own without discussing them with your doctor.) At the very least, the doctor can assure you that the medication's benefits far outweigh its side effects.

PREDNISOLONE (SYSTEMIC)

Administration Guidelines
• May be given with food or milk to prevent stomach irritation.

• If your child is taking only 1 dose of this drug a day, try to give it before 9:00 A.M. This will mimic the body's normal production of this chemical.

• Missed doses: It is important not to miss a dose of this drug. If you do miss a dose, follow these guidelines:

  1. If usually given more than once a day, give as soon as possible and return to the regular schedule. If it is already time for the next dose, double the dose given.

  2. If usually given once a day, give the missed dose as soon as possible. If you do not remember until the next day, do not give the missed dose at all, just follow the regular dosing schedule. Do not give double doses.

  3. If usually given every other day, give as soon as you remember. If you miss the scheduled time by a whole day, give it when you remember and then skip a day before giving the next dose. Do not give double doses. If you miss more than 1 dose, contact your child's doctor.

• Do not suddenly stop giving this drug before speaking with the doctor.

Side Effects
Tell your child's doctor about any side effects that are persistent or particularly bothersome.

More Common. Dizziness, false sense of well-being, fatigue, increased appetite, increased sweating, indigestion, leg cramps, menstrual irregularities, muscle weakness, nausea, swelling of the skin on the face, restlessness, sleep disorders, or weight gain

Less Common. It is important to tell the doctor if your child experiences abdominal enlargement or pain; acne; back or rib pain; bloody or black, tarry stools; blurred vision; convulsions; eye pain; fever and sore throat; headaches; slow healing of wounds; increased thirst and urination; depression; mood changes; muscle wasting; nightmares; peptic ulcers; rapid weight gain (3 to 5 pounds in a week); rash; shortness of breath; unusual bleeding or bruising; or unusual weakness.

Brand Names: Cortolone, Delta-Cortef, Pediapred, Prelone

Generic Available: Yes

Type of Drug: Adrenocorticosteroid hormone

Use: Treats a variety of disorders, including endocrine and rheumatic disorders; asthma; blood diseases; certain cancers; eye disorders; gastrointestinal disturbances such as ulcerative colitis; respiratory diseases; and inflammatory diseases such as arthritis, dermatitis, and poison ivy.

Time Required for Drug to Take Effect: Varies based on the illness being treated. It may take several days before this drug takes effect.

Dosage Forms and Strengths: Tablets (5 mg); Syrup (15 mg per 5 mL, with 5% alcohol); Liquid (5 mg per 5 mL)

Storage: Store at room temperature in tightly closed containers.

How This Drug Works: How this drug works is not completely understood. It is similar to the cortisonelike chemicals naturally produced by the adrenal gland. These chemicals are involved in various regulatory processes.

Possible Drug Interactions

• Aspirin and anti-inflammatory medications such as ibuprofen, indomethacin, and ketoprofen may increase the stomach problems caused by this drug.

• Cholestyramine and colestipol can bind to this drug in the stomach and prevent its absorption.

Tell Your Child's Doctor If

• Your child is taking any other medications.

• Your child has had allergic reactions to this drug or other adrenocorticoids such as betamethasone, cortisone, dexamethasone, fluocinolone, hydrocortisone, methylpred-nisolone, prednisone, or triamcinolone.

• Your child has recently been exposed to or currently has chicken pox or measles.

• Your child has any medical problems such as diabetes, glaucoma, fungal infections, heart disease, high blood pressure, peptic ulcers, thyroid disease, tuberculosis, ulcerative colitis, kidney disease, or liver disease.

• Your daughter is or becomes pregnant.

• Your daughter is breast-feeding her baby.

Special Instructions

• Do not have your child vaccinated or immunized while taking this drug. This drug decreases the effectiveness of vaccines and can lead to infection if a live virus vaccine is given.

Symptoms of Overdose: Severe restlessness

Special Notes

• With long-term use, the doctor may want your child to be on a low-salt and potassium-rich diet. The doctor may also want your child's eyes examined periodically during treatment with this drug to detect glaucoma and cataracts.

• With long-term use, your doctor may need to increase your child's dose during times of stress such as a serious infection, injury, or surgery.

PREDNISONE (SYSTEMIC)

Administration Guidelines

- May be given with food or milk to prevent stomach irritation.

- If your child is taking only 1 dose a day, try to give it before 9:00 A.M. This will mimic the body's normal production of this chemical.

- Missed doses: It is important not to miss a dose. If you do miss a dose, follow these guidelines:

  1. If usually given more than once a day, give as soon as possible and return to the regular schedule. If it is already time for the next dose, double the dose given.

  2. If usually given once a day, give as soon as possible. If you do not remember until the next day, do not give the missed dose at all, just follow the regular dosing schedule. Do not give double doses.

  3. If usually given every other day, give as soon as you remember. If you miss the scheduled time by a whole day, give it when you remember, then skip a day before giving the next dose. Do not give double doses. If you miss more than 1 dose, contact your child's doctor.

- Do not suddenly stop giving this drug before speaking with the doctor.

Side Effects

Tell your child's doctor about any side effects that are persistent or particularly bothersome.

More Common. Dizziness, false sense of well-being, fatigue, increased appetite, increased sweating, indigestion, leg cramps, menstrual irregularities, muscle weakness, nausea, swelling of the skin on the face, restlessness, sleep disorders, or weight gain

Less Common. It is important to tell the doctor if your child experiences abdominal enlargement or pain; acne; back or rib pain; bloody or black, tarry stools; blurred vision; convulsions; eye pain; fever and sore throat; headaches; slow healing of wounds; increased thirst and urination; depression; mood changes; muscle wasting; nightmares; peptic ulcers; rapid weight gain (3 to 5 pounds in a week); rash; shortness of breath; unusual bleeding or bruising; or unusual weakness.

Brand Names: Deltasone, Liquid Pred, Meticorten, Orasone, Panasol-S, Prednicen-M

Generic Available: Yes

Type of Drug: Adrenocorticosteroid hormone

Use: Treats a variety of disorders, including endocrine and rheumatic disorders; asthma; blood diseases; certain cancers; eye disorders; gastrointestinal disturbances such as ulcerative colitis; respiratory diseases; and inflammatory diseases such as arthritis, dermatitis, and poison ivy.

Time Required for Drug to Take Effect: Varies with illness being treated. It may be several days before this drug takes effect.

Dosage Forms and Strengths: Tablets (1 mg, 2.5 mg, 5 mg, 10 mg, 20 mg, 25 mg, 50 mg); Syrup (5 mg per 5 mL, with 5% alcohol); Solution (5 mg per 5 mL, with 5% alcohol); Solution, concentrated (5 mg per mL, with 30% alcohol)

Storage: Store at room temperature in tightly closed containers.

How This Drug Works: How this drug works is not completely understood.

Possible Drug Interactions

• Aspirin and anti-inflammatory medications such as ibuprofen, indomethacin, and ketoprofen may increase the stomach problems caused by this drug.

• Cholestyramine and colestipol can bind to this drug in the stomach and prevent its absorption.

Tell Your Child's Doctor If

• Your child is taking any other medications.

• Your child has had allergic reactions to this drug or other adrenocorticosteroids such as betamethasone, cortisone, dexamethasone, fluocinolone, hydrocortisone, methylpred-nisolone, prednisolone, and triamcinolone.

• Your child has recently been exposed to or currently has chicken pox or measles.

• Your child has any medical problems such as diabetes, glaucoma, fungal infections, heart disease, high blood pressure, peptic ulcers, thyroid disease, tuberculosis, ulcerative colitis, kidney disease, or liver disease.

• Your daughter is or becomes pregnant.

• Your daughter is breast-feeding her baby. This drug can pass into breast milk; however, the American Academy of Pediatrics considers it compatible with breast-feeding in most cases.

Special Instructions

• Do not have your child vaccinated or immunized while taking this drug. This drug decreases the effectiveness of vaccines and can lead to infection if a live virus vaccine is given.

Symptoms of Overdose: Your child may show severe restlessness.

Special Notes

• With long-term use, the doctor may want your child to be on a low-salt and potassium-rich diet. The doctor may also want your child's eyes examined periodically during treatment to detect glaucoma and cataracts.

• With long-term use, the doctor may need to increase your child's dose during times of stress such as serious infection, injury, or surgery.

PRIMIDONE

Administration Guidelines

- Usually given 2 or 3 times a day. Try to give at the same times each day.

- May be taken on an empty stomach or with food, but be consistent.

- Shake suspension thoroughly for several minutes before measuring each dose.

- Do not stop giving this drug without first speaking with your child's doctor. Stopping this drug abruptly could lead to severe seizures called status epilepticus.

- Missed doses: Give as soon as possible and stagger remaining doses for that day at regular intervals. However, if it's within 3 hours of the next dose, skip the missed dose and give the next regular dose. Do not give double doses.

- Ask the pharmacist to dispense the same brand for each prescription.

Side Effects

Tell your child's doctor about any side effects that are persistent or particularly bothersome.

More Common. Dizziness, fatigue, upset stomach, excitement, agitation. Contact the doctor if your child develops a skin rash.

Less Common. Mood changes, irritability, low blood counts, constipation. Contact the doctor if your child experiences unusual bleeding or bruising, an increasing number of convulsions, difficulty breathing, yellowing of the eyes or skin, swelling of the face or eyes, fever, sore throat, or mouth sores.

Possible Drug Interactions

- Acetazolamide, carbamazepine, ethosuximide, and rifampin can decrease blood concentrations of this drug and higher doses may be required.

- Phenytoin, valproic acid, and isoniazid may increase blood concentrations of this drug, and lower doses may be required.

- Alcohol, antihistamines, tranquilizers, muscle relaxants, and pain medications may increase drowsiness.

- May decrease the effectiveness of warfarin, beta blockers, carbamazepine, clonazepam, oral contraceptives, corticosteroids, quinidine, theophylline, and verapamil.

Brand Name: Mysoline

Generic Available: Yes

Type of Drug: Anticonvulsant, anti-epileptic

Use: Treats seizure disorders (epilepsy)

Time Required for Drug to Take Effect: Several days to several weeks.

Dosage Forms and Strengths: Tablets (50 mg, 250 mg); Suspension (250 mg/5 mL)

Storage: Store at room temperature in tightly closed, light-resistant containers.

How This Drug Works: Controls abnormal impulses in the brain that cause convulsions.

Tell Your Child's Doctor If

• Your child has had allergic reactions to or is taking any other medications.

• Your child has liver or kidney disease, porphyria, or any other diseases.

• Your daughter is or becomes pregnant. Seizure disorders should be controlled by a doctor during pregnancy.

• Your daughter is breast-feeding her baby. This drug can pass into breast milk and cause drowsiness and other side effects in the infant.

Symptoms of Overdose: Clumsiness, slurred speech, confusion, drunken appearance

Special Notes

• Partially converted to phenobarbital in the body, which also helps control seizures. Your child will require blood tests for this drug and phenobarbital levels while taking this drug.

• Make sure you know how your child is reacting to this drug before allowing participation in activities that require alertness, such as riding a bicycle.

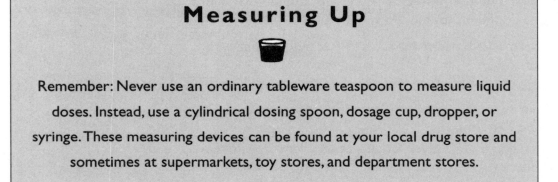

Measuring Up

Remember: Never use an ordinary tableware teaspoon to measure liquid doses. Instead, use a cylindrical dosing spoon, dosage cup, dropper, or syringe. These measuring devices can be found at your local drug store and sometimes at supermarkets, toy stores, and department stores.

PROCAINAMIDE

Administration Guidelines

• Can be given with food.

• Do not crush or allow your child to chew the sustained-release tablets. They should be swallowed whole.

• Usually given 4 or more times daily. Try to give at the same time each day.

• Missed doses: Give as soon as possible if you remember within 2 hours (4 hours for sustained-release tablets). However, if it's almost time for the next dose, skip the missed dose and give the next regular dose. Do not give double doses.

• Do not stop giving this drug or give more than the prescribed amount without first speaking with your child's doctor.

Side Effects

Tell your child's doctor about any side effects that are persistent or particularly bothersome.

More Common. Upset stomach, loss of appetite, nausea, vomiting, bitter taste. Contact the doctor if your child experiences palpitations, fever, chills, skin rash, or dizziness.

Less Common. Tremor, low blood counts, weakness. Contact the doctor if your child experiences sore throat, mouth sores, swelling of the feet or ankles, fainting, dark urine, yellowing of the eyes or skin, hallucinations, or chest pain.

Possible Drug Interactions

• Beta blockers, cimetidine, ranitidine, quinidine, and trimethoprim (found in Septra and Bactrim) increase the effects of this drug.

Tell Your Child's Doctor If

• Your child has had allergic reactions to or is taking any other medications.

• Your child has liver, kidney, or heart disease; lupus; or any other diseases.

• Your daughter is or becomes pregnant.

• Your daughter is breast-feeding her baby. This drug can pass into breast milk; however, the American Academy of Pediatrics considers it compatible with breast-feeding in most cases.

Symptoms of Overdose: Increased number and severity of palpitations, fainting

Brand Names: Pronestyl, Procan-SR, Pronestyl SR

Generic Available: Yes

Type of Drug: Antiarrhythmic

Use: Treats abnormal heart rhythms.

Time Required for Drug to Take Effect: Several days

Dosage Forms and Strengths: Tablets (250 mg, 375 mg, 500 mg); Capsules (250 mg, 375 mg, 500 mg); Tablets, sustained-release (250 mg, 500 mg, 750 mg, 1000 mg); Injection (100 mg/ml, 500 mg/ml). A special liquid formulation can be prepared by the pharmacist if necessary.

Storage: Store at room temperature in tightly closed, light-resistant containers. Refrigerate the special liquid.

How This Drug Works: Controls electrical impulses in the heart.

Special Notes

• Partially converted in the body to N-acetyl procainamide (NAPA), which also helps control abnormal rhythms. Your child will need blood tests for procainamide and NAPA levels while taking this drug.

• It is normal to see empty tablets in the stools of children taking sustained-release tablets.

• Your child will need to have weekly blood tests to check red blood cells, white blood cells, and platelets for the first 3 months of therapy and periodically thereafter.

Teach Your Children Well

Let's face it. Kids can be pretty stubborn when it comes to accepting medication. When appropriate, try giving your child information about his or her condition and how the medicine works. In a nonthreatening voice, talk about the consequences of not taking the medication, reminding the child perhaps of how uncomfortable he or she was before beginning the medication. Use reasoning when possible, but don't scare the child. Children who understand the importance of antibiotics for infection, insulin for diabetes, or inhalants for asthma are more likely to take the medication without objection.

PROCHLORPERAZINE

Administration Guidelines

- Give with food or a full glass of water or milk to decrease stomach upset.

- Do not spill syrup on skin or clothing. It can cause a skin rash.

- Do not use syrup if markedly discolored. A slight yellowing of color is acceptable.

- Do not break, crush, or allow your child to chew extended-release capsules.

- Missed doses: Give as soon as you remember. If on a regular schedule, give any remaining doses for that day at regularly spaced intervals. Do not give double doses.

- Do not give within 2 hours of giving antacids or medicine for diarrhea.

- Do not give this drug to children who weigh less than 22 pounds (10 kg) or who are younger than 2 years of age.

- Do not stop giving this drug without first checking with the doctor if your child is taking it for problems other than nausea and vomiting. The doctor may want to gradually reduce the dose.

Side Effects

Tell your child's doctor about any side effects that are persistent or particularly bothersome.

More Common. Constipation, decreased sweating, dizziness, drowsiness, dry mouth, stuffy nose, low blood pressure, stomach upset, nausea, vomiting, weight gain, blurred vision, difficulty urinating, changes in menstrual period. Contact the doctor immediately if your child experiences lip smacking or puckering, puffing of cheeks, rapid or fine wormlike tongue movements, uncontrolled chewing movements, uncontrolled arm or leg movements, blurred vision, change in color perception, difficulty seeing at night, difficulty in speaking or swallowing, fainting, inability to move eyes, loss of balance, masklike face, muscle spasms, restlessness or need to keep moving, shuffling walk, stiffness of arms or legs, twitching movements, trembling and shaking, twisting body movements, weakness of arms and legs, skin rash, or severe sunburn.

Less Common. Contact the doctor immediately if your child experiences sore throat, seizures, difficult or fast breathing, fast or irregular heartbeat, fever, high or low blood pressure, increased sweating, loss of bladder control, severe muscle stiffness, pale skin, or unusual fatigue or weakness.

Brand Name: Compazine

Generic Available: Yes (in tablet form only)

Type of Drug: Antiemetic; antipsychotic agent, phenothiazine class

Use: Treats severe and prolonged nausea and vomiting that has a known cause. Also treats acute and chronic psychoses.

Time Required for Drug to Take Effect: 1 hour for nausea and vomiting. It may take 6 weeks to 6 months to achieve full benefit for mental disorders.

Dosage Forms and Strengths: Tablets (5 mg, 10 mg, 25 mg); Capsules, long-acting (10 mg, 15 mg, 30 mg); Syrup (5 mg / 5 mL); Suppository (2.5 mg, 5 mg, 25 mg); Injection (5 mg/mL)

Storage: Store at room temperature in tightly closed, light-resistant containers. Do not freeze the syrup.

How This Drug Works: Causes complex changes in the central nervous system producing antiemetic and tranquilizing effects.

Possible Drug Interactions

• Central nervous system depressants such as alcohol, antihistamines, cold preparations, muscle relaxants, tranquilizers, and some pain medications may cause extreme drowsiness when used with this drug.

• Cough and cold products may increase the chance of heat stroke, dizziness, dry mouth, blurred vision, and constipation.

• Antidepressants, monoamine oxidase (MAO) inhibitors, or lithium can cause an increase in side effects of both drugs. These medications need to be dosed carefully when used with this drug.

• Medications to lower blood pressure may lead to blood pressure that is too low.

• Epinephrine may cause low blood pressure.

Tell Your Child's Doctor If

• Your child has had an allergic reaction to this drug or any other medication.

• Your child has taken or is taking any other prescription or nonprescription medicine.

• Your child has lung or heart disease, seizures, glaucoma, liver or kidney disease, difficult urination, stomach ulcers, a bone marrow or blood disorder, Reye syndrome, or any other medical condition.

• The blurred vision continues beyond the first few weeks or gets worse.

• Your child develops a rash from the sun.

• Your child is taking this drug before having surgery or any medical or dental treatment.

• Your child continues to have a dry mouth after 2 weeks. Continued dry mouth can lead to cavities.

• Your child develops side effects after this drug has been stopped.

• Your child abuses alcohol.

• Your daughter is or becomes pregnant.

• Your daughter is breast-feeding her baby. This drug can pass into breast milk, and the American Academy of Pediatrics is concerned about its effect on the baby.

Special Instructions

• Give this drug only as directed by the doctor.

• Protect your child from overheating during exercise, play, or hot weather as this drug decreases sweating and can cause an increase in body temperature. Hot baths, hot tubs, or saunas may make your child dizzy or faint.

• Dress your child warmly as this drug increases sensitivity to cold weather.

• This drug may cause a skin rash or severe sunburn from exposure to sunlight or ultraviolet light. Your child should avoid sunlamps and wear an effective sunscreen, protective clothing, and sunglasses when out-of-doors.

• Do not allow your child to drink alcohol while taking this drug.

• Do not give other medicines that may make your child sleepy.

• Have your child stand up slowly to prevent dizziness or light-headedness.

• Do not give your child cough or cold products without checking with the doctor.

Symptoms of Overdose: Deep sleep, coma, low blood pressure, increased severity of side effects listed above

Special Notes

• Safer antiemetics should be tried before giving this drug. It has a very high incidence of adverse reactions in children.

• Make sure you know how your child is reacting to this drug before allowing participation in any activity that requires alertness and coordination, such as riding a bicycle. This drug may cause your child to be dizzy, drowsy, less alert, or to have blurred vision.

- With long-term use, this drug may cause serious side effects that may not go away after this drug is stopped. Discuss this with the doctor.

- Some products contain tartrazine dye. Ask the pharmacist for a tartrazine-free product if your child is allergic to this dye or aspirin.

- Doses for antipsychotic effect are increased slowly to decrease the side effects.

- Your child's progress should be checked regularly by the doctor.

- With long-term use, the effects of this drug may last up to 1 week after you stop giving it.

Keep a Lid on It

Pharmacists are required to put drugs in bottles that have child-resistant caps. Don't switch to a bottle that's easier for you to open—children may also find it easier to open. Remember, too, that child-resistant does not mean childproof. Children older than five years may be able to open most medicine bottles. That's why it's essential for you to teach them that drugs can be harmful if not taken correctly and that children need supervision before taking anything. And, just to be on the safe side, keep all medicines out of your child's reach.

Brand Names: Phenergan, Anergan, Phenazine, Phencen, Prometh, Prorex, V-Gan

Generic Available: Yes

Type of Drug: Antihistamine, antiemetic, antivertigo agent, sedative

Use: Treats allergic conditions, nausea, vomiting, and motion sickness. Provides sedation for test procedures or surgery.

Time Required for Drug to Take Effect: 15 to 60 minutes for oral administration; 20 minutes for rectal administration

Dosage Forms and Strengths: Tablets (12.5 mg, 25 mg, 50 mg); Suppository (12.5 mg, 25 mg, 50 mg); Syrup (6.25 mg/5mL, 25 mg/5mL; Injection (25 mg/mL, 50 mg/mL). Also found in some prescription cough and cold products.

Storage: Store tablets, syrup, and injection at room temperature in tightly closed, light-resistant containers. Refrigerate suppository. Do not freeze syrup or injection.

How This Drug Works: Blocks histamine receptors in the body and the dopaminergic and alpha-adrenergic receptors in the brain.

PROMETHAZINE

Administration Guidelines

- Give with food or a full glass of water or milk to decrease stomach upset.

- For motion sickness, give 30 to 60 minutes before your child begins to travel.

- Missed doses: If you remember within 1 hour, give the missed dose. Otherwise skip the missed dose and go back to the regular schedule. Do not give double doses.

Side Effects

Tell your child's doctor about any side effects that are persistent or particularly bothersome.

More Common. Drowsiness, thickening of mucus, headache, fatigue, nervousness, dizziness, dry mouth, abdominal pain, nausea, diarrhea, increase appetite, joint pain, sore throat

Less Common. Blurred vision, confusion, difficult urination, increased sweating, loss of appetite, nightmares, unusual excitement, ringing in ears, skin rash. Contact the doctor if your child experiences sore throat and fever, unusual bleeding or bruising, unusual fatigue, weakness, or any involuntary muscle movements.

Possible Drug Interactions

- Central nervous system depressants such as alcohol, antihistamines, cold preparations, muscle relaxants, tranquilizers, and some pain medications may cause extreme drowsiness when used with this drug.

- Cough and cold products may increase the chance of heat stroke, dizziness, dry mouth, blurred vision, and constipation.

- Antidepressants, monoamine oxidase (MAO) inhibitors, or antipsychotics may lead to increased side effects.

- Antithyroid drugs can cause an increase in rare blood disorders when used with this drug.

- Epinephrine may cause low blood pressure.

Tell Your Child's Doctor If

- Your child has had an allergic reaction to this drug or any other medication.

- Your child is taking any other prescription or nonprescription medicine.

- Your child has asthma, sleep apnea, lung disease, heart disease, seizures, glaucoma, liver or kidney disease, difficult urination, Reye syndrome, or any other medical condition.

- Your child continues to have a dry mouth after 2 weeks. Continued dry mouth can lead to cavities.

- Your daughter is or becomes pregnant.

- Your daughter is breast-feeding her baby. This medicine can pass into breast milk, and the American Academy of Pediatrics has expressed concern about the effect of similar medications on the baby.

Special Instructions

- If your child is having skin tests for allergies, tell the doctor who is doing the test that your child is taking this drug.

- Do not allow your child to drink alcohol while taking this drug.

- Do not give other medicines that may make your child sleepy.

- Do not increase the dose of this drug unless directed by the doctor.

- Your child should wear sunscreen and protective clothing when out-of-doors.

Symptoms of Overdose: Coma; clumsiness; severe drowsiness; severe dry mouth, nose, and throat; redness of face; shortness of breath or other trouble with breathing; hallucinations; seizures; trouble sleeping; muscle spasms; restlessness; shuffling walk; jerky movement of head and face; trembling and shaking of hands

Special Notes

- Make sure you know how your child is reacting to this drug before allowing participation in activities that require alertness and coordination, such as riding a bicycle. This drug may cause your child to feel dizzy, drowsy, or less alert.

- Newborns and children with dehydration, acute infections, or acute illnesses have an increased risk of severe side effects.

- This drug is not recommended for children younger than 2 years of age because of an increased risk of sudden infant death syndrome (SIDS).

- Oral solutions may contain alcohol.

Brand Names: Inderal, Inderal LA

Generic Available: Yes

Type of Drug: Beta-adrenergic blocking agent (beta blocker)

Use: Treats high blood pressure (hypertension), abnormally fast heart rhythms (tachycardia), and chest pain (angina). Has also been used to treat tremors and certain emotional disturbances and to prevent bleeding in liver disease, migraine headaches, and alcohol withdrawal symptoms.

Time Required for Drug to Take Effect: Several days to several weeks

Dosage Forms and Strengths: Tablets (10 mg, 20 mg, 40 mg, 60 mg, 80 mg, 90 mg); Capsules, sustained-release (60 mg, 80 mg, 120 mg, 160 mg); Solution (20 mg/5 mL and 40 mg/5 mL); Concentrate (80 mg/mL); Injection (1 mg/mL)

Storage: Store at room temperature in tightly closed, light-resistant containers.

How This Drug Works: Controls nerve impulses that excite the heart, causing the heart to beat more slowly.

PROPRANOLOL

Administration Guidelines

- Usually given 1 to 4 times a day. Try to give the dose(s) at approximately the same time each day.

- May be given with food or milk.

- Measure concentrate with the dropper provided, and mix with water, juice, or soda. Make sure your child drinks the full amount of the beverage in which the solution was mixed.

- Do not stop giving this drug without first speaking with your child's doctor. Stopping this drug abruptly can increase blood pressure.

- Missed doses: Give as soon as possible. However, if it's almost time for the next dose, skip the missed dose. Do not give double doses. Call the doctor or pharmacist for more specific instructions.

Side Effects

Tell your child's doctor about any side effects that are persistent or particularly bothersome.

More Common. Vivid dreams, constipation or diarrhea, upset stomach, difficulty sleeping, fatigue, dizziness, headache. Contact the doctor if your child experiences difficulty breathing or nightmares.

Less Common. Allergic reactions, cold hands or feet, dry eyes and mouth. Contact the doctor if your child experiences swelling of the feet or legs, palpitations, hallucinations, confusion, unusual bleeding or bruising, or tingling of fingers or toes.

Possible Drug Interactions

- Cimetidine (Tagamet), birth control pills, clonidine, digoxin, phenothiazine-type drugs (Compazine, Phenergan, Thorazine), and monoamine oxidase (MAO) inhibitors (Nardil, Parnate) can increase the side effects of this drug.

- Decongestants in cough, cold, allergy, asthma, weight control, and sinus medications can increase blood pressure when taken with this drug.

- Alcohol, barbiturate sedatives (phenobarbital and others), nonsteroidal anti-inflammatory drugs (indomethacin and others), and rifampin can decrease the effectiveness of this drug.

- Can offset the therapeutic effect of asthma medications such as theophylline, albuterol, terbutaline, and metaproterenol.

Tell Your Child's Doctor If

• Your child has had allergic reactions to or is taking any other medications.

• Your child has allergies; asthma; wheezing; slow heartbeat; diabetes mellitus; heart, blood vessel, liver, thyroid, or kidney disease; or any other diseases.

• Your daughter is or becomes pregnant.

• Your daughter is breast-feeding her baby. This drug can pass into breast milk; however, the American Academy of Pediatrics considers it compatible with breast-feeding in most cases.

Symptoms of Overdose: Excessively slow heartbeat and low blood pressure, difficulty breathing, unconsciousness

Special Notes

• This drug can affect blood sugar levels in children with diabetes and hide signs and symptoms of low blood sugar, such as a fast heartbeat.

• Make sure you know how your child is reacting to this drug before allowing participation in activities that require alertness, such as riding a bicycle.

Be Accurate

If you don't give medication correctly, it may be ineffective or even cause side effects. An estimated 10 to 30 percent of medications aren't effective because they have been given incorrectly. To do it right, you have to give the exact amount of medicine prescribed at the scheduled time, for the specified duration, and in the appropriate manner. Always read the label, follow the directions carefully, and use the appropriate equipment for measuring and administering the medication. Also, be sure to wash your hands before you give any medication to your child.

Brand Name: None

Generic Available: Yes

Type of Drug: Antithyroid agent

Use: Treats high blood thyroid concentrations.

Time Required for Drug to Take Effect: Onset in 24 to 36 hours, but it may take 4 or more months to normalize thyroid hormone levels.

Dosage Form and Strength: Tablets (50 mg)

Storage: Store at room temperature in tightly closed containers.

How This Drug Works: Inhibits the synthesis of thyroid hormones.

PROPYLTHIOURACIL (PTU)

Administration Guidelines

- Give with food.

- Give at the same time in relation to meals every day.

- Usually given every 8 or 12 hours around the clock.

- Missed doses: Give as soon as possible, even if it's time for the next dose. You can give the missed dose and the next dose together. If you miss more than one dose, call your child's doctor.

- Do not stop giving this drug without first checking with the doctor.

Side Effects

Tell your child's doctor about any side effects that are persistent or particularly bothersome.

More Common. Dizziness, nausea, vomiting, stomach pain. Contact the doctor if your child experiences fever, skin rash, or itching.

Less Common. Contact the doctor if your child experiences chills; a general feeling of discomfort, illness, or weakness; hoarseness; mouth sores; pain, swelling, or redness in the joints; throat infection; yellow eyes or skin; backache; black stools; blood in urine or stools; shortness of breath; increased bleeding or bruising; an increase or decrease in urination; numbness or tingling of fingers, toes, or face; pinpoint red spots on the skin; swelling of feet or lower legs; swollen lymph nodes; swollen salivary glands; changes in menstrual periods; coldness; constipation; dry, puffy skin; headache; sleepiness; fatigue; weight gain.

Possible Drug Interactions

- Increases the effect of warfarin. Dosage of warfarin may need to be decreased.

Tell Your Child's Doctor If

- Your child has had an allergic reaction to this drug or any other medication.

- Your child has been or is taking any other prescription or nonprescription medicine.

- Your child develops a new medical condition.

- Your child has heart, liver, or kidney disease, or any other medical condition.

- Your daughter is or becomes pregnant.

- Your daughter is breast-feeding her baby. The American Academy of Pediatrics considers this drug compatible with breast-feeding, but the baby may need to have the thyroid function measured.

Special Instructions

• Give this drug only as directed by the doctor.

• Do not let your child have surgery or any medical or dental treatment unless you tell the doctor or dentist that your child is taking this drug.

• Do not give any other medication without first checking with the pharmacist or doctor.

Symptoms of Overdose: Nausea, vomiting, joint pain, headache, fever, excitement or depression, heartburnlike pain

Special Notes

• Your child's progress should be checked with regular visits to the doctor.

• The doctor may perform routine tests to monitor the effects of this drug in your child's blood cells, liver, and thyroid.

Just Call

If you have any concerns about any side effects, even minor ones, you should be sure to discuss them with your child's doctor. The doctor may be able to minimize or eliminate the side effects by prescribing a different medication or changing your child's dosage, dosing schedule, or the way the drug is given. (Do not make adjustments on your own without discussing them with your doctor.) At the very least, the doctor can assure you that the medication's benefits far outweigh its side effects.

Brand Names: Afrinol,* Cenafed,* Decofed Syrup,* Drixoral Non-Drowsy,* Neofed,* Novafed,* PediaCare Oral,* Sudafed,* Sudafed 12 Hour,* Sufedrin,* Triaminic AM Decongestant Formula.* Also available in combination with other products. (*available over the counter)

Generic Available: Yes

Type of Drug: Decongestant

Use: Temporarily relieves nasal congestion due to the common cold, upper respiratory allergies, and sinusitis; also promotes nasal or sinus drainage.

Time Required for Drug to Take Effect: 15 to 30 minutes

Dosage Forms and Strengths: Capsules (60 mg); Capsules, timed-release, as hydrochloride (120 mg); Drops (7.5 mg/0.8 mL); Liquid (15 mg/5 mL, 30 mg/5 mL); Tablets (30 mg, 60 mg); Tablets, timed-release, as hydrochloride (120 mg); Tablets, extended-release, as sulfate (120 mg).

Storage: Store at room temperature in tightly closed, light-resistant containers.

How This Drug Works: Constricts blood vessels in the nasal passages.

PSEUDOEPHEDRINE
Administration Guidelines
• Give on an empty stomach or with food or milk to avoid stomach irritation.

• Do not break, crush, or allow your child to chew timed-release tablets.

• Missed doses: Give as soon as possible. However, if it is within 30 to 90 minutes of a dose given every 6 hours, or 2 to 3 hours for doses given every 12 hours, skip the missed dose and return to your regular dosing schedule. Do not give double doses.

• Do not use longer than 3 to 5 days.

Side Effects
Tell your child's doctor about any side effects that are persistent or particularly bothersome.

More Common. Rapid or pounding heartbeat, nervousness, excitation, dizziness, insomnia, drowsiness, headache

Less Common. Nausea, vomiting, tremors, difficult urination

Possible Drug Interactions
• Monoamine oxidase (MAO) inhibitors such as isocarboxazid, pargyline, phenelzine, and tranylcypromine may prolong and intensify the effects of this drug.

• May reduce the antihypertensive effects of methyldopa, mecamylamine, and reserpine; this may cause an increase in blood pressure.

• Beta blockers may increase the effects of this drug, causing an increase in its side effects.

• Digoxin and nonprescription asthma, allergy, cough, cold, diet, or sinus preparations may increase the side effects of this drug.

Tell Your Child's Doctor If
• Your child is taking any medications, especially any of those listed above.

• Your child has had unusual or allergic reactions to any medications, especially to this drug or other adrenergic agents such as albuterol, amphetamines, ephedrine, epinephrine, isoproterenol, metaproterenol, norepinephrine, phenylpropanolamine, and terbutaline.

• Your child has or ever had diabetes mellitus, epilepsy, heart or blood-vessel disease, high blood pressure, obstructed bladder or intestinal tract, peptic ulcers, or thyroid disease.

Special Instructions

• Make sure you know how your child is reacting to this drug before allowing participation in activities that require alertness, such as riding a bicycle.

Symptoms of Overdose: Sleepiness, sedation, or coma. Sedation may be accompanied by profuse sweating, low blood pressure, or shock.

Keep It Out of Reach

Do not rely on a child-resistant cap to deter your child from opening a bottle of medication. Child-resistant does not mean childproof. Legally, a cap can be called child-resistant if 80 percent of all five-year-olds need more than five minutes to open it. That means the other 20 percent could get into it in even less time. Put the bottle in a hard-to-reach cabinet with a childproof lock. Do not keep it on the countertop, kitchen table, or nightstand.

Brand Names: Metamucil,* Fiberall Powder,* Fiberall Wafer,* Modane Bulk,* Perdiem Fiber,* Konsyl,* Reguloid,* Serutan,* Syllact,* Natural Vegetable* (*available over the counter)

Generic Available: Yes

Type of Drug: Laxative, bulk-forming

Use: Treats and prevents constipation; also treats irritable bowel syndrome.

Time Required for Drug to Take Effect: 12 to 24 hours; peak effect in 2 to 3 days

Dosage Forms and Strengths: Powder (3.5 gm); Granules (4 gm); Powder, effervescent (3.5 gm/ packet); Wafers, chewable (1.7 gm, 3.4 gm)

Storage: Store at room temperature in tightly-closed containers

How This Drug Works: Adsorbs water in the intestine to increase the volume of the stool, promoting its movement through the intestine.

PSYLLIUM

Administration Guidelines

• Mix powder with water or juice. Give immediately after mixing with water as this drug thickens quickly. One full glass (8 oz.) of liquid must be consumed with every dose, including the amount in which the powder is mixed.

• Have your child chew the wafer well and drink a full glass of liquid with it.

• Increase your child's intake of water or other fluids.

• Usually given 1 to 4 times a day.

• Granules should not be chewed.

• Do not give within 3 hours of other medications.

• Do not give to children younger than 6 years of age unless prescribed by your child's doctor.

• Do not give regularly for more than 1 week unless prescribed by the doctor.

Side Effects

Tell your child's doctor about any side effects that are persistent or particularly bothersome.

More Common. Diarrhea, constipation, abdominal cramps. Contact the doctor if your child experiences difficulty swallowing or intestinal blockage.

Less Common. Contact the doctor if your child experiences runny nose, watery eyes, or wheezing.

Possible Drug Interactions

• Decreases the absorption of digoxin and warfarin.

Tell Your Child's Doctor If

• Your child has had an allergic reaction to this drug or any other medication.

• Your child has taken or is taking any other prescription or nonprescription medicine.

• Your child has a history of taking medication for treatment of constipation.

• Your child has kidney, liver, or heart disease; intestinal blockage; other intestinal problems; diabetes mellitus; high blood pressure; rectal bleeding; or any other medical condition.

- Your child experiences a sudden change in bowel movements that either lasts longer than 2 weeks or returns intermittently.

- Your daughter is or becomes pregnant.

Special Instructions
- Do not give if your child has abdominal pain, appendicitis, intestinal blockage, nausea, vomiting, or rectal bleeding.

Symptoms of Overdose: Abdominal pain, diarrhea, constipation

Special Notes
- Inhaling the powder can cause asthmalike symptoms or allergic reactions in some children.

- Many products contain sugars and will increase blood sugars in children with diabetes. Ask the pharmacist for a sugar-free product.

- Some products may contain aspartame and cannot be used if your child has phenylketonuria. Ask the pharmacist for a product that does not contain aspartame.

- If this drug is not mixed with enough water, it can obstruct the esophagus and intestine. If your child does not drink plenty of fluids during the day, constipation or intestinal obstruction also can occur.

- Available in regular, orange, lemon-lime, strawberry, and other fruit flavors.

- Some products are sugar free.

Over-the-Counter Wisdom

Keep in mind that even a medication that is available without a doctor's prescription may still be harmful and should be given appropriately and only when necessary. Talk to your pediatrician about what to do if your child gets sick. Some illnesses can be treated at home, some require a call to the pediatrician's office, and some will require a visit to the doctor. In addition, ask the doctor what situations constitute an emergency. If you're not sure if it's safe or appropriate to give your child a particular over-the-counter medication, be sure to talk to the doctor first.

Brand Name: None

Generic Available: Yes

Type of Drug: Antitubercular antibiotic

Use: Treats tuberculosis infections.

Time Required for Drug to Take Effect: Adequate treatment requires several months.

Dosage Form and Strength: Tablets (500 mg)

Storage: Store at room temperature in tightly closed, light-resistant containers.

How This Drug Works: Slows the growth of the tuberculosis organism.

PYRAZINAMIDE

Administration Guidelines

• Usually given once a day. Under some circumstances, it may be given 2 times a week.

• Don't stop giving this drug even if your child is feeling better. To be effective, tuberculosis treatment must be continued for several months.

• Missed doses: Give as soon as possible. However, if it's within 6 hours of the next dose, skip the missed dose and give the next regular dose. Do not give double doses.

Side Effects

Tell your child's doctor about any side effects that are persistent or particularly bothersome.

More Common. Nausea, vomiting, loss of appetite, muscle and joint pains. Contact the doctor if your child experiences yellowing of the eyes or skin or flulike symptoms.

Less Common. Fever, anemia, itching. Contact the doctor if your child experiences weakness, swelling, pains in the hands or feet (gout), rashes, or difficulty urinating.

Tell Your Child's Doctor If

• Your child has had allergic reactions to any medications.

• Your child has any other diseases.

• Your child has been or is taking any other medications.

• Your child has liver or kidney disease.

• Your daughter becomes pregnant. It is not known if this drug affects the fetus.

• Your daughter is breast-feeding her baby. This drug can pass into breast milk and should be used with caution in nursing mothers.

Special Notes

• Usually used in combination with 3 to 4 other antitubercular antibiotics.

• Your child should have periodic blood tests for liver function while taking this drug.

PYRETHRIN

Administration Guidelines
• Apply enough gel, shampoo, or solution to cover the affected hairy and adjacent areas.

• Do not use near the eyes or allow to come in contact with mucous membranes. Flush eyes thoroughly with water if they come in contact with this drug.

• Do not apply to inflamed skin or raw, oozing surfaces.

• Shake containers before using.

Side Effects
Tell your child's doctor about any side effects that are persistent or particularly bothersome.

Less Common. Local irritation (flushing of the skin; itching; allergic reaction in which red, round wheals develop on the skin; swelling; inflammation of the skin; corneal erosion)

Tell Your Child's Doctor If
• Your daughter is pregnant or is breast-feeding her baby. This drug is recommended for the treatment of lice in infants, children 2 years of age and younger, and pregnant or lactating women instead of lindane (G-well, Kwell, Scabene).

Special Instructions
• Do not use to treat lice in the eyelashes.

• Remove all clothing and bed linen that may have been contaminated by your child. Machine wash in hot water and dry in a hot dryer or dry-clean following treatment.

Symptoms of Overdose: Nausea, vomiting, diarrhea, central nervous system depression

Special Notes
• Contains pyrethrins with piperonyl butoxide.

Brand Names: Blue Gel, Tisit Blue Gel, Clear Lice Elimination System Kit, Licide, Pyrinyl Plus, R&C Shampoo, RID Lice Killing Shampoo, Tisit Shampoo, Triple X, A-200 Pediculicide, Pronto Lice-Killing Shampoo Kit, Barc Liquid, Tisit Liquid, Pyrinyl II

Generic Available: Yes

Type of Drug: Pediculicide

Use: Treats lice infestations.

Time Required for Drug to Take Effect: Treatments take 10 minutes each; should be repeated after 7 to 10 days.

Dosage Forms and Strengths: Gel (pyrethrins 0.3% with piperonyl butoxide 3%); Shampoo (pyrethrins 0.3% with piperonyl butoxide 3%, pyrethrins 0.33% with piperonyl butoxide 4%); Solution (pyrethrins 0.18% with piperonyl butoxide 2.2%, pyrethrins 0.3% with piperonyl butoxide 2%, pyrethrins 0.3% with piperonyl butoxide 3%)

Storage: Store in tightly closed containers at room temperature (below 40°C or 104°F).

How This Drug Works: Blocks nerve impulse transmissions of arthropods; paralysis and death of lice follow.

Brand Name: Daraprim

Generic Available: No

Type of Drug: Antimalarial agent

Use: Suppresses malaria due to susceptible strains of plasmodia.

Time Required for Drug to Take Effect: For protection, begin giving this drug 2 weeks before exposure; this drug should be continued during and for 6 to 10 weeks after exposure to malaria.

Dosage Form and Strength: Tablets (25 mg)

Storage: Store in tightly closed, light-resistant containers.

How This Drug Works: Interferes with the synthesis of tetrahydrofolic acid in malarial parasites.

PYRIMETHAMINE

Administration Guidelines
• Take with meals to minimize vomiting.

Side Effects
Tell your child's doctor about any side effects that are persistent or particularly bothersome.

MORE COMMON. Anorexia, vomiting

LESS COMMON. Insomnia, headache, light-headedness, dryness of the mouth or throat, fever, malaise (general feeling of being unwell), dermatitis (inflammation of the skin), abnormal skin pigmentation, depression, seizures

Possible Drug Interactions
• Antifolic drugs such as methotrexate and sulfonamides such as Septra, Bactrim, Cotrim, and Sulfatrim inhibit the uptake of folic acid and decrease nucleoprotein synthesis.

Tell Your Child's Doctor If
• Your child experiences rash, sore throat, pallor, or glossitis (inflammation of the tongue).

• Your child has impaired renal or hepatic (liver) function, or a possible folate deficiency.

• Your daughter becomes pregnant or is breast-feeding her baby.

Special Instructions
• Continue giving this drug for at least 6 to 10 weeks after leaving the area of potential exposure.

• Discontinue this drug and seek medical attention at the first sign of a skin rash.

• Do not miss or delay scheduled blood tests; these tests are essential for patients receiving high doses of this drug.

• Keep out of the reach of children as they are extremely susceptible to adverse effects from an overdose. Accidental ingestion of this drug has been fatal in children.

Symptoms of Overdose: Initial symptoms usually involve the gastrointestinal tract and may include abdominal pain, nausea, and severe and repeated vomiting, possibly including the vomiting of blood. Acute intoxication may involve gastrointestinal symptoms or central nervous system stimulation including excitability and generalized and prolonged convulsions; this may be followed by respiratory depression, circulatory collapse, and death within a few hours.

RANITIDINE

Administration Guidelines

• Give with food or milk.

• Usually given 1 to 4 times a day.

• Dissolve effervescent tablets and granules in 6 to 8 oz. water before use.

• At least 1 hour should separate doses of antacids from doses of this drug.

• Missed doses: Give as soon as possible. However, if it's within a couple hours of the next dose, skip the missed dose. Do not give double doses.

Side Effects

Tell your child's doctor if your child experiences any side effects that are persistent or particularly bothersome.

More Common. Constipation, diarrhea, dizziness, headache, nausea, or stomach upset

Less Common. Tell the doctor if your child experiences confusion, unusual bleeding or bruising, or weakness.

Possible Drug Interactions

• Increases the blood-sugar-lowering effects of glipizide.

• Decreases the elimination of warfarin from the body, which can increase the risk of bleeding complications.

• Causes a false-positive result with the Multistix® urine protein test.

Tell Your Child's Doctor If

• Your child is allergic to this drug.

• Your child has kidney or liver disease

• Your daughter is or becomes pregnant.

Symptoms of Overdose: Rapid respiration, muscle tremors, rapid heart rate, severe nausea, and vomiting

Special Notes

• Available over the counter.

• Consult the doctor before giving this drug to children younger than 12 years of age.

Brand Name: Zantac

Generic Available: Syrup only

Type of Drug: Gastric-acid-secretion inhibitor (decreases stomach acid)

Use: Treats duodenal and gastric ulcers. Also used in long-term treatment of excessive stomach acid secretion, prevention of recurrent ulcers, and treatment of heartburn.

Time Required for Drug to Take Effect: Within 1 to 3 hours

Dosage Forms and Strengths: Tablets (150 mg and 300 mg); Tablets, effervescent (150 mg); Syrup (15 mg per mL); Capsules (150 mg, 300 mg); Granules, effervescent (150 mg)

Storage: Store at room temperature in tightly closed, light-resistant containers.

How This Drug Works: Blocks the effects of histamine on the stomach, thereby reducing stomach-acid secretion.

Brand Names: Rifadin, Rimactane

Generic Available: No

Type of Drug: Antibiotic, antitubercular

Use: Treats tuberculosis and certain types of *Staphylococcal* infections. Also used to prevent certain types of meningitis.

Time Required for Drug to Take Effect: Several days. Treatment of tuberculosis may require up to 2 years of therapy.

Dosage Forms and Strengths: Capsules (150 mg, 300 mg); Injection (600 mg/vial). A special liquid formulation can be prepared by the pharmacist.

Storage: Store capsules at room temperature in tightly closed, light-resistant containers. Refrigerate liquids.

How This Drug Works: Stops the growth of susceptible bacteria.

RIFAMPIN

Administration Guidelines

• Give on an empty stomach either 1 hour before or 2 hours after meals.

• Usually given 1 or 2 times a day. May be given 2 or 3 times a week under some circumstances.

• Shake liquid thoroughly before measuring each dose.

• Missed doses: Give as soon as possible. However, if it's within 6 hours of the next dose, skip the missed dose and give the next regular dose. Do not give double doses.

• Give this drug for the prescribed period of time even if your child seems better. Adequate treatment of tuberculosis may take 6 months to 2 years of therapy.

Side Effects

Tell your child's doctor about any side effects that are persistent or particularly bothersome.

More Common. Upset stomach, nausea, vomiting, diarrhea. Contact the doctor if your child experiences fever, chills, or rash.

Less Common. Anemia, headache, dizziness, fatigue. Contact the doctor if your child experiences yellowing of the skin or eyes; unusual bleeding or bruising; difficulty breathing; swelling of the face, eyes, or lips; or difficulty urinating.

Possible Drug Interactions

• May decrease the effects of digoxin, warfarin, barbiturate drugs such as phenobarbital, beta blockers such as Inderal, corticosteroids such as prednisone, cyclosporine, phenytoin (Dilantin), theophylline, quinidine, ketoconazole, and verapamil.

• Regular use of alcohol can increase the risk of liver damage.

• Decreases the effectiveness of oral contraceptives. Your child should use an alternate birth control method.

Tell Your Child's Doctor If

• Your child has had allergic reactions to any medications.

• Your child has any other diseases.

• Your child is taking any other medications.

• Your child has liver disease.

• Your daughter is or becomes pregnant. This drug has caused birth defects in animals.

• Your daughter is breast-feeding her baby. This drug passes into breast milk; however, the American Academy of Pediatrics considers it compatible with breast-feeding in most cases.

Symptoms of Overdose: Nausea, vomiting, fatigue, unconsciousness

Special Notes

• Can cause a red-orange discoloration of urine, saliva, tears, sweat, or stools.

• Can permanently discolor contact lenses if they are worn while taking this drug.

• Frequently used in combination with other antibiotics.

To Each His Own

If one of your children has been prescribed an antibiotic and another child gets sick, it is not safe to give the antibiotic to the child for whom it was not prescribed. The medication may not be the appropriate one for the other child—even if the children's symptoms are similar. Treating an infection with the wrong drug may make the condition worse instead of better. What's more, children respond to the same drug differently and may need different dosages. The child who became ill first needs the drug in the amount prescribed for the time advised; otherwise, it may not be effective. If you think another child needs medication, consult the doctor.

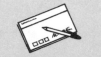

Brand Name: Serevent

Generic Available: No

Type of Drug:
Bronchodilator

Use: To maintain control of asthma and other lung diseases.

Time Required for Drug to Take Effect: 10 minutes

Dosage Form and Strength: Aerosol (21 mcg/spray)

Storage: Store at room temperature, away from excessive heat. The contents are pressurized and can explode if heated.

How This Drug Works: Relaxes the smooth muscles of the bronchial tree.

SALMETEROL

Administration Guidelines

• Shake well just before each use to distribute the ingredients evenly and equalize the doses.

• If more than 1 inhalation is prescribed, wait 1 full minute between inhalations to receive the full benefit from the first dose.

• Missed doses: If you remember within 1 hour, take the missed dose immediately, then follow the regular dosing schedule. Otherwise, wait until the next scheduled dose. Do not give double doses.

• Do not use for immediate relief of asthma symptoms. This drug has a slow onset of action and is not effective for acute symptom relief. Your child should use a short-acting bronchodilator such as albuterol for acute symptoms. Discuss this with your child's doctor.

• To prevent exercise-induced bronchospasm, give 30 to 60 minutes before exercise.

Side Effects

Tell your child's doctor about any side effects that are persistent or particularly bothersome.

More Common. Headache, tremor, cough

Less Common. Increased heart rate, dizziness, giddiness, unrest, depression, anxiety, cough, runny nose, flulike symptoms, stomach pain. It is especially important to tell the doctor if your child experiences chest pain, increased blood pressure, itching or rash, or awareness of a heartbeat.

Possible Drug Interactions

• The beta blockers (acebutolol, atenolol, labetalol, metoprolol, nadolol, pindolol, propranolol, timolol) decrease the effectiveness of this drug.

• Monoamine oxidase (MAO) inhibitors; tricyclic antidepressants; antihistamines; levothyroxine; and nonprescription cough, cold, asthma, allergy, diet, and sinus medications may increase the side effects of this drug.

• Other bronchodilator drugs (oral and inhalation) may increase side effects. Discuss this with the doctor.

Tell Your Child's Doctor If

• Your child is taking any other medications, especially any of those listed above.

• Your child has had unusual or allergic reactions to any medications, especially to this drug or to any related drugs such as albuterol, amphetamines, ephedrine, epinephrine, isoproterenol, metaproterenol, norepinephrine, phenylephrine, phenylpropanolamine, pseudoephedrine, or terbutaline.

• Your child has had heart disease, epilepsy, high blood pressure, thyroid disease, or diabetes mellitus.

• You notice a decrease in the control of the asthma.

• Your daughter is or becomes pregnant. The effects of this drug during pregnancy have not been well studied in humans, but it has caused side effects in the offspring of animals that received large doses during pregnancy.

• Your daughter is breast-feeding her baby. It is not known if this drug passes into breast milk.

Special Instructions

• Your child should be cautious if participating in any activity that requires alertness, such as riding a bicycle. This drug causes drowsiness.

• Do not exceed the recommended dose. Excessive use may lead to serious side effects.

• Do not puncture, break, or burn the aerosol container. The contents are under pressure and may explode.

Symptoms of Overdose: Exaggeration of the side effects listed above. Seizures, low potassium levels, hypertension, angina (a sense of suffocation)

Teach Your Children Well

Let's face it. Kids can be pretty stubborn when it comes to accepting medication. When appropriate, try giving your child information about his or her condition and how the medicine works. In a nonthreatening voice, talk about the consequences of not taking the medication, perhaps reminding the child of how uncomfortable he or she was before beginning the medication. Use reasoning when possible, but don't scare the child. Children who understand the importance of antibiotics for infection, insulin for diabetes, or inhalants for asthma are more likely to take the medication without objection.

Brand Names: Gas Relief,* Gas-X,* Mylicon,* Mylanta Gas,* Phazyme* (*available over the counter)

Generic Available: Yes

Type of Drug: Antiflatulent

Use: Relieves intestinal gas.

Time Required for Drug to Take Effect: Within minutes for stomach gas.

Dosage Forms and Strengths: Liquid, drops (40 mg/0.6 mL); Tablets (60 mg, 95 mg); Tablets, chewable (40 mg, 80 mg, 125 mg); Capsule (125 mg)

Storage: Store at room temperature in tightly closed containers. Protect the liquid from light and do not freeze.

How This Drug Works: Decreases the surface tension of foam bubbles, causing the bubbles to collapse and coalesce into larger bubbles to be expelled.

SIMETHICONE

Administration Guidelines

• Chewable tablets must be chewed thoroughly before swallowing; follow with a glass of water or other liquid.

• Give after meals and at bedtime.

• Shake the liquid well before measuring each dose.

• Liquid may be mixed with at least 30 mL of cool water, infant formula, or other liquid.

• Missed doses: Give as soon as you remember. Do not give double doses.

• For children older than 12 years of age, do not give more than 500 mg in a 24-hour period. For younger children, follow the doctor's instructions for maximum dosage.

Side Effects

Tell your child's doctor about any side effects that are persistent or particularly bothersome. This agent has few side effects when used appropriately.

Tell Your Child's Doctor If

• Your child has had an allergic reaction to this drug.

• Your child's symptoms do not get better after taking this drug for a few days.

Special Notes

• Not recommended for the treatment of infant colic. If your child has signs of colic, consult the doctor.

• Available over the counter.

SODIUM BICARBONATE (BAKING SODA)

Administration Guidelines
• Mix powder in a glass of water.

• Do not give within 2 hours of other medications.

• Do not take with large amounts of milk or milk products.

• Missed dose: Give as soon as possible, but do not give within 2 hours of the next dose. Do not give double doses.

• Do not give regularly for more than 2 weeks unless prescribed by your child's doctor.

Side Effects
Tell your child's doctor about any side effects that are persistent or particularly bothersome.

Less Common. Increased thirst, stomach cramps. Contact the doctor if your child experiences a frequent urge to urinate, irregular heartbeat, headache, loss of appetite, mood or mental changes, muscle pain or twitching, nausea or vomiting, nervousness or restlessness, slow breathing, swelling of feet or legs, unpleasant taste in the mouth, fatigue, or weakness.

Possible Drug Interactions
• Decreases the absorption of ketoconazole and tetracycline.

• Decreases the effectiveness of methenamine.

Tell Your Child's Doctor If
• Your child has had an allergic reaction to any medication.

• Your child is taking any other medications.

• Your child has kidney, liver, or heart disease; swelling of legs or feet; high blood pressure; intestinal problems; rectal bleeding; problems with urination; toxemia of pregnancy; or any other medical condition.

• Your daughter is or becomes pregnant.

Special Instructions
• Do not use if your child has abdominal pain, appendicitis, intestinal blockage, nausea, vomiting, or rectal bleeding.

Symptoms of Overdose: Nausea, vomiting, weakness, mental confusion, muscle cramping, seizures, coma

Special Notes
• Contains a large amount of sodium. If your child is on a sodium-restricted diet, talk to the doctor before giving it to your child.

Brand Names: Citrocarbonate,* Soda Mint,* Arm and Hammer Pure Baking Soda* (*available over the counter)

Generic Available: Yes

Type of Drug: Antacid, alkalinizing agent

Use: Treats occasional heartburn. Also used to make the blood and urine more alkaline.

Time Required for Drug to Take Effect: Within minutes for heartburn.

Dosage Forms and Strengths: Tablet (300 mg, 325 mg, 520 mg, 600 mg, 650 mg); Powder (3.4 gm/5mL); Powder, effervescent (780 mg with 1.82 gm sodium citrate/5 mL)

Storage: Store at room temperature in tightly closed containers.

How This Drug Works: The bicarbonate ion neutralizes the hydrogen (acid) ion to raise the blood, urine, and stomach pH.

Brand Names: Fleet's Phospho-Soda,* Fleet's Enema*
(*available over the counter)

Generic Available: Yes

Type of Drug: Laxative, saline hyperosmotic

Use: Treats constipation and cleans out the large bowel prior to surgery or medical tests. Also, treats and prevents low body phosphate levels.

Time Required for Drug to Take Effect: 2 to 5 minutes after rectal administration and 3 to 6 hours after oral administration.

Dosage Forms and Strengths: Liquid (sodium phosphate 0.9 gm and sodium biphosphate 2.4 gm/ 5 mL); Enema (67.5 mL, 135 mL)

Storage: Store at room temperature in tightly closed containers.

How This Drug Works: Draws water into the small intestine, producing distention and increased movement of stool through the intestine. Phosphates help with bone deposition and calcium metabolism.

SODIUM PHOSPHATE (PHOSPHO-SODA)

Administration Guidelines

- Give on an empty stomach for laxative effect. Give with or after meals to decrease laxative effect and stomach upset.

- Dilute liquid with at least ½ cup cool water.

- Give each dose with a large amount (4 to 8 ounces) of water or juice.

- Increase your child's intake of water or other fluids.

- Do not give to children younger than 6 years of age unless prescribed by your child's doctor.

- Do not give the enema to children younger than 2 years of age.

- Do not give an adult enema to children younger than 12 years of age.

- Do not give regularly for more than 1 week unless prescribed by the doctor.

Side Effects

Tell your child's doctor about any side effects that are persistent or particularly bothersome.

More Common. Cramping, diarrhea, gas, increased thirst

Less Common. Contact the doctor if your child experiences confusion, dizziness, light-headedness, irregular heartbeat, muscle cramps, unusual fatigue, or weakness.

Possible Drug Interactions

- Sucralfate and antacids containing magnesium, aluminum, or calcium decrease the absorption of this drug.

Tell Your Child's Doctor If

- Your child has heart failure; liver or kidney disease; intestinal blockage; increased body phosphate, sodium, or potassium levels; decreased body calcium levels; or any other medical condition.

- Your child has had an allergic reaction to this drug or any other medication.

- Your child is taking any other prescription or nonprescription medicine.

- Your child has a sudden change in bowel movements that lasts longer than 2 weeks or keeps returning intermittently.

- Your child does not have a return of the liquid or a stool after using the enema.

- Your daughter is or becomes pregnant.

Special Instructions

- Do not use if your child has abdominal pain, appendicitis, intestinal blockage, nausea, vomiting, or rectal bleeding.

- A children's product is available and should be used instead of the adult product.

Symptoms of Overdose: Gastrointestinal irritation, fast or slow heartbeat, edema, fast breathing, coma, seizures, nausea, vomiting, dehydration, confusion, dizziness, light-headedness, muscle cramps, unusual fatigue, or weakness

Special Notes

- Serious electrolyte imbalances and dehydration have been reported in children who received these enemas. Do not use more than the recommended dose.

- This drug contains sodium phosphates and sodium biphosphate.

Over-the-Counter Wisdom

Keep in mind that even a medication that is available without a doctor's prescription may still be harmful and should be given appropriately and only when necessary. Talk to your pediatrician about what to do if your child gets sick. Some illnesses can be treated at home, some require a call to the pediatrician's office, and some will require a visit to the doctor. In addition, ask the doctor what situations constitute an emergency. If you're not sure if it's safe or appropriate to give your child a particular over-the-counter medication, be sure to talk to the doctor first.

Brand Names: AK-Sulf, AK Sulf Forte, Bleph-10, Cetamide, Isopto Cetamide, Ophthacet, Sodium Sulamyd, Sulf-10, Sulfair 15, Sulten-10, Sodium Sulfacetamide (various manufacturers)

Generic Available: Yes

Type of Drug: Ophthalmic antibiotic

Use: Treats bacterial eye infections and corneal ulcers.

Time Required for Drug to Take Effect: It may take a few days for this drug to affect the infection.

Dosage Forms and Strengths: Drops (10%, 15%, 30% solution); Ointment (10%)

Storage: Store at room temperature in tightly closed containers away from light; do not freeze. Discard drops that are discolored or turn brown.

How This Drug Works: Prevents the production of the nutrients required for the growth of the infecting bacteria. It is not effective against infections that are caused by viruses or fungi.

SODIUM SULFACETAMIDE (OPHTHALMIC)

Administration Guidelines
• Wash your hands with soap and water before applying.

• Do not touch the dropper or the tip of the ointment tube with your fingers or touch them to the eyes. Do not wipe off or rinse the dropper after use.

• Missed doses: Give as soon as possible. However, if it is time for the next dose, skip the missed dose and return to the regular dosing schedule. Do not give double doses.

• Give this drug for the entire time prescribed by your child's doctor, even if the symptoms disappear. If this drug is stopped too soon, resistant bacteria can continue growing, and the infection could recur.

Side Effects
Tell your child's doctor about any side effects that are persistent or particularly bothersome.

More Common. Blurred vision, burning or stinging in the eyes immediately after application (especially the 30% solution). This effect should last only a few minutes.

Less Common. It is especially important to tell the doctor if your child experiences signs of irritation in the eyes (such as redness, swelling, or itching) that last more than several minutes, chills, fever, itching, or difficulty breathing.

Possible Drug Interactions
• Do not use with preparations containing silver, such as silver nitrate ophthalmic solution, or with gentamycin.

Tell Your Child's Doctor If
• Your child is taking any other prescription or nonprescription medications.

• Your child has had unusual or allergic reactions to any medications, especially to this drug or to any other sulfa medication such as diuretics, oral antidiabetic medications, or sulfonamide antibiotics.

• There is no change in your child's condition 2 or 3 days after starting this drug.

• Your child's symptoms are getting worse rather than improving.

• Your daughter is or becomes pregnant. The safety of this drug during pregnancy has not been established. Some of the drug may be absorbed into the bloodstream if large amounts are applied for a long period of time.

• Your daughter is breast-feeding her baby. If absorbed, small amounts of this drug may pass into breast milk and cause diarrhea in the nursing infant.

Special Instructions
• Have your child wear sunglasses as this drug causes sensitivity to bright light.

• Do not allow your child to apply makeup to the affected eye.

• Do not use the product if it is cloudy or has changed to a yellowish-brown or reddish color.

Special Notes
• May cause hives, itching, wheezing, or anaphylaxis in sulfite-sensitive patients or in patients who are allergic to sulfa drugs.

• For use in children older than 2 months of age.

Outdated Doses

Safe and proper medication disposal is essential, especially when you have children in the house. Do not keep medication—whether prescription or nonprescription—past the expiration date, even if it appears normal. Expired medication may be ineffective and can even be dangerous. Make a habit of regularly checking the expiration date on all medicines in your home. Flush leftover medication down the toilet or pour it down the sink. Rinse the container before throwing it out. If your medication does not display an expiration date, throw it out after one year.

Brand Name: Chemet

Generic Available: No

Type of Drug: Lead chelating (binding) agent

Use: Treats lead poisoning. Has also been used to treat mercury and arsenic poisoning.

Time Required for Drug to Take Effect: Several weeks

Dosage Form and Strength: Capsules (100 mg)

Storage: Store at room temperature in tightly closed, light-resistant containers.

How This Drug Works: Binds (chelates) lead in the body which is then eliminated in the urine.

SUCCIMER

Administration Guidelines
• If your child can't swallow the capsule, open it and sprinkle the beads on soft foods such as applesauce or ice cream.

• Can be given with food

• Usually given 2 or 3 times a day.

• Missed doses: Give as soon as possible and space the remaining doses for the day at equal intervals. Do not give double doses.

Side Effects
Tell your child's doctor about any side effects that are persistent or particularly bothersome.

More Common. Nausea, vomiting, diarrhea, loss of appetite, metallic taste in the mouth, headache. Contact the doctor if your child experiences skin rashes or cold or flulike symptoms.

Less Common. Drowsiness, dizziness, tingling of fingers or toes, joint pains. Contact the doctor if your child experiences difficulty urinating.

Possible Drug Interactions
• Do not give at the same time as vitamin products containing minerals or with other chelation therapies.

Tell Your Child's Doctor If
• Your child has had allergic reactions to any medications.

• Your child has any other diseases.

• Your child is taking any other medications.

• Your child has liver or kidney disease.

• Your daughter is or becomes pregnant. Extremely high doses have caused birth defects in animals.

• Your daughter is breast-feeding her baby. It is not known if this drug passes into breast milk.

Special Instructions
• In addition to treatment, you must identify and remove the source of lead causing the poisoning.

• Do not allow your child to become dehydrated while taking this drug. Give your child plenty of fluids to drink.

Symptoms of Overdose: Large overdoses caused dizziness, convulsions, and breathing difficulty in animal tests.

Special Notes

- Your child will require periodic blood tests for lead blood concentrations during and after treatment. It is common for lead concentrations to decrease during treatment and then increase afterward (rebound), which may require further treatment.

- Multiple courses of therapy may be necessary to adequately treat your child.

- Can cause false-positive urine tests for ketones in children with diabetes.

Keep a Lid on It

Pharmacists are required to put drugs in bottles that have child-resistant caps. Don't switch to a bottle that's easier for you to open—children may also find it easier to open. Remember, too, that child-resistant does not mean childproof. Children older than five years of age may be able to open most medicine bottles. That's why it's essential for you to teach them that drugs can be harmful if not taken correctly and that children need supervision before taking anything. And, just to be on the safe side, keep all medicines out of your child's reach.

Brand Name: Carafate

Generic Available: No

Type of Drug: Antiulcer

Use: Short-term treatment of ulcers

Time Required for Drug to Take Effect: Within 1 to 2 hours

Dosage Forms and Strengths: Tablets (1g); Suspension (1g/10 mL)

Storage: Store at room temperature in tightly closed, light-resistant containers.

How This Drug Works: Forms a protective coating over the damaged mucosal area.

SUCRALFATE

Administrative Guidelines

- Give on an empty stomach 1 hour before or 2 hours after a meal.

- Do not give antacids within 30 minutes before or after giving this drug.

- Shake suspension well before measuring each dose.

- Usually given 2 to 4 times a day.

- Tablets may be broken or dissolved in water.

- Missed doses: Give as soon as possible. However, if it's within a couple hours of the next dose, skip the missed dose. Do not give double doses.

Side Effects

Tell your child's doctor about any side effects that are persistent or particularly bothersome.

More Common. Back pain, constipation, diarrhea, dizziness, drowsiness, dry mouth, indigestion, nausea, or stomach pain

Less Common. Tell the doctor if your child experiences itching or develops a rash.

Possible Drug Interactions

- Decreases absorption of tetracycline, digoxin, phenytoin, theophylline, ketoconazole, ciprofloxacin, and ranitidine from the gastrointestinal tract. Wait 2 hours after giving this drug before giving any of these medications.

Tell Your Child's Doctor If

- Your child is taking any of the medications listed above.

- Your child is allergic to this drug.

- Your child has kidney disease.

- Your daughter is or becomes pregnant.

SULFADIAZINE SILVER

Administration Guidelines
- Generally applied 1 or 2 times a day, usually with a dressing change.

- Wear a sterile glove when applying. A $\frac{1}{16}$-inch strip of cream usually is sufficient. Burned area should be covered with cream at all times.

- For external use only.

- Avoid contact with the eyes.

- Use this drug for the entire time recommended by your child's doctor. If you stop giving the drug too soon, resistant bacteria can continue growing, and the infection could recur.

- Do not give to an infant younger than 1 month of age unless the doctor specifically directs you to do so.

Side Effects
Tell your child's doctor about any side effects that are persistent or particularly bothersome.

More Common. Itching, rash, redness around the site of application, pain, burning sensation

Less Common. Anemia, unusual bleeding, kidney pain, difficulty urinating

Possible Drug Interactions
- May inactivate other topical preparations that contain enzymes.

Tell Your Child's Doctor If
- Your child has had unusual or allergic reactions to any medications, especially to sulfonamide antibiotics or other sulfa drugs, including diuretics (water pills), dapsone, oral antidiabetics, and oral anti-glaucoma medication.

- Your child is taking any prescription or nonprescription medications, especially any of those listed above.

- Your child has or ever had glucose-6-phosphate dehydrogenase (G6PD) deficiency, liver disease, or kidney disease.

- Your child is taking a sulfonamide prior to surgery or any other medical or dental treatment.

- Your child's symptoms of infection seem to be getting worse rather than improving.

- Your daughter is or becomes pregnant. If given to a woman late in pregnancy, this drug can be toxic to the fetus.

- Your daughter is breast-feeding her baby. This drug can pass into

Brand Names: Flint SSD, Silvadene, Thermazene

Generic Available: Yes

Type of Drug: Sulfonamide antibiotic, topical

Use: Prevents and treats infection in second- and third-degree burns.

Time Required for Drug to Take Effect: It may take up to 1 week before maximum effect is achieved.

Dosage Form and Strength: Cream (1%)

Storage: Store in a cool, dry place in tightly closed containers.

How This Drug Works: Kills the bacteria responsible for the infection.

breast milk and may cause side effects in nursing infants who have G6PD deficiency.

Special Instructions

• This drug can increase sensitivity to sunlight. Your child should avoid prolonged exposure to sunlight and sunlamps. Make sure your child wears an effective sunscreen on areas not covered by the cream, protective clothing, and sunglasses when out-of-doors. The sunscreen should not contain para-aminobenzoic acid (PABA) since it interferes with the antibacterial activity of this drug.

Symptoms of Overdose:

Severe forms of side effects listed above. Severe nausea, vomiting, and convulsions may occur.

Special Notes

• Not recommended for use on newborns or premature infants.

Be Accurate

If you don't give medication correctly, it may be ineffective or even cause side effects. An estimated 10 to 30 percent of medications aren't effective because they have been given incorrectly. To do it right, you have to give the exact amount of medicine prescribed at the scheduled time, for the specified duration, and in the appropriate manner. Always read the label, follow the directions carefully, and use the appropriate equipment for measuring and administering the medication. Also, be sure to wash your hands before you give any medication to your child.

SULFAMETHOXAZOLE AND PHENAZOPYRIDINE COMBINATION

Administration Guidelines

• Give this drug with a full glass of water on an empty stomach, either 1 hour before or 2 hours after a meal. However, if your child experiences stomach upset, ask your child's doctor if you can give it with food or milk.

• Generally given 2 times a day.

• Works best when blood concentrations are kept within a safe and effective range. Give at evenly spaced intervals around the clock. If you are to give 2 doses a day, space them 12 hours apart.

• Missed doses: Give immediately. However, if you do not remember until it is time for the next dose, give the missed dose immediately and space the next dose about halfway through the regular interval between doses. Then return to the regular dosing schedule. Try not to skip any doses.

• Give for the entire time prescribed by the doctor, even if the symptoms disappear before the end of that period. If you stop giving the drug too soon, resistant bacteria can continue growing, and the infection could recur.

• Do not give to infants younger than 2 months of age.

Side Effects

Tell your child's doctor about any side effects that are persistent or particularly bothersome.

More Common. Abdominal pain, diarrhea, dizziness, headache, indigestion, insomnia, loss of appetite, nausea, or vomiting. These side effects should disappear as the body adjusts to this drug.

Less Common. It is especially important to tell the doctor if your child experiences aching joints and muscles, back pain, bloating, blood in the urine, chest pain, chills, confusion, convulsions, depression, difficult or painful urination, difficulty in breathing, difficulty in swallowing, fever, hallucinations, hives, itching, loss of coordination, pale skin, rash or peeling skin, ringing in the ears, sore throat, swelling of the front part of the neck, swollen ankles, unusual bleeding or bruising, unusual fatigue, or yellowing of the eyes or skin.

Possible Drug Interactions

• Can increase the blood levels of oral anticoagulants (blood thinners such as warfarin), oral antidiabetic agents, methotrexate, and

Brand Name: Azo Gantanol

Generic Available: No

Type of Drug: Antibiotic, urinary-tract analgesic

Use: Treats painful urinary tract infections.

Time Required for Drug to Take Effect: It may take a few days for this drug to become fully effective.

Dosage Form and Strength: Tablets (500 mg sulfamethoxazole and 100 mg phenazopyridine)

Storage: Store at room temperature in tightly closed, light-resistant containers.

How This Drug Works: Prevents production of the nutrients that are required for growth and proliferation of the infecting bacteria. Phenazopyridine is excreted in the urine, where it exerts a topical analgesic (pain-relieving) effect on the urinary tract.

phenytoin, which can lead to serious side effects.

• Methenamine can increase the side effects to the kidneys caused by sulfamethoxazole.

• Probenecid, phenylbutazone, oxyphenbutazone, and sulfinpyrazone can increase the blood concentration of sulfamethoxazole, which can lead to an increase in side effects.

Tell Your Child's Doctor If
• Your child is taking any prescription or nonprescription medications, especially any of those listed above.

• Your child has or had unusual or allergic reactions to any medications, especially to phenazopyridine, sulfamethoxazole, or any other sulfa drug (other sulfonamide antibiotics, diuretics, dapsone, oral antidiabetic medications, or acetazolamide).

• Your child is taking this drug before undergoing surgery or any other medical or dental treatment.

• Your child has or ever had glucose-6-phosphate dehydrogenase (G6PD) deficiency, kidney disease, liver disease, or porphyria.

• There is no improvement in your child's condition several days after starting this drug. This drug may not be effective against the particular type of bacteria causing your child's infection.

• Your child's symptoms seem to be getting worse rather than improving.

• Your daughter is or becomes pregnant. Small amounts of sulfamethoxazole cross the placenta. Avoid using this drug late in pregnancy or at term.

• Your daughter is breast-feeding her baby. Small amounts of this drug pass into breast milk and may temporarily cause diarrhea in the nursing infant. It's best to avoid using this drug if the infant is younger than 2 months of age.

Special Instructions
• Sulfamethoxazole can cause increased sensitivity to sunlight. Your child should avoid prolonged exposure to sunlight and sunlamps and wear an effective sunscreen, protective clothing, and sunglasses when out-of-doors. Do not use a sunscreen containing para-aminobenzoic acid (PABA).

Symptoms of Overdose: Very severe forms of side effects listed above. Severe symptoms of overdose may include convulsions and shortness of breath.

Special Notes
• Phenazopyridine is only useful for pain from a urinary-tract infection.

• Phenazopyridine causes urine to turn orange-red. This is not harmful; however, it may stain clothing. The urine will return to its normal color soon after the drug is discontinued.

SULFAMETHOXAZOLE AND TRIMETHOPRIM COMBINATION

Administration Guidelines

• Give with a full glass of water on an empty stomach, either 1 hour before or 2 hours after a meal. However, if your child experiences stomach upset, ask the doctor if you can give it with food or milk.

• Generally given 2 times a day.

• Works best when blood concentrations are kept within a safe and effective range. Give at evenly spaced intervals around the clock. If you are to give 2 doses a day, space them 12 hours apart.

• For best results, give your child plenty of water (8 to 12 glasses) during the day.

• Missed doses: Give immediately. However, if you do not remember until it is time for the next dose, give the missed dose and space the following dose about halfway through the regular interval between doses (wait about 6 hours if you are giving 2 doses a day). Then return to the regular dosing schedule.

• Shake the suspension well just before measuring each dose to distribute the ingredients evenly and equalize the doses.

• Give this drug for the entire time prescribed by your child's doctor (usually 7 to 14 days), even if the symptoms disappear before the end of that period. If you stop giving the drug too soon, resistant bacteria can continue growing, and the infection could recur.

• Do not use in infants younger than 2 months of age to avoid serious side effects.

Side Effects

Tell your child's doctor about any side effects that are persistent or particularly bothersome.

More Common. Abdominal pain, diarrhea, dizziness, headache, loss of appetite, nausea, sore mouth, or vomiting. These side effects should disappear as the body adjusts to this drug.

Less Common. It is especially important to tell the doctor if your child experiences bloody urine, convulsions, difficult or painful urination, difficulty in breathing, difficulty in swallowing, fever, hallucinations, itching, joint pain, lower back pain, pale skin, rash, ringing in the ears, sore throat, swelling of the front part of the neck, swollen or inflamed tongue, tingling in the hands or feet, unusual bleeding or bruising, unusual fatigue, or yellowing of the eyes or skin.

Brand Names: Bactrim, Bactrim DS, Bethaprim DS, Cotrim, Cotrim DS, Cotrim Pediatric, Septra, Septra DS, Sulfamethoxazole and Trimethoprim (various manufacturers), Sulfatrim, Sulfatrim DS

Generic Available: Yes

Type of Drug: Antibiotic

Use: Treats a broad range of infections, including urinary tract infections, certain respiratory and gastrointestinal infections, and otitis media (middle-ear infection).

Time Required for Drug to Take Effect: It may take a few days for this drug to take effect.

Dosage Forms and Strengths: Tablets (400 mg sulfamethoxazole and 80 mg trimethoprim); Tablets, double-strength (DS) (800 mg sulfamethoxazole and 160 mg trimethoprim); Suspension (200 mg sulfamethoxazole and 40 mg trimethoprim per 5 mL)

Storage: Store tablets and suspension at room temperature in tightly closed, light-resistant containers. Do not freeze.

How This Drug Works: Prevents the production of the nutrients that are required for growth of the infecting bacteria.

Possible Drug Interactions

• May increase the blood levels of oral anticoagulants (blood thinners, such as warfarin), oral antidiabetic agents, metho-trexate, and phenytoin, which can lead to increased side effects.

Tell Your Child's Doctor If

• Your child is currently taking any prescription or nonprescription medications, especially any that are listed above.

• Your child has had unusual or allergic reactions to any medications, especially to trimethoprim, sulfamethoxazole, or other sulfa drugs (other sulfonamide antibiotics, diuretics, dapsone, oral antidiabetic medications, or acetazolamide).

• Your child has or ever had glucose-6-phosphate dehydrogenase (G6PD) deficiency, kidney disease, liver disease, porphyria, or megaloblas-tic anemia (folate-deficiency anemia).

• Your child is taking this drug before having surgery or any other medical or dental treatment.

• Your child's infection seems to be getting worse rather than improving.

• Your daughter is or becomes pregnant. Small amounts of sulfamethoxazole and trimetho-prim cross the placenta. Avoid use late in pregnancy or at term. Trimethoprim has been shown to cause birth defects in the offspring of animals that received very large doses during pregnancy.

• Your daughter is breast-feeding her baby. Sulfa products should not be used in infants younger than 2 months of age. Small amounts of sulfamethoxazole pass into breast milk. This drug may temporarily alter the bacterial balance in the intestinal tract of the nursing infant, resulting in diarrhea. Also, small amounts of trimethoprim pass into breast milk, and there is a chance that it may cause anemia in the nursing infant.

Special Instructions

• If there is no improvement in your child's condition several days after starting this drug, check with the doctor. This drug may not be effective against the bacteria causing your child's infection.

• Monitor your child closely for signs of a rash. Notify the doctor immediately if you see any rash. Some forms of rashes from this drug can be life threatening.

• Can cause increased sensitivity to sunlight. Your child should avoid prolonged exposure to sunlight and sunlamps and wear an effective sunscreen and protective clothing and sun-glasses when out-of-doors. Do not use a sunscreen containing para-aminobenzoic acid (PABA).

Symptoms of Overdose: Severe forms of side effects such as nausea, vomiting, con-vulsions, and kidney and liver failure

SULFASALAZINE

Administration Guidelines

• May be given with food or after meals.

• Do not give at the same time as antacids.

• Enteric-coated tablets should be swallowed whole.

• Shake suspension well before measuring each dose.

• Missed doses: Give as soon as possible. However, if it's within a couple hours of the next dose, skip the missed dose. Do not give double doses.

Side Effects

Tell your child's doctor about any side effects that are persistent or particularly bothersome.

More Common. Urine color change (orange-yellow), dizziness, loss of appetite, mild headache, nausea, stomach upset, vomiting, increased sensitivity to sunlight.

Less Common. Tell the doctor if your child experiences blood in the urine, convulsions, depression, difficulty in swallowing, diarrhea, difficult or painful urination, fatigue, drowsiness, insomnia, fever, hallucinations, hearing loss, itching, joint pain, lower back pain, mouth sores, pale skin, rash or peeling skin, ringing in the ears, severe headache, sore throat, swelling of the front part of the neck, tingling sensations, unusual bleeding or bruising, or yellowing of the eyes or skin.

Possible Drug Interactions

• Decreases blood digoxin and folic acid levels.

• Increases the side effects of anticoagulants, antidiabetic agents, methotrexate, aspirin, and phenytoin.

Tell Your Child's Doctor If

• Your child is taking any medication, especially those listed above.

• Stomach upset, decreased appetite, and nausea or vomiting do not subside after the first few doses.

• Your child is allergic to sulfasalazine, aspirin or other salicylates, or any sulfa drug.

• Your child has blood disorders, blockage of the urinary tract or intestine, glucose-6-phosphate dehydrogenase (G6PD) deficiency, kidney or liver disease, or porphyria.

• Your daughter is or becomes pregnant.

Brand Names: Azulfidine, Azulfidine EN-Tabs, Sulfasalazine (various manufacturers)

Generic Available: Yes

Type of Drug: Sulfonamide, anti-inflammatory

Use: Treats inflammatory bowel disease and has been used to treat juvenile rheumatoid arthritis.

Time Required for Drug to Take Effect: 2 to 3 days, but may be longer in some cases

Dosage Forms and Strengths: Tablets (500 mg); Tablets, enteric-coated (500 mg); Suspension (compounded at some pharmacies)

Storage: Store at room temperature in tightly closed, light-resistant containers.

How This Drug Works: Decreases inflammation in the intestine.

Special Instructions

• Your child should drink at least 8 to 12 glasses of water or fruit juice each day to help prevent the formation of kidney stones.

Symptoms of Overdose: Severe nausea, vomiting, dizziness, headache, drowsiness, unconsciousness

Special Notes

• This drug increases sensitivity to sunlight. Your child should avoid prolonged exposure to sunlight and sunlamps. Make sure your child uses an effective sunscreen and wears protective clothing when out-of-doors. Do not use sunscreen containing PABA

• Can discolor contact lenses. Your child may want to stop wearing them while taking this drug. Discuss this with the ophthalmologist.

• May cause orange-yellow discoloration of urine and skin.

Just Call

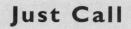

If you have any concerns about any side effects, even minor ones, you should be sure to discuss them with your child's doctor. The doctor may be able to minimize or eliminate the side effects by prescribing a different medication or changing your child's dosage, dosing schedule, or the way the drug is given. (Do not make adjustments on your own without discussing them with your doctor.) At the very least, the doctor can assure you that the medication's benefits far outweigh its side effects.

SULFATHIAZOLE, SULFACETAMIDE, AND SULFABENZAMIDE COMBINATION

Administration Guidelines
• Wash the applicator with warm water and soap, and dry it thoroughly after each use.

• Give your child large amounts of water (8 to 12 glasses each day).

• Missed doses: Insert as soon as possible. However, if it's within a couple hours of the next dose, skip the missed dose. Do not give double doses.

• Use the full course of therapy.

Side Effects
Tell your child's doctor about any side effects that are persistent or particularly bothersome.

More Common. Mild, temporary burning or stinging after each of the first few applications.

Less Common. Tell the doctor if your child experiences itching, rash, redness, swelling, or any other signs of irritation that were not present before your child started this drug.

Tell Your Child's Doctor If
• Your child is allergic to sulfathiazole, sulfacetamide, sulfabenzamide, or any other sulfa drug, including sulfonamide antibiotics, diuretics (water pills), or oral antidiabetic medicines, oral antiglaucoma medicines, or dapsone.

• Your child has kidney disease.

• Your daughter is or becomes pregnant.

• Your daughter is breast-feeding her baby. This drug can pass into breast milk and cause side effects in the infant.

Special Instructions
• Your child should not use tampons while taking this drug.

• Do not get the cream in the eyes.

• Your child should not engage in vaginal intercourse during treatment with this drug.

Symptoms of Overdose: Rare. Contact your local poison control center if taken orally.

Brand Names: Gyne-Sulf, Sultrin Triple Sulfa, Triple Sulfa Vaginal (various manufacturers), Trysul, V.V.S., Dayto Sulf

Generic Available: Yes

Type of Drug: Antibiotic

Use: Treats vaginal infections.

Time Required for Drug to Take Effect: 2 to 3 days

Dosage Forms and Strengths: Tablets, vaginal (172.5 mg sulfathiazole, 143.75 mg sulfacetamide, and 184 mg sulfabenzamide); Cream, vaginal (3.42% sulfathiazole, 2.86% sulfacetamide, and 3.7% sulfabenzamide)

Storage: Store at room temperature in tightly closed, light-resistant containers.

How This Drug Works: Destroys susceptible bacteria.

Brand Names: Gantanol, Gantrisin, Microsulfon, Neotrizine, Renoquid, Terfonyl, Thiosulfil Forte, Triple Sulfa (systemic), Urobak

Generic Available: Yes

Type of Drug: Anti-infective

Use: Treats urinary-tract infections, as well as other infections.

Time Required for Drug to Take Effect: It may take a few days for this drug to take effect.

Dosage Forms and Strengths: Tablets (250 mg, 500 mg); Suspension (500 mg per 5 mL); Syrup (500 mg per 5 mL), Suspension, pediatric (500 mg per 5 mL); Tablets, multiple sulfonamides (167 mg sulfadiazine, 167 mg sulfamerazine, and 167 mg sulfamethazine); Suspension, multiple sulfonamides (167 mg sulfadiazine, 167 mg sulfamerazine, and 167 mg sulfamethazine per 5-mL, with 2% alcohol)

Storage: Store at room temperature in the original container. Do not refrigerate this drug.

How This Drug Works: Kills the bacteria responsible for the infection.

SULFONAMIDE ANTIBIOTICS (ORAL)

Administration Guidelines

• Give with a full glass of water on an empty stomach either 1 hour before or 2 hours after a meal. Give 8 to 12 (8 oz.) glasses of water throughout the day unless your child's doctor directs you to do otherwise.

• Generally given 2 to 4 times a day.

• Work best when drug concentrations in the blood are kept constant. Give doses at evenly spaced intervals around the clock. If you are to give 4 doses a day, space them about 6 hours apart.

• Shake the suspension well before measuring each dose to distribute the ingredients evenly and equalize the doses.

• Missed doses: Give as soon as possible. However, if it is time for the next dose and you are giving 2 doses a day, give the missed dose immediately and the next dose 5 to 6 hours later. If you are giving 3 or more doses a day, give the missed dose immediately and the next dose 2 to 4 hours apart. Then return to the regular dosing schedule.

• Give the full course of therapy prescribed (usually 10 days), even if the symptoms disappear before the end of that period. If you stop giving this drug too soon, the infection could recur.

• Do not give to an infant younger than 2 months of age unless the doctor specifically directs you to do so. Avoid giving sulfacytine to children younger than 14 years of age.

Side Effects

Tell your child's doctor about any side effects that are persistent or particularly bothersome.

More Common. Diarrhea, dizziness, headache, loss of appetite, nausea, or vomiting. As the body adjusts to this drug, these side effects should disappear.

Less Common. It is especially important to tell the doctor if your child experiences aching joints and muscles; blood in the urine; difficulty swallowing; itching; lower back pain; pain while urinating; pale skin; redness, blistering, or peeling of the skin; skin rash; sore throat and fever; swelling of the front part of the neck; unusual bleeding or bruising; unusual fatigue; or yellowing of the eyes or skin.

Possible Drug Interactions

• Products such as sunscreens containing para-amino benzoic acid (PABA) can decrease the effectiveness of this drug.

• May increase the activity and side effects of anticoagulants (blood thinners such as warfarin), oral antidiabetic medications, methotrexate, aspirin, phenytoin, and thiopental.

• Oxyphenbutazone, phenylbutazone, methenamine, probenecid, and sulfinpyrazone can increase the toxicity of this drug.

Tell Your Child's Doctor If

• Your child has had unusual or allergic reactions to any medications, especially to sulfonamide antibiotics or other sulfa drugs, including diuretics (water pills), dapsone, oral anti-diabetics, and oral antiglaucoma medication.

• Your child is taking any prescription or nonprescription medications, especially any of those listed above.

• Your child has or ever had glucose-6-phosphate dehydrogenase (G6PD) deficiency, liver disease, porphyria, or kidney disease.

• Your child is taking this drug prior to surgery or any other medical or dental treatment.

• Your child's symptoms seem to be getting worse rather than improving.

• Your daughter is or becomes pregnant. Given in late pregnancy, this drug can be toxic to the fetus.

• Your daughter is breast-feeding her baby. This drug can pass into breast milk and may cause side effects in nursing infants who have G6PD deficiency.

Special Instructions

• These drugs can increase sensitivity to sunlight. Your child should avoid prolonged exposure to sunlight and sunlamps. Your child should wear an effective sunscreen, protective clothing, and sunglasses when out-of-doors. The sunscreen, however, should not contain PABA.

Symptoms of Overdose: Severe forms

of side effects listed above, severe nausea, vomiting, and convulsions.

Brand Name: Prograf

Generic Available: No

Type of Drug:
Immunosuppressant

Use: Prevents rejection of liver transplants. Also used to prevent rejection of kidney and heart transplants. May be used to prevent or treat graft versus host disease after bone marrow transplant.

Time Required For Drug to Take Effect: To be effective, this drug must be maintained at a target blood concentration. The doctor will monitor your child's tacrolimus blood concentration routinely to ensure the drug's effectiveness.

Dosage Form and Strengths: Capsules (1 mg, 5 mg)

Storage: Store at room temperature in original container.

How This Drug Works: Interferes with the body's ability to reject the foreign transplanted tissue or marrow by reducing the body's natural immunity.

TACROLIMUS

Administration Guidelines

• Give at evenly spaced intervals around the clock to maintain a constant concentration of this drug in your child's blood. If you are to give this drug 2 times a day, space the doses 12 hours apart.

• Give at the same time each day.

• Give in the same way each day to keep the blood concentration constant. If your child prefers to take this drug with meals, always give it with meals.

• Missed doses: Give as soon as you remember if it's within 2 hours of the missed dose. If more than 2 hours have passed, call your child's doctor for instructions.

Side Effects

Tell your child's doctor about any side effects that are persistent or particularly bothersome.

More Common. Headache, tremors, insomnia, nausea, diarrhea, abdominal pain, increased blood pressure, increased blood sugar

Less Common. Constipation, vomiting, decreased appetite, pruritus, rash, fever, back pain. Contact the doctor immediately if your child experiences convulsions, difficult or painful urination, tingling of the hands or feet, unusual bleeding, shortness of breath, rapid weight gain (3 to 5 pounds in 1 week), yellowing of the eyes or skin, or unusual weakness.

Possible Drug Interactions

• Phenytoin, phenobarbital, carbamazepine, and rifampin can decrease the effectiveness of this drug by decreasing its blood concentration.

• Erythromycin, clarithromycin, fluconazole, ketoconazole, diltiazem, verapamil, nicardipine, methylprednisolone, and metoclopramide can increase the side effects of this drug by increasing its blood concentration.

Tell Your Child's Doctor If

• Your child is allergic to any medications.

• Your child has any diseases or illnesses.

• Your child experiences any new side effects.

• Your daughter is or becomes pregnant.

• Your daughter is breast-feeding her baby.

Special Instructions

• Do not have your child immunized without the doctor's approval.

- Consult your child's doctor before starting any other medications.

- Other household members should not receive the oral polio vaccine while your child is taking this drug.

Symptoms of Overdose: Convulsions, severe trembling, delirium, coma

Special Notes

- The doctor will want to see your child regularly to ensure the drug is working properly and to check for unwanted side effects.

Teach Your Children Well

Let's face it. Kids can be pretty stubborn when it comes to accepting medication. When appropriate, try giving your child information about his or her condition and how the medicine works. In a nonthreatening voice, talk about the consequences of not taking the medication, perhaps reminding the child of how uncomfortable he or she was before beginning the medication. Use reasoning when possible, but don't scare the child. Children who understand the importance of antibiotics for infection, insulin for diabetes, or inhalants for asthma are more likely to take the medication without objection.

Brand Names: Brethaire, Brethine, Bricanyl

Generic Available: Yes

Type of Drug: Bronchodilator

Use: Relieves wheezing and shortness of breath caused by lung diseases such as asthma, bronchitis, and emphysema.

Time Required for Drug to Take Effect: 30 minutes for tablets; 5 to 30 minutes for the aerosol

Dosage Forms and Strengths: Aerosol (0.2 mg/inhalation); Tablets (2.5 mg, 5 mg)

Storage: Store at room temperature in tightly closed, light-resistant containers. Do not refrigerate. Keep aerosol away from heat and do not puncture, break or burn; contents is under pressure and may explode.

How This Drug Works: Relaxes the smooth muscle of the bronchi (breathing tubes).

TERBUTALINE

Administration Guidelines
• Give with food to decrease stomach upset unless your child's doctor directs you to do otherwise.

• Shake the canister well before each dose.

• Missed doses: Give immediately if you remember within 1 hour, then return to your regular schedule. If more than 1 hour has passed, do not give the missed dose at all; just return to your regular dosing schedule. Do not give double doses.

• Do not exceed the recommended dosage; excessive use may lead to an increase in side effects or a loss of effectiveness.

Side Effects
Tell your child's doctor about any side effects that are persistent or particularly bothersome.

More Common. Anxiety, bad taste in the mouth, dizziness, headache, flushing, irritability insomnia, loss of appetite, nausea, nervousness, restlessness, sweating, vomiting, or weakness. These side effects should disappear as your child's body adjusts to this drug.

Less Common. It is especially important to tell the doctor if your child experiences bluish coloration of the skin, chest pain, difficult or painful urination, increased wheezing or difficulty in breathing, muscle cramps, tremors, or an awareness of one's heartbeat.

Possible Drug Interactions
• Beta blockers (acebutolol, atenolol, betaxolol, carteolol, esmolol, labetalol, metoprolol, nadolol, penbutolol, pindolol, propranolol, and timolol) decrease the effectiveness of this drug.

• Monoamine oxidase (MAO) inhibitors; tricyclic antidepressants; antihistamines; levothyroxine; and nonprescription cough, cold, allergy, asthma, diet, and sinus medications may increase the side effects of this drug. At least 14 days should separate the use of this drug and the use of an MAO inhibitor.

• There may be a change in the dosage requirements of insulin or oral antidiabetic medications.

• Other bronchodilator drugs (oral or inhalant) can cause more intense side effects when used with this drug. Discuss this with the doctor.

Tell Your Child's Doctor If
• Your child is taking any other medications, especially any of those listed above.

- Your child has had unusual or allergic reactions to any medications, especially to this drug or any related drug such as albuterol, amphetamines, ephedrine, epinephrine, isoproterenol, norepinephrine, phenylephrine, phenylpropanolamine, pseudoephedrine, or metaproterenol.

- Your child has or ever had diabetes, glaucoma, high blood pressure, epilepsy, heart disease, or thyroid disease.

- Your child does not respond to the usual dose of this drug. It may be a sign of worsening asthma which may require additional therapy.

- Your child is taking this drug prior to surgery or any other medical or dental treatment.

- Your daughter is or becomes pregnant. Asthma should be carefully controlled by a doctor during pregnancy.

- Your daughter is breast-feeding her baby. Small amounts of this drug pass into breast milk.

Special Instructions
- Do not spray the aerosol in or near the eyes.

- To avoid difficulty in falling asleep, ask the doctor if your child can take the last dose of this drug several hours before bedtime each day.

Symptoms of Overdose: Seizures, nausea, vomiting, high blood sugar, dysrhythmias

Special Notes
- This drug can cause dizziness and may impair your child's ability to perform tasks that require alertness, such as riding a bicycle.

- Your child's mouth should be rinsed after each dose to prevent dryness or irritation of the mouth or throat.

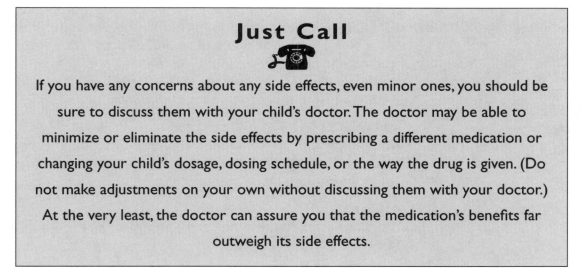

Just Call

If you have any concerns about any side effects, even minor ones, you should be sure to discuss them with your child's doctor. The doctor may be able to minimize or eliminate the side effects by prescribing a different medication or changing your child's dosage, dosing schedule, or the way the drug is given. (Do not make adjustments on your own without discussing them with your doctor.) At the very least, the doctor can assure you that the medication's benefits far outweigh its side effects.

Brand Name: Seldane

Generic Available: No

Type of Drug: Long-acting antihistamine

Use: Treats symptoms of allergic response, including sneezing, runny nose, itching, and eye tearing.

Time Required for Drug to Take Effect: 1 to 3 hours

Dosage Form and Strength: Tablets (60 mg)

Storage: Store at room temperature in a tightly closed container. Do not expose to high temperatures (above 40°C or 104°F), direct sunlight, or moisture during storage.

How This Drug Works: Blocks the action of histamine, a chemical that is released by the body during an allergic reaction.

TERFENADINE

Administration Guidelines

• Can be given on an empty stomach or with food or milk unless your child's doctor directs otherwise.

• Give only as needed to control the symptoms of allergy.

• Missed doses: If you are giving it on a regular schedule, give the missed dose as soon as possible. However, if it is almost time for the next dose, skip the missed dose and return to your regular dosing schedule. Do not give double doses.

Side Effects

Tell your child's doctor about any side effects that are persistent or particularly bothersome.

More Common. Abdominal pain; cough; dizziness; drowsiness; dry mouth, nose, or throat; fatigue; headache; increased appetite; insomnia; nausea; nervousness; nosebleeds; sore throat; sweating; vomiting; or weakness. These side effects should disappear as your child's body adjusts to this drug.

Less Common. It is especially important to tell the doctor if your child experiences depression, hair loss, itching, menstrual disorders, tingling of the fingers or toes, tremors, urinary frequency, visual disturbances, or yellowing of the skin or eyes. Hypotension (low blood pressure), palpitations, and dizziness could reflect undetected ventricular arrhythmias (deviations from the normal rhythm of the heart). In some patients, cardiac arrest and irregular heartbeat have been preceded by episodes of fainting.

Possible Drug Interactions

• Ketoconazole or itraconazole and selected antibiotics (erythromycin, troleandomycin, clarithromycin) can cause cardiac toxicity when used with this drug.

Tell Your Child's Doctor If

• Your child is taking any other medications, especially any of those listed above.

• Your child has had unusual or allergic reactions to any medications, especially to this drug.

• Your child has or ever had asthma, high blood pressure, heart disease, liver disease, or arrhythmias.

• Your daughter is or becomes pregnant. This drug's safety in human pregnancy has not been established.

• Your daughter is breast-feeding her baby. The effects of this drug on nursing infants are not yet known.

Symptoms of Overdose: Effects may vary from mild central nervous system depression (sedation, temporary cessation from breathing, diminished mental alertness) and cardiovascular collapse to stimulation (insomnia, hallucinations, tremors or convulsions), especially in children. Toxic effects are seen within 30 minutes to 2 hours.

Special Notes

• For dizziness or light-headedness, have your child sit or lie down for a while. Your child should get up slowly from a sitting or reclining position and be careful on stairs.

• This drug causes less drowsiness than other antihistamines. However, you should still be cautious about having your child perform tasks that require alertness, such as riding a bicycle, until you see how the drug affects your child.

• Serious and adverse cardiovascular effects, such as deviation from the normal rhythm of the heart, low blood pressure, cardiac arrest, and death, have been reported following high doses of this drug.

Keep a Lid on It

Pharmacists are required to put drugs in bottles that have child-resistant caps. Don't switch to a bottle that's easier for you to open—children may also find it easier to open. Remember, too, that child-resistant does not mean childproof. Children older than five years of age may be able to open most medicine bottles. That's why it's essential for you to teach them that drugs can be harmful if not taken correctly and that children need supervision before taking anything. And, just to be on the safe side, keep all medicines out of your child's reach.

Brand Names: Sumycin, Achromycin, Tetracyn, Tetracycline (various manufacturers)

Generic Available: Yes

Type of Drug: Antibiotic

Use: Treats bacterial infections, including acne.

Time Required for Drug to Take Effect: 1 to 2 days

Dosage Forms and Strengths: Tablets (250 mg, 500 mg); Suspension (125 mg/5mL); Capsules (100 mg, 250 mg, 500 mg)

Storage: Store at room temperature in tightly closed, light-resistant containers.

How This Drug Works: Destroys susceptible bacteria.

TETRACYCLINE

Administration Guidelines

• Do not give to children younger than 8 years of age as this drug may damage developing teeth and bone.

• Give on an empty stomach, 1 hour before or 2 hours after meals.

• Shake suspension well before measuring each dose.

• Usually given 1 to 4 times a day.

• Usually given for 7 to 10 days for acute infection or once a day for acne treatment on a continuous basis.

• Missed doses: Give as soon as possible. However, if it's within a couple hours of the next dose, skip the missed dose. Do not give double doses.

• Do not give antacids or calcium supplements within 1 to 2 hours of a dose of this drug to ensure its adequate absorption.

• Do not give iron products within 2 to 3 hours of a dose of this drug.

Side Effects

Tell your child's doctor about any side effects that are persistent or particularly bothersome.

More Common. Increased sensitivity to the sun, stomach upset, nausea, diarrhea, dizziness, headache

Less Common. Loss of appetite. Tell the doctor if your child experiences rash, yellowing of the skin, or visual changes.

Possible Drug Interactions

• Barbiturates, cimetidine, carbamazepine, and phenytoin may decrease the effectiveness of this drug.

• May increase serum levels of digoxin.

• May decrease insulin requirements.

• May increase or decrease lithium levels.

• May decrease the effectiveness of birth control pills. Your daughter should use an additional form of protection.

Tell Your Child's Doctor If

• Your child is allergic to this drug.

• Your child has kidney disease.

• Your daughter is or becomes pregnant. This drug should be avoided during pregnancy.

• Your daughter is breast-feeding her baby. This drug will permanently discolor the baby's teeth.

Special Instructions
• Discard this drug if it changes color or taste, if it looks different, or if it has expired.

• Your child should wear an effective sunscreen and protective clothing when out-of-doors as this drug can cause increased sensitivity to sunlight.

Symptoms of Overdose: Severe nausea, vomiting, headache, rapid heart rate

To Each His Own

If one of your children has been prescribed an antibiotic and another child gets sick, it is not safe to give the antibiotic to the child for whom it was not prescribed. The medication may not be the appropriate one for the other child—even if the children's symptoms are similar. Treating an infection with the wrong drug may make the condition worse instead of better. What's more, children respond to the same drug differently and may need different dosages. The child who became ill first needs the drug in the amount prescribed for the time advised; otherwise, it may not be effective. If you think another child needs medication, consult the doctor.

Brand Names: Aerolate III, Aerolate JR, Aerolate SR, Aquaphyllin, Asmalix, Bronkodyl, Elixicon, Elixophyllin, Elixophyllin SR, Quibron T, Quibron T/SR, Respbid, Slo-bid, Slo-Phyllin, Sustaire, Theo-24, Theobid, Theochron, Theoclear LA, Theo-Dur, Theo-Dur Sprinkle, Theolair, Theospan SR, Theovent, Theox, Uniphyl

Generic Available: Yes

Type of Drug: Bronchodilator

Use: Treats symptoms of reversible airway obstruction due to chronic asthma, bronchitis, or obstructive pulmonary disease (COPD).

Time Required for Drug to Take Effect: 2 to 3 hours

Dosage Forms and Strengths: Capsules, immediate-release; Capsules, timed-release; Tablets, immediate-release; Tablets, controlled release (all available in a variety of strengths); Elixir (80 mg/15 mL); Solution (80 mg/15 mL); Syrup (80 mg/15 mL)

Storage: Store at room temperature in tightly closed, light-resistant containers. Do not freeze.

How This Drug Works: Relaxes the smooth muscles of the bronchi and pulmonary blood vessels.

THEOPHYLLINE

Administration Guidelines

• Give on an empty stomach 30 to 60 minutes before a meal or 2 hours after a meal. If this drug causes stomach irritation, you can give it with food or a full glass of water or milk unless your child's doctor directs you to do otherwise.

• Do not give antidiarrheal medications or antacids for at least 1 hour before or 1 hour after giving this drug.

• Timed-release tablets and timed-release capsules should be swallowed whole. Chewing, crushing, or crumbling the tablets or capsules destroys their timed-release activity and may increase side effects. If the tablet is scored for breaking, you can break it along these scored lines. If the regular capsules are too large to swallow, open them and sprinkle the contents on jam, jelly, or applesauce. Your child should swallow the mixture without chewing the little beads.

• The sprinkle capsules can be swallowed whole. You also can open the capsule and sprinkle the beads on a spoonful of soft food such as applesauce or pudding. The mixture should be swallowed immediately without chewing the beads. Do not subdivide the capsule contents.

• Works best when blood levels are kept constant. Give at evenly spaced intervals around the clock. For example, if you are to give 4 doses a day, space the doses 6 hours apart. Try to give this drug at the same time(s) each day.

• Missed doses: Maintaining a safe and effective blood concentration of this drug is crucial. Therefore, if you miss giving a dose, call your child's doctor for specific instructions.

Side Effects
Tell your child's doctor about any side effects that are persistent or particularly bothersome.

More Common. Diarrhea, dizziness, flushing, headache, heartburn, increased urination, insomnia, irritability, loss of appetite, nausea, nervousness, stomach pain, or vomiting. These side effects should disappear as your child's body adjusts to this drug.

Less Common. It is especially important to tell the doctor if your child experiences black, tarry stools; confusion; convulsions; difficulty in breathing; fainting; muscle twitches; palpitations; rash; severe abdominal pain; or unusual weakness.

Possible Drug Interactions
• Can increase the diuretic effect of furosemide.

- Reserpine can cause rapid heart rate when used with this drug.

- Beta blockers (acebutolol, atenolol, betaxolol, carteolol, esmolol, labetalol, metoprolol, nadolol, penbutolol, pindolol, propranolol, or timolol) can decrease the effectiveness of this drug.

- Can increase the side effects of nonprescription sinus, cough, cold, asthma, allergy, and diet products; digoxin; and oral anticoagulants (blood thinners, such as warfarin).

- Can decrease the effectiveness of phenytoin and lithium.

- Phenobarbital, carbamazepine, and rifampin can increase the elimination of this drug from the body, decreasing its effectiveness.

- Cimetidine, ciprofloxacin, erythromycin, norfloxacin, troleandomycin, oral contraceptives (birth control pills), allopurinol, and thiabendazole can decrease the elimination of this drug from the body and increase its side effects.

- Verapamil can increase the side effects of this drug.

Tell Your Child's Doctor If
- Your child is taking any other medications.

- Your child has had unusual or allergic reactions to any medications, especially to this drug, aminophylline, caffeine, dyphylline, oxtriphylline, or theobromine.

- Your child has or ever had heart or kidney disease, low or high blood pressure, liver disease, stomach ulcers, or thyroid disease.

- Your child has experienced any episodes of high fever or prolonged diarrhea while taking this drug.

- Your child is taking this drug before the child receives any vaccinations, especially those to prevent the flu.

- Your child is taking this drug before having surgery or dental treatment.

- Your child smokes cigarettes or marijuana. Smoking may decrease this drug's effectiveness by decreasing blood concentrations. However, your child should not quit smoking without first informing the doctor as dosage adjustments may be necesary.

- Your daughter is or becomes pregnant. Although this drug appears to be safe during pregnancy, extensive studies in humans have not been conducted. Asthma should be controlled by a doctor during pregnancy.

- Your daughter is breast-feeding her baby. Small amounts of this drug pass into breast milk and may cause irritability, fretfulness, or insomnia in nursing infants.

Special Instructions
- Your child should avoid drinking large amounts of caffeine-containing beverages, such as coffee, cocoa, tea, or cola drinks, and avoid eating large amounts of chocolate. These products may increase the side effects of this drug.

- Do not change your child's diet without first consulting the doctor. A high-protein, low-carbohydrate diet or char-broiled foods may affect the action of this drug.

- Do not give any nonprescription asthma, allergy, cough, cold, sinus, or diet product without first speaking to the doctor or pharmacist. These products increase the side effects of this drug.

- Do not change brands or dosage forms of this drug without the doctor's permission. If your refill looks different, check with the doctor or pharmacist. Not all brands are interchangeable.

Symptoms of Overdose: Anorexia, nausea, vomiting, nervousness, insomnia, agitation, irritability, headache, rapid heartbeat, convulsions. Convulsions or abnormal rhythm of the heart may be the first signs of toxicity.

Special Notes
• Young children may be more sensitive to the effects of this drug.

• The doctor may require periodic blood tests to be sure the blood concentration of this drug is within a safe and effective range.

Be Accurate

If you don't give medication correctly, it may be ineffective or even cause side effects. An estimated 10 to 30 percent of medications aren't effective because they have been given incorrectly. To do it right, you have to give the exact amount of medicine prescribed at the scheduled time, for the specified duration, and in the appropriate manner. Always read the label, follow the directions carefully, and use the appropriate equipment for measuring and administering the medication. Also, be sure to wash your hands before you give any medication to your child.

THIABENDAZOLE

Administration Guidelines

• Give with food. This decreases stomach irritation and increases its absorption.

• Tablets may be crushed and mixed with food, chewed, or swallowed whole.

• Generally given 1 to 2 times a day.

• The duration of treatment varies with the type of infection: 2 to 4 consecutive days for trichinosis; 3 days for strongyliasis and dracunculiasis; 2 to 5 or 5 to 7 days for cutaneous and visceral larva migrans.

• Give at evenly spaced intervals around the clock. This drug works best when blood concentrations are kept within a safe and effective range.

• Missed doses: Give immediately. However, if you do not remember until it is time for the next dose, give the missed dose and space the next dose about halfway through the regular interval between doses; then return to the regular schedule. Do not skip any doses.

• Give this drug for the entire time prescribed by your child's doctor, even if the symptoms disappear before the end of that period. If the drug is stopped too soon, the infection could recur.

Side Effects

Tell your child's doctor about any side effects that are persistent or particularly bothersome.

More Common. Dizziness, drowsiness, fever, headache, rash, itching, hair loss, diarrhea, abdominal pain, nausea, vomiting, ringing noise in the ears

Less Common. It is especially important to tell the doctor if your child experiences blood in the urine, persistent fever or headache, body rash (Steven-Johnson syndrome), itching, or blurred vision.

Possible Drug Interactions

• Increases the concentration of theophylline in the bloodstream.

Tell Your Child's Doctor If

• Your child has or ever had unusual or allergic reactions to any medications, especially to this drug.

• Your child has any liver, kidney, or blood disease.

• Symptoms of infection are getting worse rather than improving.

Brand Name: Mintezol

Generic Available: No

Type of Drug: Anthelmintic

Use: Treats helmintic infections of the skin and gastrointestinal tract such as strongyliasis, cutaneous and visceral larva migrans, dracunculosis, and trichinosis.

Time Required for Drug to Take Effect: It may take a few days to achieve maximum effect.

Dosage Forms and Strengths: Tablets, chewable (500 mg); Suspension (500 mg/5mL)

Storage: Store tablets and suspension in tightly closed containers in a cool, dry place.

How This Drug Works: Deprives the infecting worms of nutrition, causing their eradication.

- Your daughter is or becomes pregnant. The safety of this drug in pregnancy has not been established in humans.

- Your daughter is breast-feeding her baby. The safety of this drug during breast-feeding has not been established.

Symptoms of Overdose: Severe forms of side effects listed above.

Keep It Out of Reach

Do not rely on a child-resistant cap to deter your child from opening a bottle of medication. Child-resistant does not mean childproof. Legally, a cap can be called child-resistant if 80 percent of all five-year-olds need more than five minutes to open it. That means the other 20 percent could get into it in even less time. Put the bottle in a hard-to-reach cabinet with a childproof lock. Do not keep it on the countertop, kitchen table, or nightstand.

THIETHYLPERAZINE

Administration Guidelines

• Give with food, water, or milk to decrease stomach upset.

• Your child must remain lying down for 1 hour after an intramuscular shot.

• Give only as directed by your child's doctor.

• Missed doses: Give as soon as possible, but do not give within 3 hours of the next dose. Do not give double doses.

Side Effects

Tell your child's doctor about any side effects that are persistent or particularly bothersome.

More Common. Drowsiness, dizziness, dry mouth and nose

Less Common. Constipation, decreased sweating, fever, headache, light-headedness, unusual weakness or fatigue, nightmares, restlessness, irritability, ringing or buzzing in the ears, skin rash. Contact the doctor immediately if your child experiences lip smacking or puckering; puffing of cheeks; rapid or fine wormlike tongue movements; uncontrolled chewing movements; uncontrolled arm or leg movements; aching muscles and joints; blurred vision; change in color perception; difficulty seeing at night; difficulty in speaking or swallowing; fainting; inability to move the eyes; loss of balance; masklike face; muscle spasms; shuffling walk; stiffness of arms or legs; twitching movements; trembling and shaking; twisting movements of body, weakness of arms and legs; seizures; fast heartbeat; confusion; fever and chills; nausea; vomiting; diarrhea; sore throat and fever; skin itching; swelling of arms, hands and face; unusual bruising or bleeding; yellow skin or eyes; abdominal or stomach pains; skin rash; or severe sunburn.

Possible Drug Interactions

• Central nervous system depressants such as alcohol, antihistamines, cold preparations, muscle relaxants, tranquilizers, and some pain medications may cause extreme drowsiness, low blood pressure, or a decrease in respiratory rate when used with this drug.

• Cough and cold products may increase the chance of heat stroke, dizziness, dry mouth, blurred vision, and constipation.

• Epinephrine may cause low blood pressure.

• Increases the cardiac toxicity of quinidine.

Brand Name: Torecan

Generic Available: No

Type of Drug: Antiemetic, phenothiazine

Use: Treats nausea and vomiting

Time Required for Drug to Take Effect: Up to 30 minutes

Dosage Forms and Strengths: Injection (5 mg/mL); Suppository (10 mg); Tablet (10 mg)

Storage: Store at room temperature in tightly closed, light-resistant containers

How This Drug Works: Causes complex changes in the central nervous system, producing antiemetic effects.

Tell Your Child's Doctor If

• Your child has had an allergic reaction to this drug or any other medication.

• Your child is taking any other prescription or nonprescription medicine.

• Your child abuses alcohol or has asthma, sleep apnea, lung disease, heart disease, seizures, glaucoma, liver or kidney disease, difficult urination, chicken pox, nausea and vomiting, measles, Reye syndrome, or any other medical condition.

• Your child continues to have a dry mouth after 2 weeks. Continued dry mouth can lead to cavities.

• Your child develops a rash from the sun.

• Your daughter is or becomes pregnant.

• Your daughter is breast-feeding her baby. This drug can pass into breast milk. The American Academy of Pediatrics has concerns about the effect of similar medications on the baby.

Special Instructions

• Do not stop giving this drug without first talking with the doctor if your child has been taking it for a long time. The doctor may want to gradually reduce the dose.

• Do not allow your child to drink alcohol while taking this drug.

• Do not give other medicines that may make your child sleepy.

• To prevent dizziness or light-headedness, your child should stand up slowly.

• Do not give your child cough or cold products without first checking with the doctor.

• Do not give any other medications without first asking the pharmacist or the doctor.

• Your child should avoid exposure to sunlight and sunlamps. This drug may cause a skin rash or severe sunburn with exposure to direct sunlight or ultraviolet light. Make sure your child wears an effective sunscreen when out-of-doors.

Symptoms of Overdose: Deep sleep, coma, low blood pressure, increased severity of side effects

Special Notes

• Make sure you know how your child is reacting to this drug before allowing participation in an activity that requires alertness and coordination, such as riding a bicycle. This drug may cause your child to have blurred vision, dizziness, drowsiness, or to be less alert.

• The safety and efficacy of this drug has not been established in children younger than 12 years of age.

• Children, especially those with chicken pox, infections, measles, diarrhea, vomiting, or dehydration, are more prone to serious side effects.

• With long-term use, your child's progress should be checked by regular visits to the doctor.

THIORIDAZINE

Administration Guidelines

- Shake the suspension well before measuring each dose.

- Give with food or a full glass of water or milk to decrease stomach upset.

- Dilute concentrate in distilled water, or orange or grapefruit juice before giving.

- Suspension does not need to be diluted.

- Do not spill suspension or concentrate on skin or clothing. These forms can be irritating and cause a skin rash.

- Missed doses: Give as soon as you remember. Then give any remaining doses for that day at regularly spaced intervals. Do not give double doses.

- Do not give within 2 hours of giving antacids or medicine for diarrhea.

- Do not stop giving this drug without first checking with your child's doctor. The doctor may want to gradually reduce the dose before stopping it.

- Give this drug only as directed by the doctor.

Side Effects

Tell your child's doctor about any side effects that are persistent or particularly bothersome.

More Common. Constipation, decreased sweating, dizziness, drowsiness, dry mouth, stuffy nose, low blood pressure, stomach upset, nausea, vomiting, weight gain, blurred vision, difficulty urinating, changes in menstrual period. Contact the doctor immediately if your child experiences lip smacking or puckering, puffing of cheeks, rapid or fine wormlike tongue movements, uncontrolled chewing movements, uncontrolled arm or leg movements, blurred vision, change in color perception, difficulty seeing at night, difficulty in speaking or swallowing, fainting, inability to move the eyes, loss of balance, masklike face, muscle spasms, restlessness or need to keep moving, shuffling walk, stiffness of arms or legs, twitching movements, trembling and shaking, twisting movements of body or weakness of arms and legs, skin rash, or severe sunburn.

Less Common. Contact the doctor immediately if your child experiences seizures, difficult or fast breathing, fast or irregular heartbeat, fever, high or low blood pressure, increased sweating, loss of bladder control, severe muscle stiffness, pale skin, or unusual fatigue or weakness.

Brand Names: Mellaril, Mellaril-S

Generic Available: Yes

Type of Drug: Antipsychotic agent, phenothiazine

Use: Treats nervous, mental, emotional, and behavioral disorders such as psychoses and mania.

Time Required for Drug to Take Effect: It may take 6 weeks to 6 months to achieve full benefit for mental and emotional disorders.

Dosage Forms and Strengths: Tablets (10 mg, 15 mg, 25 mg, 50 mg, 100 mg, 150 mg, 200 mg); Suspension (25 mg/ 5 mL, 100 mg/5 mL); Concentrate (30 mg/mL, 100 mg/mL)

Storage: Store at room temperature in tightly closed, light-resistant containers. Do not freeze the concentrate or suspension.

How This Drug Works: Causes complex changes in the central nervous system, producing tranquilizing effects.

Possible Drug Interactions

- Central nervous system depressants such as alcohol, antihistamines, cold preparations, muscle relaxants, tranquilizers, and some pain medications may cause extreme drowsiness when used with this drug.

- Cough and cold products may increase the chance of heat stroke, dizziness, dry mouth, blurred vision, and constipation.

- Antidepressants, monoamine oxidase (MAO) inhibitors, or lithium lead to increased side effects. These medications need to be dosed carefully when used together.

- Medications that lower blood pressure may lead to blood pressure that's too low when given with this drug.

- Antithyroid drugs lead to an increase in rare blood disorders when given with this drug.

- Epinephrine may cause low blood pressure.

Tell Your Child's Doctor If

- Your child has had an allergic reaction to this drug or any other medication.

- Your child has taken or is taking any other prescription or nonprescription medicine.

- Your child abuses alcohol or has lung or heart disease, seizures, glaucoma, liver or kidney disease, difficulty urinating, stomach ulcers, bone marrow or blood disorders, Reye syndrome, or any other medical condition.

- The blurred vision continues beyond the first few weeks or gets worse.

- Your child develops a new medical problem.

- Your child develops a rash from the sun.

- Your child continues to have a dry mouth after 2 weeks. Continued dry mouth can lead to cavities.

- Your child develops side effects after the drug has been stopped.

- Your daughter is or becomes pregnant.

- Your daughter is breast-feeding her baby. This drug can pass into breast milk, and the American Academy of Pediatrics is concerned about the effects of similar medications on the baby.

Special Instructions

- Protect your child from overheating during exercise, play, or hot weather. This drug decreases sweating and can cause an increase in body temperature. Hot baths, hot tubs, or saunas may make your child dizzy or faint.

- Dress your child warmly as this drug increases sensitivity to cold weather.

- Your child should avoid exposure to sunlight and sunlamps. This drug may cause a skin rash or severe sunburn with exposure to direct sunlight or ultraviolet light. Make sure your child wears an effective sunscreen and sunglasses that block ultraviolet light.

- Do not give any medication with this drug before talking to the pharmacist or doctor.

- Do not let your child have surgery or any medical treatment or dental work unless the doctor or dentist is aware that your child is taking this drug.

- Do not allow your child to drink alcohol while taking this drug.

- Do not give other medicines that may make your child sleepy.

- Do not give your child cough or cold products without first checking with the doctor.

- Your child should stand up slowly to prevent dizziness or light-headedness.

Symptoms of Overdose: Deep sleep, coma, low blood pressure, increased severity of side effects

Special Notes

- Make sure you know how your child is reacting to this drug before allowing participation in an activity that requires alertness and coordination, such as riding a bicycle. This drug may cause your child to have blurred vision, dizziness, drowsiness, or to be less alert.

• This drug may cause serious side effects that may not go away after this drug is stopped. Discuss this with the doctor.

• Doses are increased slowly to decrease side effects.

• The effects of this drug may last up to a week after you stop giving it.

• Appropriate dosage for children younger than 2 years of age has not been established.

• May turn urine a pink or reddish-brown color.

• Your child's progress should be checked by regular visits to the doctor.

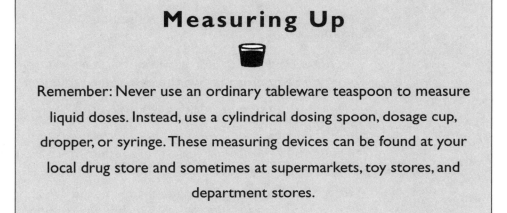

Measuring Up

Remember: Never use an ordinary tableware teaspoon to measure liquid doses. Instead, use a cylindrical dosing spoon, dosage cup, dropper, or syringe. These measuring devices can be found at your local drug store and sometimes at supermarkets, toy stores, and department stores.

Brand Name: Navane

Generic Available: Yes

Type of Drug: Antipsychotic agent

Use: Treats nervous, mental, emotional, and behavioral disorders such as psychoses or mania.

Time Required for Drug to Take Effect: It may take 6 weeks to 6 months to achieve full benefit for mental and emotional disorders.

Dosage Forms and Strengths: Capsules (1 mg, 2 mg, 5 mg, 10 mg, 20 mg); Concentrate (5 mg/mL)

Storage: Store at room temperature in tightly closed, light-resistant containers. Protect concentrate from freezing.

How This Drug Works: Causes complex changes in the central nervous system, producing tranquilizing effects.

THIOTHIXENE

Administration Guidelines

• Give with food or a full glass of water or milk to decrease stomach upset.

• Dilute concentrate with 1 cup tomato or fruit juice, milk, water, soup, or carbonated beverage before giving.

• Do not spill the concentrate on skin or clothing. It can cause a skin rash.

• Missed doses: Give as soon as you remember, then give any remaining doses for that day at regularly spaced intervals. Do not give double doses.

• Do not give within 2 hours of giving antacids or medicine for diarrhea.

• Do not stop giving this drug without first checking with your child's doctor. The doctor may want to gradually reduce the dose.

• Give this drug to your child only as directed by the doctor.

Side Effects

Tell your child's doctor about any side effects that are persistent or particularly bothersome.

More Common. Constipation, decreased sweating, drowsiness, dry mouth, increased appetite, weight gain, stuffy nose, dizziness, light-headedness, fainting. Contact the doctor if your child experiences severe restlessness, the need to keep moving, difficulty speaking, inability to move the eyes, muscle spasms, twitching body movements, loss of balance, masklike face, shuffling walk, stiffness of arms and legs, trembling, lip smacking or puckering, puffing of cheeks, rapid or wormlike movements of the tongue, chewing movements, uncontrolled movements of arms and legs

Less Common. Changes in menstrual period, swelling of breasts. Contact the doctor if your child experiences skin rash; difficulty urinating; blurred vision; fainting; skin discoloration; sore throat and fever; unusual bleeding or bruising; hot, dry skin; lack of sweating; muscle weakness; yellow skin or eyes; seizures; difficulty breathing; increased sweating; fast heartbeat; pale skin; fatigue; increased blinking or spasms of the eyelids; or uncontrolled twisting of the neck, arms, legs, or trunk.

Possible Drug Interactions

• Central nervous system depressants such as alcohol, antihistamines, cold preparations, muscle relaxants, tranquilizers, and some pain medications may cause extreme drowsiness when used with this drug.

- Epinephrine may cause low blood pressure.

- Increases the cardiac toxicity of quinidine.

Tell Your Child's Doctor If
- Your child has had an allergic reaction to this drug or any other medication.

- Your child has taken or is taking any other prescription or nonprescription medicine.

- Your child abuses alcohol or has lung or heart disease, seizures, glaucoma, liver or kidney disease, difficulty urinating, stomach ulcers, bone marrow or blood disorders, Reye syndrome, or any other medical condition.

- The blurred vision continues beyond the first few weeks or gets worse.

- Your child develops a new medical problem.

- Your child develops a rash from the sun.

- Your child continues to have a dry mouth after 2 weeks. Continued dry mouth can lead to cavities.

- Your child develops side effects after this drug has been stopped.

- Your daughter is or becomes pregnant.

- Your daughter is breast-feeding her baby. This drug can pass into breast milk, and the American Academy of Pediatrics is concerned about the effects of similar medications on the baby.

Special Instructions
- Protect your child from overheating during exercise, play, or hot weather as this drug decreases sweating and can cause an increase in body temperature. Hot baths, hot tubs, or saunas may make your child dizzy or faint.

- Your child should avoid exposure to sunlight and sunlamps. This drug may cause a skin rash or severe sunburn with exposure to direct sunlight or ultraviolet light. Make sure your child wears an effective sunscreen when out-of-doors.

- Do not give any other medication before talking to the pharmacist or doctor.

- Do not let your child have surgery or any medical treatment or dental work unless the doctor or dentist is aware that your child is taking this drug.

- Do not allow your child to drink alcohol while taking this drug.

- Do not give other medicines that may make your child sleepy.

- Do not give your child cough or cold products without first checking with the doctor.

- Your child should stand up slowly to prevent dizziness or light-headedness.

- Limit your child's caffeine intake.

Symptoms of Overdose: Seizures, difficulty breathing, drowsiness, coma, fast heartbeat, fever, low blood pressure, muscle trembling, jerking, stiffness, uncontrolled movements, small pupils, excitement, fatigue, weakness

Special Notes
- Make sure you know how your child is reacting to this drug before allowing participation in activities that require alertness and coordination, such as riding a bicycle. This drug may cause your child to have blurred vision, dizziness, drowsiness, or to be less alert.

- This drug may cause side effects that are serious or may not go away after stopping it. Talk this over with the doctor.

- The safety and efficacy of this drug in children younger than 12 years of age has not been established.

- Doses are increased slowly to decrease the side effects.

- Your child's progress should be checked by regular visits to the doctor.

Brand Names: Armour Thyroid, S-P-T, Thyrar

Generic Available: Yes

Type of Drug: Thyroid Hormone

Use: Treats low thyroid hormone levels and other thyroid problems.

Time Required for Drug to Take Effect: Onset within 3 to 5 days; full effect in 3 to 4 weeks.

Dosage Forms and Strengths: Tablets (15 mg, 30 mg, 60 mg, 90 mg, 120 mg, 180 mg, 240 mg, 300 mg); Capsules (60 mg, 120 mg, 180 mg, 300 mg)

Storage: Store at room temperature in tightly closed containers.

How This Drug Works: Replaces thyroid hormone.

THYROID HORMONE

Administration Guidelines

• Usually given once a day.

• Give only as directed by your child's doctor.

• Missed doses: If you miss a once-a-day dose, give the dose as soon as you remember on the day missed. Otherwise, skip the dose and go back to the regular schedule. Do not give double doses.

• Do not suddenly stop giving this drug before speaking to the doctor.

Side Effects

Tell your child's doctor about any side effects that are persistent or particularly bothersome.

More Common. Temporary decrease in performance, especially in school, due to short attention, hyperactivity, insomnia, irritability, and behavior difficulties.

Less Common. Contact the doctor if your child develops a headache, hives, skin rash, chest pain, rapid or irregular heartbeat, or shortness of breath.

Possible Drug Interactions

• Increases the effect of warfarin.

• Cholestyramine and colestipol decrease the absorption of this drug.

Tell Your Child's Doctor If

• Your child has thyroid, heart, or adrenal gland disease; high blood pressure; diabetes mellitus; diabetes insipidus; asthma; lung disease; or any other medical condition.

• Your child has taken or is taking any other prescription or nonprescription medicine.

• Your child has had an allergic reaction to this drug or to any other medications, foods, preservatives, or dyes.

• Your child has changes in appetite, diarrhea, fever, hand tremors, headache, irritably, leg cramps, an increase or decrease in weight, nervousness, sweating, trouble sleeping, vomiting, or changes in menstrual periods. The dose may need to be changed.

• Your child develops a new medical problem.

• Your child is taking this drug before having any medical tests, surgery, or dental work.

• Your daughter is or becomes pregnant.

Special Instructions
• Do not use a different brand of this drug without first checking with the doctor. Not all brands are interchangeable.

Symptoms of Overdose: Acute overdose: Fever, low blood sugar, or heart failure. Chronic overdose: Weight loss, nervousness, sweating, fast heart rate, insomnia, heat intolerance, fever, or psychosis.

Special Notes
• Children with long-standing, severe thyroid underactivity will experience temporary behavioral changes if thyroid hormone is replaced too fast. These children need to be started at a low dose, increasing it slowly to decrease these side effects.

• Most children are started on levothyroxine instead of this drug because the hormone content of thyroid varies between manufacturing lots.

• Your child may always have to take this drug.

• Doses may be gradually increased to decrease behavioral side effects.

• Thyroid blood tests (T_4 and TSH blood concentrations) are measured to determine the dose needed.

• Your child's progress should be checked regularly by the doctor.

☎ Just Call

If you have any concerns about any side effects, even minor ones, you should be sure to discuss them with your child's doctor. The doctor may be able to minimize or eliminate the side effects by prescribing a different medication or changing your child's dosage, dosing schedule, or the way the drug is given. (Do not make adjustments on your own without discussing them with your doctor.) At the very least, the doctor can assure you that the medication's benefits far outweigh its side effects.

Brand Names: AKTob, Tobrex

Generic Available: No

Type of Drug: Antibiotic

Use: Treats superficial ophthalmic infections.

Time Required for Drug to Take Effect: Approximately 2 days.

Dosage Forms and Strengths: Ointment (0.3%); Solution (0.3%)

Storage: Store at room temperature in tightly closed containers. Discard any that you no longer need.

How This Drug Works: Kills the offending bacteria by inhibiting protein synthesis in the bacteria.

TOBRAMYCIN (OPHTHALMIC)

Side Effects
Tell your child's doctor about any side effects that are persistent or particularly bothersome.

More Common. Blurred vision, burning, or stinging. These side effects should disappear as your child's body becomes accustomed to this drug.

Less Common. It is especially important to tell the doctor if your child experiences disturbed or reduced vision, eye pain, itching or swelling, severe irritation, or body rash.

Tell Your Child's Doctor If
• Your child has had allergic or unusual reactions to drugs, especially to this drug or to any other aminoglycoside antibiotics such as amikacin, gentamicin, kanamycin, neomycin, netilmicin, paromomycin, or streptomycin.

• Your child has or ever had kidney disease or fungal or viral infections of the eye.

• There is no change in your child's condition 2 or 3 days after starting this drug. It may not be effective for your child's infection.

• Your daughter is pregnant.

• Your daughter is breast-feeding her baby. Small amounts of this drug may pass into breast milk.

Special Instructions
• Your child should not apply makeup to the affected eye.

Symptoms of Overdose: Inflammation of the tear duct and cornea, abnormal flushing of the skin, production of excess tears, swelling of the lid or area around the eyes, and lid itching

TOLMETIN

Administration Guidelines

• Give with a full glass of water.

• Give with food or immediately after meals to avoid stomach upset.

• Give on a regular basis if your child is taking this drug for arthritis.

• Missed doses: Give as soon as you remember if it's within 2 hours of the missed dose. Otherwise, skip the missed dose and give the next dose at the scheduled time. Do not give double doses.

Side Effects

Tell your child's doctor about any side effects that are persistent or particularly bothersome.

More Common. Heartburn, nausea, vomiting, stomach pain, dizziness, drowsiness, light-headedness, indigestion

Less Common. Bitter taste, constipation, decreased appetite, flushing. Contact the doctor if your child experiences bloody or black, tarry stools; changes in vision; spitting up or vomiting of blood, severe stomach upset; skin rash; hives; trouble breathing; wheezing; ringing in the ears; or difficult or painful urination.

Possible Drug Interactions

• Other anti-inflammatory medications and aspirin can increase stomach upset when used with this drug.

• May decrease the effect of diuretics.

• Blood thinners such as warfarin may increase bleeding complications when used with this drug.

Tell Your Child's Doctor If

• Your child has had allergic reactions to any medications, especially other nonsteroidal anti-inflammatory drugs or aspirin.

• Your child has any diseases, especially asthma, stomach problems, or liver or kidney disease.

• Your daughter is or becomes pregnant.

• Your daughter is breast-feeding her baby. This drug can pass into breast milk; however, the American Academy of Pediatrics considers it compatible with breast-feeding in most cases.

Special Instructions

• Before your child has any medical or dental surgery, tell the doctor performing the procedure your child is taking this drug.

Symptoms of Overdose: Fainting, fast or irregular breathing, confusion, ringing in the ears, convulsions, sweating, blurred vision

Brand Name: Tolectin

Generic Available: No

Type of Drug: Nonsteroidal anti-inflammatory analgesic.

Use: Relieves mild to moderate pain and inflammation (swelling and stiffness) of arthritis.

Time Required for Drug to Take Effect: 1 to 2 hours for pain relief. Begins to relieve inflammation of arthritis in 1 to 2 weeks, with full effect in 4 weeks.

Dosage Forms and Strengths: Tablets (200 mg, 600 mg); Capsules (400 mg)

Storage: Store at room temperature in tightly closed, light-resistant containers.

How This Drug Works: Decreases the production of the chemical prostaglandin.

Brand Names: Absorbine Antifungal, Aftate, NP-27, Quinsana Plus, Tinactin, Ting, Zeasorb-AF

Generic Available: Yes

Type of Drug: Topical antifungal

Use: Treats certain fungal infections of the skin such as athlete's foot, jock itch, ringworm, and tinea versicolor. Can also be used to prevent athlete's foot.

Time Required for Drug to Take Effect: Several days to several weeks.

Dosage Forms and Strength: Cream; Solution; Gel; Powder; Spray Powder; Spray Liquid (all 1%)

Storage: Store at room temperature in tightly closed, light-resistant containers.

How This Drug Works: Destroys certain types of skin fungus.

TOLNAFTATE

Administration Guidelines
• For external use only. Avoid contact with the eyes.

• Wash infected area thoroughly and dry before applying.

• Usually applied 2 times a day.

• Treatment for several weeks may be necessary to clear the infection. Continue to treat for approximately 2 weeks after signs and symptoms of infection disappear.

• Discontinue use if irritation or inflammation occurs.

Tell Your Child's Doctor If
• Your child has had allergic reactions to any medications

• Your child has any other diseases.

• Your child is taking any other medications.

Special Notes
• This product usually is not effective for fingernail, toenail, or scalp infections.

TRAZODONE

Administration Guidelines

- Give with or shortly after a meal or snack to decrease light-headedness and sedation.

- Usually given 2 to 3 times a day. A larger dose may be given at bedtime.

- The 150 mg tablet can be broken into thirds or halves, yielding doses of 50 mg or 75 mg. The 300 mg tablet can be broken into thirds or halves, yielding doses of 100 mg or 150 mg.

- Missed doses: Give as soon as possible, but do not give within 4 hours of the next dose. Do not give double doses.

- Give only as directed by your child's doctor.

- Do not stop giving this drug without first checking with the doctor. The doctor may want to gradually decrease the dose before stopping it.

Side Effects

Tell your doctor about any side effects that are persistent or particularly bothersome.

More Common. Dizziness, light-headedness, drowsiness, insomnia, dry mouth, headache, nausea, vomiting, unpleasant taste in the mouth

Less Common. Blurred vision, constipation, diarrhea, muscle aches or pains, unusual fatigue, weakness. Contact the doctor if your child experiences confusion; seizures; muscle tremors; skin rash; fast or slow heartbeat; fainting; excitement; or priapism (prolonged, inappropriate, and painful penile erection).

Possible Drug Interactions

- Central nervous system depressants such as alcohol, antihistamines, cold or hay fever preparations, medicine for seizures, muscle relaxants, tranquilizers, and some pain medications may cause extreme drowsiness when used with this drug.

- Medications that lower blood pressure may lead to blood pressure that's too low. These medications need to be dosed carefully when used together.

Tell Your Child's Doctor If

- Your child has had an allergic reaction to this drug or any other medication.

- Your child has been or is taking any other prescription or nonprescription medicine.

Brand Names: Desyrel, Trazon, Trialodine

Generic Available: Yes

Type of Drug: Antidepressant

Use: Treats mental depression.

Time Required for Drug to Take Effect: 2 to 6 weeks

Dosage Form and Strengths: Tablets (50 mg, 100 mg, 150 mg, 300 mg)

Storage: Store at room temperature in tightly closed, light-resistant containers.

How This Drug Works: Increases the concentration of serotonin in the central nervous system.

- Your child abuses alcohol; has heart, liver, or kidney disease; or any other medical condition.

- Your child continues to have a dry mouth after 2 weeks. Continued dry mouth can lead to cavities.

- Your daughter is or becomes pregnant.

- Your daughter is breast-feeding her baby. This drug can pass into breast milk, and the American Academy of Pediatrics is concerned about its effect on the baby.

Special Instructions

- Do not allow your child to drink alcohol while taking this drug.

- Do not give other medicines that may make your child sleepy.

- Your child should stand up slowly to prevent dizziness or light-headedness.

- Do not let your child have surgery or any medical or dental treatment unless you tell the doctor or dentist the child is taking this drug.

- Do not give any other medication without first checking with the pharmacist or the doctor.

Symptoms of Overdose: Drowsiness, loss of muscle coordination, nausea, vomiting, low blood pressure

Special Notes

- Make sure you know how your child is reacting to this drug before allowing participation in an activity that requires alertness and coordination, such as riding a bicycle. This drug may cause your child to have blurred vision, dizziness, drowsiness, or to be less alert.

- Doses for children younger than 6 years of age have not been established.

- Priapism (prolonged, painful, and inappropriate penile erection) is a medical emergency. Contact the doctor or an emergency room immediately.

- Doses may be increased slowly to decrease the side effects.

- Your child's progress should be checked with regular visits to the doctor.

TRIAMCINOLONE (SYSTEMIC)

Administration Guidelines
• May be given with food or milk to prevent stomach irritation.

• If your child is taking only 1 dose of this drug a day, try to give it before 9:00 A.M. This will mimic the body's normal production of this chemical.

• Missed doses: It is important not to miss a dose of this drug. If you do miss a dose, follow these guidelines:

1. If usually given more than once a day, give as soon as possible and return to the regular schedule. If it is already time for the next dose, double the dose given.

2. If usually given once a day, give as soon as possible. If you do not remember until the next day, do not give the missed dose at all, just follow the regular dosing schedule. Do not give double doses.

3. If usually given every other day, give as soon as you remember. If you miss the scheduled time by a whole day, give it when you remember, then skip a day before you give the next dose. Do not give double doses. If you miss more than one dose, contact your child's doctor.

• Do not suddenly stop giving this drug before speaking with the doctor.

Side Effects
Tell your child's doctor about any side effects that are persistent or particularly bothersome.

More Common. Dizziness, false sense of well-being, fatigue, increased appetite, increased sweating, indigestion, leg cramps, menstrual irregularities, muscle weakness, nausea, swelling of the skin on the face, restlessness, sleep disorders, or weight gain

Less Common. It is important to tell the doctor if your child experiences abdominal enlargement or pain; acne; back or rib pain; bloody or black, tarry stools; blurred vision; convulsions; eye pain; fever and sore throat; headaches; slow healing of wounds; increased thirst and urination; depression; mood changes; muscle wasting; nightmares; peptic ulcers; rapid weight gain (3 to 5 pounds in a week); rash; shortness of breath; unusual bleeding or bruising; or unusual weakness.

Possible Drug Interactions
• Aspirin and anti-inflammatory medications such as ibuprofen, indomethacin, and ketoprofen may increase the stomach problems caused by this drug.

Brand Names: Aristocort A, Kenacort

Generic Available: Yes

Type of Drug: Adrenocorticosteroid hormone

Use: Treats a variety of disorders, including endocrine and rheumatic disorders; asthma; blood diseases; certain cancers; eye disorders; gastrointestinal disturbances such as ulcerative colitis; respiratory diseases; and inflammatory diseases such as arthritis, dermatitis, and poison ivy.

Time Required for Drug to Take Effect: Varies depending on the illness being treated. It may be several days before this drug takes effect.

Dosage Forms and Strengths: Tablets (1mg, 2 mg, 4 mg, 8 mg); Syrup (2 mg and 4 mg per 5 mL).

Storage: Store at room temperature in tightly closed containers.

How This Drug Works: How this drug works is not completely understood. It is similar to the cortisonelike chemicals naturally produced by the adrenal gland that are involved in various regulatory processes in the body.

• Cholestyramine and colestipol can bind to this drug in the stomach and prevent its absorption.

Tell Your Child's Doctor If:

• Your child is taking any other medications.

• Your child has had allergic reactions to this drug or other adrenocorticoids such as betamethasone, cortisone, dexamethasone, fluocinolone, hydrocortisone, methylpred-nisolone, prednisone, or prednisolone.

• Your child has recently been exposed to or currently has chicken pox or measles.

• Your child has any medical problems such as diabetes, glaucoma, fungal infections, heart disease, high blood pressure, peptic ulcers, thyroid disease, tuberculosis, ulcerative colitis, or kidney or liver disease before starting this drug.

• Your daughter is or becomes pregnant.

• Your daughter is breast-feeding her baby.

Special Instructions

• Do not have your child vaccinated or immunized while taking this drug. This drug decreases the effectiveness of vaccines and can lead to infection if a live virus vaccine is given.

Symptoms of Overdose: Severe restlessness

Special Notes

• With long-term use, the doctor may want your child to be on a low-salt and potassium-rich diet. The doctor may also want your child's eye examined periodically during treatment to detect glaucoma and cataracts.

• With long-term use, the doctor may need to increase your child's dose during times of stress, such as serious infection, injury, or surgery.

TRIAMTERENE

Administration Guidelines
- Give with a glass of milk or with a meal to decrease stomach irritation (unless your child's doctor directs you to do otherwise).

- Generally given once a day.

- Try to give at the same time(s) every day. Avoid giving a dose after 6:00 P.M.; otherwise, your child may have to get up during the night to urinate.

- Missed doses: Give as soon as possible. However, if it is time for the next dose, do not give the missed dose at all. Wait until the next scheduled dose. Do not give double doses.

Side Effects
Tell your child's doctor about any side effects that are persistent or particularly bothersome.

More Common. Diarrhea, dizziness, drowsiness, dry mouth, headache, increased thirst, increased urination, nausea, fatigue, upset stomach, or vomiting. These side effects should disappear as your child's body adjusts to this drug.

Less Common. It is especially important to tell the doctor if your child experiences anxiety; back or flank (side) pain; confusion; cracking at the corners of the mouth; difficulty in breathing; extreme weakness; fever; mouth sores; numbness or tingling in the hands, feet, or lips; painful urination; palpitations; rash; a red or inflamed tongue; sore throat; unusual bleeding or bruising; or unusual fatigue.

Possible Drug Interactions
- Antihypertensives such as benazepril, fosinopril, lisinopril, and ramipril, or spironolactone, amiloride, potassium salts, low-salt milk, salt substitutes, captopril, enalapril, or laxatives can cause serious side effects from hyperkalemia (high levels of potassium in the blood) when used with this drug.

- Nonprescription medications for weight control or for allergy, asthma, cough, cold, or sinus problems can cause an increase in blood pressure.

- May decrease the effectiveness of antigout medications, insulin, and oral antidiabetic medications.

- May increase the side effects of lithium.

- Indomethacin may decrease the diuretic effects of this drug.

Brand Name: Dyrenium

Generic Available: No

Type of Drug: Diuretic and antihypertensive

Use: Treats high blood pressure. Also reduces fluid accumulation in the body caused by conditions such as heart failure, cirrhosis of the liver, kidney disease, and the long-term use of some medications.

Time Required for Drug to Take Effect: It may be 1 to 2 weeks before this drug becomes fully effective.

Dosage Form and Strengths: Capsules (50 mg, 100 mg)

Storage: Store at room temperature in tightly closed, light-resistant containers.

How This Drug Works: Reduces fluid accumulation by increasing the elimination of salt and water through the kidneys.

Tell Your Child's Doctor If

• Your child is taking any prescription or nonprescription medications, especially any of those listed above.

• Your child has had unusual or allergic reactions to any medications, especially to this drug or to any other diuretics.

• Your child has or ever had kidney disease, kidney stones, urination problems, hyperkalemia, diabetes mellitus, liver disease, acidosis, or gout.

• Your child is taking quinidine (an antiarrhythmia heart medication). This drug may interfere with the laboratory determination of your child's blood quinidine concentration.

• Your child has any illness that causes severe or continuous nausea, vomiting, or diarrhea, as this drug can cause severe water loss (dehydration).

• Your daughter is or becomes pregnant. This drug crosses the placenta, and its safety in human pregnancy has not been thoroughly investigated. However, effects have been reported in the fetuses of animals that received large doses of this drug during pregnancy.

• Your daughter is breast-feeding her baby. Small amounts of this drug pass into breast milk.

Special Instructions

• Do not give your child any nonprescription medications for weight control or for allergy, asthma, cough, cold, or sinus problems unless you first check with the doctor. Some of these products can lead to an increase in blood pressure.

• This drug can cause increased sensitivity to sunlight. Your child should avoid prolonged exposure to sunlight and sunlamps and wear an effective sunscreen and protective clothing when out-of-doors.

Symptoms of Overdose: Severe
dehydration, loss of consciousness, convulsions due to excessive loss of electrolytes

Special Notes

• This drug does not cure high blood pressure, but it will help to control the condition as long as your child continues to take it.

• This drug may cause the urine to turn bluish; this is a harmless side effect.

• This drug can cause hyperkalemia (high blood concentrations of potassium). Signs of hyperkalemia include palpitations; confusion; numbness or tingling in the hands, feet, or lips; anxiety; or unusual fatigue or weakness. To avoid this problem, do not alter your child's diet, and do not use salt substitutes unless the doctor tells you to do so.

• The doctor may schedule regular office visits to monitor your child's progress and adjust the dosage if necessary.

TRIFLUOPERAZINE

Administration Guidelines
- Give with food or a full glass of water or milk to decrease stomach upset.

- Dilute concentrate in juice, milk, water, soup, pudding, or carbonated beverage before giving it.

- Do not spill liquid or injection on skin or clothing. These forms can cause a skin rash.

- Missed doses: Give as soon as you remember, then give any remaining doses for that day at regularly spaced intervals. Do not give double doses.

- Do not give within 2 hours of giving antacids or medicine for diarrhea.

- Give only as directed by your child's doctor.

- Do not stop giving this drug without first checking with the doctor. The doctor may want to gradually reduce the dose first.

Side Effects
Tell your child's doctor about any side effects that are persistent or particularly bothersome.

More Common. Constipation, decreased sweating, dizziness, drowsiness, dry mouth, stuffy nose, low blood pressure, stomach upset, nausea, vomiting, weight gain, blurred vision, difficulty urinating, changes in menstrual period. Contact the doctor immediately if your child experiences lip smacking or puckering, puffing of cheeks, rapid or fine wormlike tongue movements, uncontrolled chewing movements, uncontrolled arm or leg movements, blurred vision, change in color perception, difficulty seeing at night, difficulty in speaking or swallowing, fainting, inability to move the eyes, loss of balance, masklike face, muscle spasms, restlessness or the need to keep moving, shuffling walk, stiffness of arms or legs, twitching movements, trembling and shaking, twisting movements of body or weakness of arms and legs, skin rash, or severe sunburn.

Less Common. Contact the doctor immediately if your child experiences seizures, difficult or fast breathing, fast or irregular heartbeat, fever, high or low blood pressure, increased sweating, loss of bladder control, severe muscle stiffness, pale skin, or unusual fatigue or weakness.

Possible Drug Interactions
- Central nervous system depressants such as alcohol, antihistamines, cold preparations, muscle relaxants, tranquilizers, and some

Brand Name: Stelazine

Generic Available: Yes

Type of Drug: Antipsychotic agent, phenothiazine, antiemetic

Use: Treats nervous, mental, emotional, and behavioral disorders such as psychoses or mania. Also treats severe nausea and vomiting.

Time Required for Drug to Take Effect: It may take 6 weeks to 6 months to achieve full benefit for mental and emotional disorders. Onset within 1 hour for nausea and vomiting.

Dosage Forms and Strengths: Tablets (1 mg, 2 mg, 5 mg, 10 mg); Concentrate (10 mg/mL); Injection (2 mg/mL)

Storage: Store at room temperature in tightly closed, light-resistant containers. Do not freeze the concentrate or injection.

How This Drug Works: Causes complex changes in the central nervous system, producing tranquilizing effects.

pain medications may cause extreme drowsiness when used with this drug.

- Cough and cold products may increase the chance of heat stroke, dizziness, dry mouth, blurred vision, and constipation.

- Antidepressants, monoamine oxidase (MAO) inhibitors, and lithium lead to an increase in side effects. These medications need to be dosed carefully when used together.

- Medications that lower blood pressure may lead to blood pressure that is too low when given with this drug.

- Antithyroid drugs lead to an increase in rare blood disorders when given with this drug.

- Epinephrine may cause low blood pressure.

Tell Your Doctor If
- Your child has had an allergic reaction to this drug or any other medication.

- Your child has taken or is taking any other prescription or nonprescription medicine.

- Your child abuses alcohol or has lung or heart disease, seizures, glaucoma, liver or kidney disease, difficulty urinating, stomach ulcers, bone marrow or blood disorders, Reye syndrome, or any other medical condition.

- The blurred vision continues beyond the first few weeks or gets worse.

- Your child develops a new medical problem.

- Your child develops a rash from the sun.

- Your child continues to have a dry mouth after 2 weeks. Continued dry mouth can lead to cavities.

- Your child develops side effects after the drug has been stopped.

- Your daughter is or becomes pregnant.

- Your daughter is breast-feeding her baby. This drug can pass into breast milk, and the American Academy of Pediatrics is concerned

about the effect of similar medications on the baby.

Special Instructions
- Protect your child from overheating during exercise, play, or hot weather as this drug decreases sweating and can cause an increase in body temperature. Hot baths, hot tubs, or saunas may make your child dizzy or faint.

- Dress your child warmly as this drug increases sensitivity to cold weather.

- Your child should avoid exposure to sunlight and sunlamps. This drug may cause a skin rash or severe sunburn with exposure to direct sunlight or ultraviolet (UV) light. Make sure your child wears an effective sunscreen when out-of-doors. Your child may also need to wear sunglasses that block UV light.

- Do not give any other medication before talking to the pharmacist or doctor.

- Do not let your child have surgery or any medical treatment or dental work unless the doctor or dentist is aware that your child is taking this drug.

- Do not allow your child to drink alcohol while taking this drug.

- Do not give other medicines that may make your child sleepy.

- Do not give cough or cold products without first checking with the doctor.

- Have your child stand up slowly after sitting or lying down to prevent dizziness or light-headedness.

Symptoms of Overdose: Deep sleep, coma, low blood pressure, increased severity of side effects listed above

Special Notes
- Make sure you know how your child is reacting to this drug before allowing participation in activities that require alertness and coordination, such as riding a bicycle. This drug may

cause your child to have blurred vision, dizziness, drowsiness, or to be less alert.

- This drug may cause serious side effects that may not go away after it is stopped. Discuss this with the doctor.

- Doses are increased slowly to decrease side effects.

- The effects of this drug may last for up to a week after you stop giving it.

- Doses for children younger than 6 years of age have not been established.

- The liquid may turn a light yellow color; this is not cause for concern.

- Your child's progress should be checked regularly by the doctor.

Outdated Doses

Safe and proper medication disposal is essential, especially when you have children in the house. Do not keep medication—whether prescription or nonprescription—past the expiration date, even if it appears normal. Expired medication may be ineffective and can even be dangerous. Make a habit of regularly checking the expiration date on all medicines in your home. Flush leftover medication down the toilet or pour it down the sink. Rinse the container before throwing it out. If your medication does not display an expiration date, throw it out after one year.

Brand Names: Arrestin, Tebamide, T-Gen, Tigan, Triban, Trimethobenzamide (various manufacturers)

Generic Available: Yes

Type of Drug: Antiemetic (antinauseant)

Use: Controls nausea and vomiting.

Time Required for Drug to Take Effect: 10 to 40 minutes

Dosage Forms and Strength: Capsules (100 mg, 250 mg); Suppositories (100 mg, 200 mg)

Storage: Store at room temperature in tightly closed containers.

How This Drug Works: Acts directly on the vomiting center in the brain.

TRIMETHOBENZAMIDE

Administration Guidelines

• Give capsules with a full glass of water.

• Usually given 2 to 4 times a day as needed.

• Your child should try to avoid having a bowel movement for 1 hour or longer after you insert the suppository. This will allow enough time for the drug to be absorbed.

• Missed doses: Give as soon as possible. However, if it's within a couple hours of the next dose, skip the missed dose. Do not give double doses.

Side Effects

Tell your child's doctor about any side effects that are persistent or particularly bothersome.

More Common. Diarrhea, dizziness, drowsiness, headache, or muscle cramps

Less Common. Tell the doctor if your child experiences back pain, blurred vision, convulsions, depression, disorientation, mouth sores, rash, tremors, unusual bleeding or bruising, unusual hand or face movements, or yellowing of the eyes or skin.

Possible Drug Interactions

• Central nervous system depressants can cause extreme drowsiness when used with this drug.

Tell Your Child's Doctor If

• Your child is allergic to this drug, benzocaine, or other local anesthetics if you are using the suppository form.

• Your child has acute fever, dehydration, electrolyte imbalance, intestinal infection, or viral infection.

• Your daughter is or becomes pregnant.

Special Instructions

• Your child should avoid participating in activities that require alertness.

• Do not give for acute vomiting; it may mask vomiting due to Reye syndrome.

• Do not give to premature infants or neonates.

Symptoms of Overdose: Severe drowsiness, muscle cramps, increased nausea

TRIMIPRAMINE

Administration Guidelines

• May be given with water or food to decrease the chance of stomach irritation, unless your child's doctor tells you to do otherwise.

• Give exactly as prescribed.

• Missed doses: Give as soon as possible, then return to the regular dosing schedule. However, if you miss a once-a-day bedtime dose, do not give that dose in the morning; check with your doctor instead. If the dose is given in the morning, it may cause unwanted side effects. Do not give double doses.

• Do not stop giving this drug suddenly. Stopping it abruptly can cause nausea, headache, stomach upset, fatigue, or a worsening of the condition.

Side Effects

Tell your child's doctor about any side effects that are persistent or particularly bothersome.

More Common. Agitation, anxiety, blurred vision, confusion, constipation, cramps, diarrhea, dizziness, drowsiness, dry mouth, fatigue, heartburn, insomnia, loss of appetite, nausea, peculiar tastes in the mouth, restlessness, sweating, vomiting, weakness, or weight gain or loss. As your child's body adjusts to this drug, these side effects should disappear.

Less Common. It is especially important to tell the doctor if your child experiences chest pain, convulsions, difficulty in urinating, enlarged or painful breasts (in both sexes), fainting, fever, hair loss, hallucinations, headaches, impotence, mood changes, mouth sores, nervousness, nightmares, numbness or tingling in the fingers or toes, palpitations, rapid weight gain or loss (3 to 5 pounds within a week), ringing in the ears, seizures, skin rash, sleep disorders, sore throat, tremors, uncoordinated movements or balance problems, unusual bleeding or bruising, or yellowing of the eyes or skin.

Possible Drug Interactions

• Central nervous system depressants including alcohol, antihistamines, barbiturates, benzodiazepine tranquilizers, muscle relaxants, narcotics, pain medications, phenothiazine tranquilizers, and sleeping medications, or other tricyclic antidepressants can cause extreme drowsiness when used with this drug.

• May decrease the effectiveness of antiseizure medications.

Brand Name: Surmontil

Generic Available: Yes

Type of Drug: Tricyclic antidepressant

Use: Relieves the symptoms of mental depression.

Time Required for Drug to Take Effect: The effects may not become apparent for at least 2 or 3 weeks.

Dosage Form and Strength: Capsules (25 mg, 50 mg, 100 mg)

Storage: Store at room temperature in a tightly closed container.

How This Drug Works: Thought to relieve depression by increasing the concentration of certain chemicals necessary for nerve transmission in the brain.

- May block the blood-pressure-lowering effects of clonidine and guanethidine.

- Oral contraceptives (birth control pills) and estrogen-containing drugs can increase the side effects and reduce the effectiveness of this drug.

- May increase the side effects of thyroid medication and over-the-counter (nonprescription) cough, cold, allergy, asthma, sinus, and diet medications.

- Monoamine oxidase (MAO) inhibitors may cause fever, convulsions, or high blood pressure when used with this drug. At least 14 days should separate the use of this drug and the use of a MAO inhibitor.

Tell Your Child's Doctor If

- Your child is taking any prescription or nonprescription medications.

- Your child has had unusual or allergic reactions to any medications, especially to this drug or other tricyclic antidepressants (such as amitriptyline, imipramine, doxepin, amoxapine, protriptyline, desipramine, maprotiline, and nortriptyline).

- Your child has a history of asthma, high blood pressure, liver or kidney disease, heart disease, heart attack, circulatory disease, stomach problems, intestinal problems, alcoholism, difficulty in urinating, enlarged prostate gland, epilepsy, glaucoma, thyroid disease, or mental illness, or has ever received electroshock therapy.

- Your child is taking this drug before having surgery or any other medical or dental treatment.

- Your daughter is or becomes pregnant.

- Your daughter is breast-feeding her baby. Small amounts of this drug can pass into breast milk and may cause unwanted effects, such as irritability or sleeping problems, in nursing infants.

Special Instructions

- This drug may cause increased sensitivity to sunlight. Your child should avoid prolonged exposure to sunlight and sunlamps and wear an effective sunscreen, protective clothing, and sunglasses when out-of-doors.

- The effects of this drug may last as long as 7 days after your child has stopped taking it, so continue to observe all precautions during that period.

Symptoms of Overdose: Severe breathing problems, confusion, delirium and, in some cases, seizures

TRIPROLIDINE

Administration Guidelines
• Usually given as needed up to 4 times a day.

• May be given with food if upset stomach occurs.

Side Effects
Tell your child's doctor about any side effects that are persistent or particularly bothersome.

More Common. Drowsiness, dizziness, upset stomach

Less Common. Excitation, increased sensitivity to sunlight, confusion, nervousness, nausea, vomiting, diarrhea, difficulty sleeping. Contact the doctor if your child experiences difficulty urinating, difficulty breathing, worsening allergy symptoms, palpitations, fainting, hallucinations, yellowing of eyes or skin, unusual bleeding or bruising.

Possible Drug Interactions
• Other sedative agents such as alcohol, barbiturate tranquilizers (such as phenobarbital), phenothiazine-type drugs (Thorazine, Compazine, Phenergan, and others), and other antihistamines (such as Benadryl) will increase this drug's sedative effects.

• Monoamine oxidase (MAO) inhibitors (such as Nardil or Parnate) may increase the anti-cholinergic side effects (fast heartbeat, flushing of the skin, constipation, dry eyes and mouth, blurred vision, fever) of this drug.

Tell Your Child's Doctor If
• Your child has had allergic reactions to any medications.

• Your child has any other diseases.

• You child is taking any other medications.

• Your child has heart, liver, or kidney disease or urinary problems.

• Your daughter is or becomes pregnant. It is not known if this drug affects the fetus.

• Your daughter is breast-feeding her baby. This drug can pass into breast milk; however, the American Academy of Pediatrics considers it compatible with breast-feeding in most cases.

Symptoms of Overdose:
Sedation or excitability, unconsciousness, convulsions, palpitations, drunken appearance

Special Notes
• This drug is frequently used in combination with the decongestant pseudoephedrine (Actifed and others).

Brand Name: Actidil

Generic Available: Yes

Type of Drug: Antihistamine

Use: Treats common allergy symptoms (runny nose, sneezing, watery eyes). Relieves some cold symptoms (runny nose).

Time Required for Drug to Take Effect: 1 to 2 hours

Dosage Forms and Strengths: Tablets (2.5 mg); Syrup (1.25 mg/5 mL)

Storage: Store at room temperature in tightly closed, light-resistant containers.

How This Drug Works: Blocks the effects of histamine, a substance in the body that causes allergic symptoms.

Brand Names: Depakene, Depakote, Myproic Acid

Generic Available: Yes

Type of Drug: Anticonvulsant

Use: Treats convulsions or seizures.

Time Required for Drug to Take Effect: It may take about 1 week to achieve complete effectiveness.

Dosage Forms and Strengths: Capsules (250 mg); Capsules, sprinkle (125 mg); Tablets, enteric-coated (125 mg, 250 mg, 500 mg); Syrup (250 mg per 5 mL)

Storage: Store at room temperature in tightly closed, light-resistant containers.

How This Drug Works: Increases concentrations of the chemical gamma amino-butyric acid in the brain.

VALPROIC ACID

Administration Guidelines

• Give with food or milk to avoid stomach upset.

• Capsules or enteric-coated tablets should be swallowed whole.

• Syrup may be mixed with fluid or food to improve the taste.

• Open sprinkle capsules and place the contents on a teaspoonful of applesauce or pudding. The mixture should be swallowed immediately, not chewed.

• Give at evenly spaced intervals around the clock to maintain a constant concentration of this drug in your child's bloodstream. If this drug is to be given 4 times a day, space the doses 6 hours apart.

• Missed doses: Give as soon as you remember, then stagger subsequent doses evenly for the rest of the day. Do not give double doses. Contact the doctor if you miss giving 2 or more doses.

• Do not suddenly stop giving this drug. Abruptly stopping it could cause seizures.

Side Effects

Tell your child's doctor about any side effects that are persistent or particularly bothersome.

More Common. Mild stomach cramps, change in menstrual periods, diarrhea, hair loss, loss of appetite, nausea, trembling of hands and arms, unusual weight gain or loss

Less Common. Clumsiness, unsteadiness, constipation, dizziness, drowsiness, headache, skin rash, unusual excitement, restlessness, irritability. Contact the doctor immediately if your child experiences severe stomach cramps, behavioral changes, uncontrolled back and forth or rolling eye movements, double vision, increase in seizures, spots in front of the eyes, swelling of the face, unusual fatigue or weakness, unusual bleeding or bruising, yellow eyes or skin, or severe vomiting.

Possible Drug Interactions

• Other central nervous system depressants such as alcohol, antihistamines, muscle relaxants, pain medications, tranquilizers, sleeping medications, or antidepressants can cause extreme drowsiness.

Tell Your Child's Doctor If

• Your child is taking any other medications.

• Your child has any diseases.

• Your child has had allergic reactions to any medications.

- Your daughter is or becomes pregnant.

- Your daughter is breast-feeding her baby. This drug can pass into breast milk; however, the American Academy of Pediatrics considers it compatible with breast-feeding in most cases.

Special Instructions
- Before your child has surgery or any medical or dental treatment, tell the doctor performing the treatment that your child is taking this drug.

Symptoms of Overdose: Severe
dizziness or clumsiness, severe drowsiness, blurred or double vision, seizures or abnormal twitching, severe vomiting, abnormal eye movements, staggered walk, slurred speech

Special Notes
- This drug can interfere with urine tests for ketones. Check with the doctor before adjusting insulin doses.

Keep a Lid on It

Pharmacists are required to put drugs in bottles that have child-resistant caps. Don't switch to a bottle that's easier for you to open—children may also find it easier to open. Remember, too, that child-resistant does not mean childproof. Children older than five years of age may be able to open most medicine bottles. That's why it's essential for you to teach them that drugs can be harmful if not taken correctly and that children need supervision before taking anything. And, just to be on the safe side, keep all medicines out of your child's

Brand Names: Calan, Calan SR, Isoptin, Isoptin SR, Verelan

Generic Available: Yes

Type of Drug: Calcium channel blocker

Use: Treats high blood pressure (hypertension), chest pain (angina), and abnormally fast heart rhythms (tachycardia). Has also been used to prevent migraine headaches.

Time Required for Drug to Take Effect: Within a few minutes for injection; several days to several weeks for full effect when given orally.

Dosage Forms and Strengths: Tablets (40 mg, 80 mg, 120 mg); Tablets, sustained-release (120 mg, 180 mg, 240 mg); Capsules, sustained-release (120 mg, 180 mg, 240 mg); Injection (5 mg/2 mL)

Storage: Store at room temperature in tightly closed, light-resistant containers.

How This Drug Works: Limits electrical impulses that stimulate the heart to beat.

VERAPAMIL

Administration Guidelines

- Usually given 3 times a day. Sustained-release forms are generally given 1 or 2 times a day. Try to give at the same time(s) each day.

- May be given on an empty stomach or with meals, but be consistent.

- Missed doses: Give as soon as possible and space out the remaining doses equally over the rest of the day. Do not give additional doses within 4 hours.

- Do not stop giving this drug abruptly without speaking with the doctor.

Side Effects

Tell your child's doctor about any side effects that are persistent or particularly bothersome.

More Common. Dizziness, light-headedness, headache, nausea, constipation, sweating. Contact the doctor if your child experiences swelling of feet or ankles or difficulty breathing.

Less Common. Difficulty sleeping, weakness, confusion, dry mouth, difficulty urinating, irregular menstrual periods, muscle cramps. Contact the doctor if your child experiences palpitations, fainting, unusual bleeding or bruising, yellowing of the eyes or skin, or skin rashes.

Possible Drug Interactions

- Barbiturate drugs such as phenobarbital, phenytoin (Dilantin), rifampin, and large amounts of calcium supplements or vitamin D supplements can decrease the effects of this drug.

- Dantrolene (Dantrium) can increase serum potassium and make congestive heart failure worse when used with this drug.

- Quinidine or cimetidine (Tagamet) can increase the effects of this drug.

- Beta blockers (Inderal and others) can make congestive heart failure worse when used with this drug.

- Can increase blood levels of carbamazepine (Tegretol), cyclosporine, digoxin, prazosin (Minipress), and theophylline, requiring dosage adjustment of these medications and increased risk of toxicity.

- Alcohol can cause an excessive drop in blood pressure.

Tell Your Child's Doctor If

• Your child has had allergic reactions to any medications.

• Your child has any other diseases.

• Your child is taking any other medications.

• Your child has liver, kidney, or heart disease.

• Your daughter is or becomes pregnant. This drug has caused birth defects in animal studies.

• Your daughter is breast-feeding her baby. This drug can pass into breast milk; however, the American Academy of Pediatrics considers it compatible with breast-feeding in most cases.

Symptoms of Overdose: Nausea, weakness, dizziness, drowsiness, confusion, drunken appearance, palpitations, fainting, excessively low heart rate and blood pressure

Teach Your Children Well

Let's face it. Kids can be pretty stubborn when it comes to accepting medication. When appropriate, try giving your child information about his or her condition and how the medicine works. In a nonthreatening voice, talk about the consequences of not taking the medication, perhaps reminding the child of how uncomfortable he or she was before beginning the medication. Use reasoning when possible, but don't scare the child. Children who understand the importance of antibiotics for infection, insulin for diabetes, or inhalants for asthma are more likely to take the medication without objection.

Brand Names: Triple-Vita-Flor, Tri-Vi-Flor, Tri-Vitamin with Fluoride Drops, Vi-Daylin/F ADC Drops

Generic Available: Yes

Type of Drug: Multivitamin, fluoride supplement

Use: Protects against tooth decay and vitamin deficiencies.

Dosage Forms and Strengths: Tablets, chewable (2,500 IU vitamin A, 400 IU vitamin D, 60 mg vitamin C, and 1 mg fluoride); Drops (1,500 IU vitamin A, 400 IU vitamin D, 35 mg vitamin C, and 0.25 mg or 0.5 mg fluoride)

Storage: Store tablets at room temperature in tightly closed, light-resistant containers. Store drops at room temperature in the original plastic container (glass containers interact with and destroy the fluoride in the solution). Do not refrigerate or freeze.

How This Drug Works: Provides partial, and in some cases complete, levels of the recommended dietary allowances of vitamins A, D, and C necessary for good nutrition. Fluoride strengthens teeth and helps prevent tooth decay.

VITAMINS A, D, & C WITH FLUORIDE

Administration Guidelines

• Tablets should be chewed or crushed before swallowing.

• Give tablets at bedtime after teeth have been brushed for maximum protection.

• Your child should not eat anything for at least 15 minutes after chewing the tablets to allow the fluoride to work on the teeth.

• Drops can be given directly from the bottle or mixed with juice or foods. Measure the dose carefully with the dropper provided.

• Do not give with milk or dairy products as they prevent the absorption of fluoride from the gastrointestinal tract.

• Missed doses: Give as soon as possible within the same day. Do not give double doses.

Side Effects

Tell your child's doctor about any side effects that are persistent or particularly bothersome.

More Common. This drug seldom causes side effects, but can occasionally cause constipation, diarrhea, drowsiness, fatigue, loss of appetite, nausea, vomiting, or weakness. These side effects should disappear as your child's body adjusts to this drug.

Less Common. It is especially important to tell the doctor if your child experiences bloody or black, tarry stools; difficulty in swallowing; discoloration of the teeth; excessive drooling; excitation; mouth sores; rash; stomach cramps; or tremors.

Possible Drug Interactions

• This product should not interact with other medications if it is used according to directions.

Tell Your Child's Doctor If

• Your child has had unusual or allergic reactions to vitamins, fluoride, or any medications.

• Your child has or ever had heart, kidney, or thyroid disease.

Special Instructions

• Do not use the chewable tablets if the fluoride content of your drinking water is 0.7 parts per million or more.

• Do not give the drops to children younger than 3 years of age in areas where the fluoride content of the drinking water is 0.3 parts per million or more. If you are unsure of the fluoride content of your drinking water, ask the doctor or call the county health department.

• Do not refer to this drug as "candy" or "candy-flavored vitamins." Your child may take you literally and swallow too many.

Symptoms of Overdose: Fluoride
overdose may cause mottling (varying shades of color) of tooth enamel. Manifestations of toxicity depend on the child's age, dosage, and the duration of administration.

Special Notes
• A slight darkening in the color of the drops does not indicate that the vitamins or fluoride have lost potency; the drops still can be used safely.

• Vitamins with fluoride often are prescribed for infants who are not being given any fluoridated water. Once your infant is given fluoridated water consistently, ask the doctor if you should continue giving this drug.

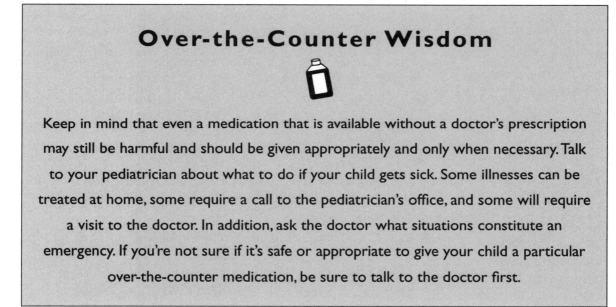

Over-the-Counter Wisdom

Keep in mind that even a medication that is available without a doctor's prescription may still be harmful and should be given appropriately and only when necessary. Talk to your pediatrician about what to do if your child gets sick. Some illnesses can be treated at home, some require a call to the pediatrician's office, and some will require a visit to the doctor. In addition, ask the doctor what situations constitute an emergency. If you're not sure if it's safe or appropriate to give your child a particular over-the-counter medication, be sure to talk to the doctor first.

Brand Names: Florvite, Multi-Vita Drops with Fluoride, Poly-Vi-Flor, Polyvitamin with Fluoride Drops, Polyvite with Fluoride Drops, Vi-Daylin/F

Generic Available: Yes

Type of Drug: Multivitamin, fluoride supplement

Use: Protects against tooth decay and vitamin deficiencies in children.

Dosage Forms and Strengths: Tablets, chewable tablets, and drops are all available in a variety of strengths.

Storage: Store all tablets at room temperature in tightly closed, light-resistant containers. Store drops at room temperature in the original plastic container (glass containers interact with and destroy the fluoride in the solution). Do not refrigerate or freeze.

How This Drug Works: Provides partial, and in some cases complete, levels of the recommended dietary allowances of the vitamins necessary for good nutrition. Fluoride strengthens teeth and helps prevent tooth decay.

VITAMINS, MULTIPLE WITH FLUORIDE

Administration Guidelines

• Chewable tablets should either be chewed or crushed before swallowing.

• Give tablets at bedtime after the teeth have been brushed for maximum protection. Your child should eat nothing for at least 15 minutes after chewing the tablets to allow the fluoride to work on the teeth.

• Give drops directly from the bottle or mix them with juice or food. Measure the dose carefully with the dropper provided.

• Do not give with milk or dairy products as they prevent the absorption of fluoride from the gastrointestinal tract.

• Missed doses: Give as soon as possible within the same day. Do not give double doses.

Side Effects

Tell your child's doctor about any side effects that are persistent or particularly bothersome.

More Common. This product occasionally causes constipation, diarrhea, drowsiness, fatigue, loss of appetite, nausea, vomiting, or weakness. These side effects should disappear as your child's body adjusts to this drug.

Less Common. It is especially important to tell the doctor if your child experiences bloody or black, tarry stools; difficulty in swallowing; discoloration of the teeth; excessive drooling; excitation; mouth sores; rash; stomach cramps; or tremors.

Possible Drug Interactions

• This product should not interact with other medications if it is used according to directions.

Tell Your Child's Doctor If

• Your child has had unusual or allergic reactions to vitamins, fluoride, or any medications.

• Your child has or ever had bone, heart, kidney, or thyroid disease.

Symptoms of Overdose: The manifestations of vitamin toxicity depend on the child's age, the dosage, and the duration of administration. Fluoride may cause mottling (various shades of color) of tooth enamel.

Special Notes

• These products contain vitamins A, D, E, C, B$_6$, B$_{12}$, folic acid, riboflavin, niacin, fluoride, and thiamine.

• A slight darkening in the color of the drops does not indicate that the vitamins or fluoride have lost potency; the drops can still be used safely.

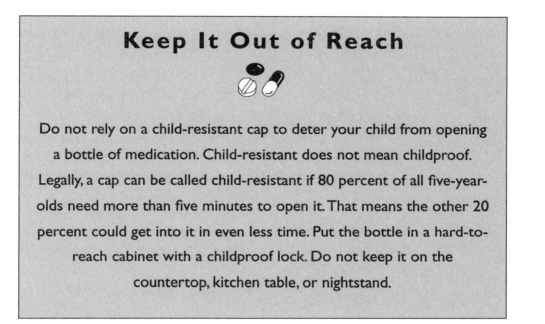

Keep It Out of Reach

Do not rely on a child-resistant cap to deter your child from opening a bottle of medication. Child-resistant does not mean childproof. Legally, a cap can be called child-resistant if 80 percent of all five-year-olds need more than five minutes to open it. That means the other 20 percent could get into it in even less time. Put the bottle in a hard-to-reach cabinet with a childproof lock. Do not keep it on the countertop, kitchen table, or nightstand.

Brand Names: Coumadin, Panwarfin, Sofarin

Generic Available: Yes

Type of Drug: Anticoagulant (blood thinner)

Use: Prevents the formation of blood clots in persons with previous blood clots in the legs or lungs, and those with artificial heart valves.

Time Required for Drug to Take Effect: Several days

Dosage Form and Strengths: Tablets (1 mg, 2 mg, 2.5 mg, 5 mg, 7.5 mg, 10 mg)

Storage: Store at room temperature in tightly closed, light-resistant containers.

How This Drug Works: Slows production of clotting compounds by the liver.

WARFARIN

Administration Guidelines

• Usually given once a day. Try to give it at the same time each day.

• Give exactly as prescribed. It is common to give different doses on alternate days.

• Missed doses: Give as soon as possible. However, if it's within 8 hours of the next dose, skip the missed dose and give the next regular dose. Do not give double doses.

Side Effects

Tell your child's doctor about any side effects that are persistent or particularly bothersome.

More Common. Bleeding episodes, which may be severe. Contact the doctor if your child experiences unusual bleeding or bruising; dark, tarry stools; bloody stools; nosebleeds; red/orange urine; or if your child coughs up blood.

Less Common. Upset stomach, diarrhea. Contact the doctor if your child experiences changes in skin color, skin rash, fever, chills, sore throat, severe headache, chest pain, stomach pain, or difficulty breathing.

Possible Drug Interactions

• This drug interacts with many medications. Do not give your child any additional prescription, nonprescription, or vitamin products without first checking with the doctor or pharmacist. Do not, however, stop giving any medication your child is currently taking without first checking with the doctor or pharmacist.

• Alcohol or salicylate-type drugs (such as aspirin) can increase the risk of bleeding when taken with this drug.

Tell Your Child's Doctor If

• Your child has had allergic reactions to any medications.

• Your child has any other diseases.

• Your child is taking any other medications.

• Your daughter is or becomes pregnant. This drug can cause severe birth defects and should not be given to pregnant women.

• Your daughter is breast-feeding her baby. This drug can pass into breast milk; however the American Academy of Pediatrics considers it compatible with breast-feeding in most cases.

Special Instructions

• Ask the pharmacist always to dispense the same brand of this drug. Switching brands may require additional dosage adjustment and increase the risk of bleeding or loss of effect.

Symptoms of Overdose: Severe bleeding or bruising

Special Notes

• It is important to maintain a consistent diet while taking this drug. Vitamin K, found in green leafy vegetables and other foods, decreases the effectiveness of this drug but it can't (and shouldn't) be eliminated from the diet. A steady amount of Vitamin K in the diet makes adjusting doses of this drug much easier.

• Your child should avoid contact sports such as football and hockey.

• Dosing may require frequent adjustment at first but will eventually stabilize.

• Your child will require regular blood tests to measure blood clotting times. These are referred to as prothrombin times (PT) or INR.

Be Accurate

If you don't give medication correctly, it may be ineffective or even cause side effects. An estimated 10 to 30 percent of medications aren't effective because they have been given incorrectly. To do it right, you have to give the exact amount of medicine prescribed at the scheduled time, for the specified duration, and in the appropriate manner. Always read the label, follow the directions carefully, and use the appropriate equipment for measuring and administering the medication. Also, be sure to wash your hands before you give any medication to your child.

Brand Name: Hivid

Generic Available: No

Type of Drug: Antiviral, antiretroviral

Use: Treats infections from human immunodeficiency virus (HIV), the virus that causes acquired immunodeficiency syndrome (AIDS).

Time Required for Drug to Take Effect: Must be given indefinitely.

Dosage Form and Strengths: Tablets (0.375 mg and 0.75 mg)

Storage: Store at room temperature in tightly closed, light-resistant containers.

How This Drug Works: Inhibits the growth of HIV.

ZALCITABINE (DIDEOXYCYTIDINE, ddC)

Administration Guidelines

- Give only on an empty stomach.

- Usually given 3 times a day. Try to space the doses about 8 hours apart.

- Do not give more than the prescribed dose.

- Do not stop giving this drug without first speaking with your child's doctor.

- Missed doses: Give as soon as possible. Space the remaining doses for that day at regular intervals. Do not give double doses.

Side Effects

Tell your child's doctor about any side effects that are persistent or particularly bothersome.

More Common. Diarrhea, mouth sores, headache, difficulty swallowing, cough, runny nose, rash, itching, fever, fatigue. Contact the doctor if your child experiences numbness or burning sensations in the hands or feet, skin rash, or yellowing of the eyes or skin.

Less Common. Liver damage, nausea, vomiting, constipation, low blood sugar, joint pain, muscle weakness, dizziness, confusion, night sweats, hair loss, anemia, flulike symptoms. Contact the doctor if your child experiences symptoms of pancreatitis (nausea, vomiting, stomach pain) or swelling of the feet or legs.

Possible Drug Interactions

- Antacids will decrease the absorption of this drug from the gastrointestinal tract if given at the same time.

- Cimetidine (Tagamet) may decrease the metabolism of this drug, which will increase blood levels and the risk of toxic effects.

- Didanosine (ddI) increases the risk of nerve damage when used in combination with this drug.

Tell Your Child's Doctor If

- Your child has had allergic reactions to any medications.

- Your child has any other diseases.

- Your child is taking any other medications.

- Your child has liver or kidney disease or any type of nerve damage.

- Your daughter is or becomes pregnant. This drug has caused birth defects in animal tests.

• Your daughter is breast-feeding her baby. It is not known if this drug passes into breast milk. Mothers with HIV infections are generally advised not to breast-feed.

Symptoms of Overdose: Drowsiness, vomiting

Special Notes
• This drug does not cure AIDS or prevent transmission of HIV.

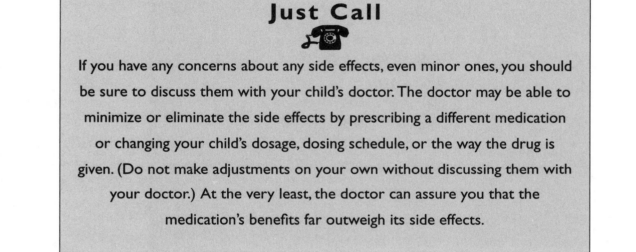

Just Call

If you have any concerns about any side effects, even minor ones, you should be sure to discuss them with your child's doctor. The doctor may be able to minimize or eliminate the side effects by prescribing a different medication or changing your child's dosage, dosing schedule, or the way the drug is given. (Do not make adjustments on your own without discussing them with your doctor.) At the very least, the doctor can assure you that the medication's benefits far outweigh its side effects.

Brand Name: Retrovir

Generic Available: No

Type of Drug: Antiviral, antiretroviral

Use: Treats infections caused by human immunodeficiency virus (HIV), which is the virus that causes acquired immunodeficiency syndrome (AIDS). Zidovudine doesn't cure HIV infections or AIDS but may slow progression of the infection.

Time Required for Drug to Take Effect: Several weeks to months

Dosage Forms and Strengths: Capsules (100 mg); Syrup (50 mg/5 mL); Injection (10 mg/mL)

Storage: Store at room temperature in tightly closed, light-resistant containers.

How This Drug Works: Slows the growth of human immunodeficiency virus.

ZIDOVUDINE (AZT, AZIDOTHYMIDINE)

Administration Guidelines
• Usually given 4 or 5 times daily. Try to give at the same times each day.

• Do not exceed prescribed dosage.

• Do not stop giving this drug without speaking with your child's doctor. This drug must be given indefinitely when treating HIV infection.

• Missed doses: Give as soon as possible and space the remaining doses for the day at equal intervals.

Side Effects
Tell your child's doctor about any side effects that are persistent or particularly bothersome.

More Common. Anemia, headache, fever, dizziness, difficulty sleeping, nausea, diarrhea, vomiting, upset stomach, muscle aches. Contact the doctor if your child experiences stomach pain, severe nausea or vomiting, or skin rash.

Less Common. Acne, changes in skin color, constipation, nervousness, difficulty urinating. Contact the doctor if your child experiences difficulty breathing; swelling of face, eyes, or lips; convulsions; or yellowing of the eyes or skin.

Possible Drug Interactions
• Proper treatment of HIV infection and complications of AIDS may require the use of this drug in combination with the following interacting drugs. Adjustment of dosage may limit the development of side effects.

• Acetaminophen, rifampin, or phenytoin may decrease the effectiveness of this drug.

• Fluconazole or trimethoprim may necessitate lowering the dosage of this drug.

• Ganciclovir or interferon can further decrease blood counts.

• Acyclovir can cause fatigue and lethargy when used in combination with this drug.

Tell Your Child's Doctor If
• Your child has had allergic reactions to any medications.

• Your child has any other diseases.

• Your child is taking any other medications.

- Your child has liver or kidney disease.

- Your daughter is or becomes pregnant. It is unknown whether this drug causes birth defects.

- Your daughter is breast-feeding her baby. It is unknown whether this drug passes into breast milk.

Symptoms of Overdose: Nausea, vomiting, headache, dizziness, drowsiness

Special Notes
- This drug does not cure AIDS or prevent its transmission.

- Your child will periodically require blood counts while taking this drug.

- This drug is frequently used in combination with other antiviral drugs.

Measuring Up

Remember: Never use an ordinary tableware teaspoon to measure liquid doses. Instead, use a cylindrical dosing spoon, dosage cup, dropper, or syringe. These measuring devices can be found at your local drug store and sometimes at supermarkets, toy stores, and department stores.

Brand Names: Component of DTP, DTaP, Acel-Imune, Tripedia, Tir-Immunol, DT, DTwP

Generic Available: No

Use: Immunizes against diphtheria

Time Required for Vaccine to Take Effect: 2 to 4 weeks after immunization

Dosage Form: Injection

How This Vaccine Works: Causes your child's body to produce its own protection (antibodies) against diphtheria.

DIPHTHERIA TOXOID VACCINE

Administration Guidelines

• Only given by or under the supervision of your child's doctor or another authorized health care professional.

• Give acetaminophen 45 minutes before vaccination and every 4 hours for 24 hours following vaccination to help prevent pain and fever.

• Usually given when your baby is 2, 4, and 6 months of age and as a booster at 12 to 15 months of age and at 4 to 6 years of age.

• Given as a component of DTP (diphtheria, tetanus, pertussis) for vaccination at 2, 4, and 6 months of age.

• Given as a component of a DTaP (acellular) booster when your child is 12 to 15 months of age and at 4 to 6 years of age.

• Usually given into a muscle.

Side Effects

Tell your child's doctor about any side effects that are persistent or particularly bothersome.

More Common. Fever of up to 102°F, ongoing crying for 3 hours or more, unusual high-pitched cry, irritability, loss of appetite, redness and/or tenderness at site of injection, fatigue

Less Common. Tell the doctor if your child experiences fever higher than 102°F; difficulty breathing or swallowing; hives; itching; swelling of eyes, face, or inside of nose; reddening of skin (especially around ears); diarrhea; hard lump, swelling, or warm feeling at site of injection; skin rash; or vomiting.

Possible Drug Interactions

• Immunosuppressants may decrease the effectiveness of the immunization.

Tell Your Child's Doctor If

• Your child has had an allergic reaction to DTP, DTaP, pertussis, or any other vaccine.

• Your child has a severe illness.

• Your child has ever had a seizure.

• Your child is allergic to preservatives such as thimersol.

• Your child has any serious medical problem.

HAEMOPHILUS b (Hib) VACCINE

Administration Guidelines

• Only given by or under the supervision of your child's doctor or another authorized health care professional.

• Give acetaminophen 45 minutes before vaccination and every 4 hours for 24 hours following vaccination to help prevent pain and fever.

• Usually given when your baby is 2, 4, and 6 months of age and as a booster at 12 to 15 months of age.

• Usually given into a muscle.

Side Effects

Tell your child's doctor about any side effects that are persistent or particularly bothersome.

More Common. Fever up to 102°F, irritability, loss of appetite, redness and/or tenderness at site of injection, fatigue

Less Common. Tell the doctor if your child experiences fever over 102°F; difficulty breathing or swallowing; hives; itching; swelling of eyes, face, or inside of nose; reddening of skin (especially around ears); diarrhea; hard lump; swelling or warm feeling at the site of injection; skin rash; or vomiting.

Tell Your Child's Doctor If

• Your child is treated for a severe infection during the 2 weeks after the vaccination is given.

• Your child has had an allergic reaction to this vaccine or any other vaccine.

• Your child has allergies to any preservatives.

Brand Names: ProHIBit, HibTITER, PedvaxHIB, Act-Hib

Generic Available: No

Use: Immunizes against *Haemophilus influenzae* type b

Time Required for Vaccine to Take Effect: 2 to 4 weeks after immunization

Dosage Form: Injection

How This Vaccine Works: Causes your child's body to produce its own protection (antibodies) against the disease.

Brand Name: Engerix-B, Recombivax HB, Recombivax HB Dialysis

Generic Available: No

Use: Immunizes against hepatitis B infection

Time Required for Vaccine to Take Effect: 2 to 4 weeks after immunization

Dosage Form: Injection

How This Vaccine Works: Causes your child's body to produce its own protection (antibodies) against the disease.

HEPATITIS B VACCINE

Administration Guidelines
• Only given by or under the supervision of your child's doctor or another authorized health care professional.

• Give acetaminophen 45 minutes before vaccination and every 4 hours for 24 hours following vaccination to help prevent pain and fever.

• The first dose is usually given at birth; the second dose between 1 and 4 months of age; and the third dose between 6 and 18 months of age.

• Usually given into a muscle.

Side Effects
Tell your child's doctor about any side effects that are persistent or particularly bothersome.

More Common. Fever up to 102°F, ongoing crying for 3 hours or more, unusual high-pitched cry, irritability, loss of appetite, redness and/or tenderness at the site of injection, fatigue

Less Common. Tell the doctor if your child experiences fever higher than 102°F; difficulty breathing or swallowing; hives; itching; swelling of eyes, face, or inside of nose; reddening of skin (especially around ears); diarrhea; hard lump, swelling, or warm feeling at the site of injection; skin rash; or vomiting.

Tell Your Child's Doctor If
• Your child has had an allergic reaction to hepatitis B vaccine or any other vaccine.

• Your child has a severe illness.

• Your child has lung or heart disease.

• Your child has an immune deficiency condition.

Special Notes
• Recommended for all adolescents who have not previously received 3 doses. The first dose can be given at 11 to 12 years of age, the second dose 1 month later, and the third dose at least 4 months after the first dose.

INFLUENZA VIRUS VACCINE

Administration Guidelines

• Only given by or under the supervision of your child's doctor or another authorized health care professional.

• Give acetaminophen 45 minutes before vaccination and every 4 hours for 24 hours following vaccination to help prevent pain and fever.

• Usually given to children older than 6 months of age.

• Usually given once a year in early October.

• Usually given into a muscle.

Side Effects

Tell your child's doctor about any side effects that are persistent or particularly bothersome.

More Common. Fever up to 102°F, ongoing crying for 3 hours or more, irritability, loss of appetite, redness and/or tenderness at the site of injection, fatigue

Less Common. Tell the doctor if your child experiences fever higher than 102°F; difficulty breathing or swallowing; hives; itching; swelling of eyes, face, or inside of nose; reddening of skin (especially around ears); diarrhea; hard lump, swelling, or warm feeling at the site of injection; skin rash; or vomiting.

Tell Your Child's Doctor If

• Your child has had an anaphylactic reaction to eggs.

• Your child has had an allergic reaction to this vaccine or any other vaccine.

• Your child has had an allergic reaction to gentamicin, streptomycin, or other aminoglycosides.

• Your child has had an anaphylactic reaction to preservatives, especially thimerosal.

• Your child was ever paralyzed by Guillain-Barré syndrome.

• Your child has moderate to severe illness.

• Your child has a sulfite sensitivity

• Your daughter is or becomes pregnant.

Special Notes

• This vaccine contains a killed virus so your child cannot get influenza from it.

Brand Names: Fluogen, FluShield, Fluzone

Generic Available: No

Use: Immunizes against influenza

Time Required for Vaccine to Take Effect: 1 to 2 weeks after immunization

Dosage Form: Injection

How This Vaccine Works: Causes your child's body to produce its own protection (antibodies) against the disease.

Brand Name: Attenuvax, also component of MMR (Measles Mumps Rubella)

Generic Available: No

Use: Immunizes against measles

Time Required for Vaccine to Take Effect: 2 to 4 weeks after immunization

Dosage Form: Injection

How This Vaccine Works: Causes the body to produce its own protection (antibodies) against the disease.

MEASLES VACCINE

Administration Guidelines
- Only given by or under the supervision of your child's doctor or another authorized health care professional.

- Give acetaminophen 45 minutes before vaccination and every 4 hours for 24 hours following vaccination to help prevent pain and fever.

- Usually given at 12 to 18 months of age and again as a booster at 4 to 6 months of age or at 11 to 12 years of age, depending on state school immunization requirements.

- Usually given as an injection under the skin.

Side Effects
Tell your child's doctor about any side effects that are persistent or particularly bothersome.

More Common. The following side effects may not occur for 1 to 3 weeks after this vaccine has been given: Fever up to 102°F, ongoing crying for 3 hours or more, unusual high-pitched cry, irritability, loss of appetite, purple color or redness at the site of injection, tenderness at site of injection, fatigue

Less Common. Tell the doctor if your child experiences fever higher than 102°F; difficulty breathing or swallowing; hives; itching; swelling of eyes, face, or inside of nose; reddening of skin (especially around ears); diarrhea; hard lump, swelling, or warmth at the site of injection; skin rash; or vomiting.

Possible Drug Interactions
- Immunosuppressants, immune globulins, or interferon may decrease the effectiveness of this vaccine.

Tell Your Child's Doctor If
- Your child has had an allergic reaction to measles vaccine, MMR, or any other vaccine.

- Your child has a severe illness.

- Your child has ever had a seizure or a brain or head injury.

- Your child is receiving cancer medications or treatment with X rays.

- Your child has an immune deficiency.

- Your child receives any other live vaccine within 1 month of receiving this vaccine.

- Your child has a blood transfusion or receives gamma globulins or other globulins within 2 weeks after receiving this vaccine.

MUMPS VACCINE

Administration Guidelines
• Only given by or under the supervision of your child's doctor or another authorized health care professional.

• Give acetaminophen 45 minutes before vaccination and every 4 hours for 24 hours following vaccination to help prevent pain and fever.

• Usually given at 12 to 18 months of age and again as a booster at 4 to 6 or 11 to 12 years of age, depending on state school immunization requirements.

• Usually given as an injection under the skin

Side Effects
Tell your child's doctor about any side effects that are persistent or particularly bothersome.

More Common. The following side effects may not occur for 1 to 3 weeks after this vaccine has been given: Fever up to 102°F, ongoing crying for 3 hours or more, unusual high-pitched cry, irritability, loss of appetite, redness and/or tenderness at the site of injection, fatigue.

Less Common. Tell the doctor if your child experiences fever higher than 102°F; difficulty breathing or swallowing; hives; itching; swelling of eyes, face, or inside of nose; reddening of skin (especially around ears); diarrhea; hard lump, swelling, or warmth at the site of injection; skin rash; or vomiting.

Possible Drug Interactions
• X-ray treatment or cancer drugs may decrease the effectiveness of this vaccine.

• Immunosuppressants, immune globulins, or interferon may decrease the effectiveness of this vaccine.

Tell Your Child's Doctor If
• Your child is allergic to eggs or has had an allergic reaction to MMR, Mumpsvax, or any other vaccine.

• Your child has a severe illness.

• Your child has ever had a seizure.

• Your child receives any other live vaccine within 1 month of receiving this vaccine.

• Your child has a blood transfusion or receives gamma globulins or other globulins within 2 weeks after receiving this vaccine.

Brand Name: Mumpsvax, also component of MMR (Measles Mumps Rubella)

Generic Available: No

Use: Immunizes against mumps

Time Required for Vaccine to Take Effect: 2 to 4 weeks after immunization

Dosage Form: Injection

How This Vaccine Works: Causes the body to produce its own protection (antibodies) against the disease.

Brand Names: Component of DTP, DTaP, Acel-Imune, Tripedia, Tir-Immunol

Generic Available: No

Use: Immunizes against pertussis

Time Required for Vaccine to Take Effect: 2 to 4 weeks after immunization

Dosage Form: Injection

How This Vaccine Works: Causes the body to produce its own protection (antibodies) against the disease.

PERTUSSIS VACCINE

Administration Guidelines
• Only given by or under the supervision of your child's doctor or another authorized health care professional.

• Give acetaminophen 45 minutes before vaccination and every 4 hours for 24 hours following vaccination to help prevent pain and fever.

• Usually given at 2, 4, 6, and 12 to 15 months of age; a booster dose is usually given at 4 to 6 years of age.

• Usually given into a muscle.

Side Effects
Tell your child's doctor about any side effects that are persistent or particularly bothersome.

More Common. Fever up to 102°F, ongoing crying for 3 hours or more, unusual high-pitched cry, irritability, loss of appetite, redness and/or tenderness at the site of injection, fatigue

Less Common. Tell the doctor if your child experiences fever higher than 102°F; difficulty breathing or swallowing; hives; itching; swelling of eyes, face, or inside of nose; reddening of skin (especially around ears); diarrhea; hard lump, swelling, or warmth at the site of injection; skin rash; or vomiting.

Tell Your Child's Doctor If
• Your child has had an allergic reaction to DTP, DTaP, pertussis, or any other vaccine.

• Your child has a severe illness.

• Your child has ever had a seizure.

• Your child has an allergy to preservatives.

PNEUMOCOCCAL VACCINE

Administration Guidelines

- Only given by or under the supervision of your child's doctor or another authorized health care professional.

- Give acetaminophen 45 minutes before vaccination and every 4 hours for 24 hours following vaccination to help prevent pain and fever.

- Usually given to children 2 years of age and older as a one-time vaccination.

- Usually given under the skin or into a muscle.

- Usually given only to children who are at high risk for pneumococcal infection such as those with chronic illness, human immunodeficiency virus (HIV), sickle-cell anemia, or those who are waiting for an organ transplant or who have had their spleen removed.

Side Effects

Tell your child's doctor about any side effects that are persistent or particularly bothersome.

More Common. Fever up to 102°F, ongoing crying for 3 hours or more, unusual high-pitched cry, irritability, loss of appetite, redness and/or tenderness at the site of injection, fatigue

Less Common. Tell the doctor if your child experiences fever higher than 102°F; difficulty breathing or swallowing; hives; itching; swelling of eyes, face, or inside of nose; reddening of skin (especially around ears); diarrhea; hard lump, swelling, or warmth at the site of injection; skin rash; or vomiting

Tell Your Child's Doctor If

- Your child has had an allergic reaction to this vaccine or any other vaccine.

- Your child has a severe illness.

- Your child has thrombocytopenic purpura or any blood disorder.

- Your child is allergic to any preservatives, especially thimerosal.

Brand Names: Pneumovax, Pnu-Imune

Generic Available: No

Use: Immunizes against pneumococcal bacterial infection

Time Required for Vaccine to Take Effect: 2 to 4 weeks after immunization

Dosage Form: Injection

How This Vaccine Works: Causes the body to produce its own protection (antibodies) against the disease.

Brand Names: Orimune, OPOL, Poliovax, IPV, OPV

Generic Available: No

Use: Immunizes against polio

Time Required for Vaccine to Take Effect: 2 to 4 weeks after immunization

Dosage Forms: Injection, Suspension

How This Vaccine Works: Causes the body to produce its own protection (antibodies) against the disease.

POLIO VACCINE

Administration Guidelines

• Only given by or under the supervision of your child's doctor or another authorized health care professional.

• Give acetaminophen 45 minutes before immunization and every 4 hours for 24 hours following vaccination to help prevent pain and fever.

• Usually given at 2, 4, and 15 to 18 months of age and again at 4 to 6 years of age as a booster (the booster is optional).

• Given either orally or into a muscle.

• The suspension may be given on a sugar cube for ease of administration.

Side Effects

Tell your doctor about any side effects that are persistent or particularly bothersome.

More Common. The following side effects may not occur for 1 to 3 weeks after this vaccine has been given: Fever up to 102°F, ongoing crying for 3 hours or more, unusual high-pitched cry, irritability, loss of appetite, redness and/or tenderness at the site of injection, fatigue.

Less Common. Tell the doctor if your child experiences fever higher than 102°F; difficulty breathing or swallowing; hives; itching; swelling of eyes, face, or inside of nose; reddening of skin (especially around ears); diarrhea; hard lump, swelling, or warmth at the site of injection; skin rash; or vomiting.

Possible Drug Interactions

• Immunosuppressants, including corticosteroids or radiation therapy, decrease the effectiveness of this vaccine.

Tell Your Child's Doctor If

• Your child has had an allergic reaction to this vaccine or any other vaccine.

• Your child has a severe illness.

• Your child is allergic to neomycin, streptomycin, or polymixin B.

• Your child has any major health problems.

• Your family has a history of immune deficiency.

RESPIRATORY SYNCYTIAL VIRUS (RSV) IMMUNE GLOBULIN VACCINE

Administration Guidelines
• Only administered in a doctor's office or clinic under the direct supervision of a physician.

• Must be given once a month for 5 months during RSV season (usually November to April).

Side Effects
Tell your child's doctor about any side effects that are persistent or particularly bothersome.

More Common. Dizziness, flushing, abdominal cramps, blood pressure changes

Less Common. Chest pain, skin rash, shortness of breath

Possible Drug Interactions
• If your child has received a live virus vaccine (such as measles, mumps, or rubella) within 10 months of a RSV-IVIG infusion, the child may need to be reimmunized. Consult the doctor.

Brand Name: RespiGam

Generic Available: No

Type of Drug: Immune Globulin

Use: Prevents serious lower respiratory tract infection caused by Respiratory Syncytial Virus (RSV) in patients younger than 24 months of age, with bronchopulmonary dysplasia (BPD) or a history of premature birth.

Time Required for Vaccine to Take Effect: 30 days

Dosage Form and Strength: Injection (2500 mg)

How This Vaccine Works: Increases levels of neutralizing antibody to RSV.

Brand Names: Meruvax II, Fluvirin, also component of MMR (Measles Mumps Rubella)

Generic Available: No

Use: Immunizes against rubella

Time Required for Vaccine to Take Effect: 2 to 4 weeks after immunization

Dosage Form: Injection

How This Vaccine Works: Causes the body to produce its own protection (antibodies) against the disease.

RUBELLA VACCINE
Administration Guidelines
• Only given by or under the supervision of your child's doctor or another authorized health care professional.

• Give acetaminophen 45 minutes before vaccination and every 4 hours for 24 hours after vaccination to help prevent pain and fever.

• Usually given at 12 to 18 months of age and again as a booster at 4 to 6 or 11 to 12 years of age, depending on state school immunization requirements.

• Usually given as an injection under the skin.

Side Effects
Tell your child's doctor about any side effects that are persistent or particularly bothersome.

More Common. The following side effects may not occur for 1 to 3 weeks after this vaccine has been given: Fever of up to 102°F, ongoing crying for 3 hours or more, unusual high-pitched cry, irritability, loss of appetite, redness and/or tenderness at the site of injection, fatigue.

Less Common. Tell the doctor if your child experiences fever higher than 102°F; difficulty breathing or swallowing; hives; itching; swelling of eyes, face, or inside of nose; reddening of the skin (especially around ears); diarrhea; hard lump, swelling, or warmth at the site of injection; skin rash; or vomiting.

Possible Drug Interactions
• Immunosuppressants, immune globulins, or interferon may decrease the effectiveness of this vaccine.

Tell Your Child's Doctor If
• Your child has had an allergic reaction to MMR or any other vaccine.

• Your child has a severe illness.

• Your child has ever had a seizure.

• Your child is receiving cancer medications or treatment with X rays.

• Your child has an immune deficiency.

• Your child has or had a brain or head injury.

• Your child receives any other live vaccine within 1 month of receiving this vaccine.

• Your child has a blood transfusion or receives gamma globulins or other globulins within 2 weeks after receiving this vaccine.

TETANUS TOXOID VACCINE

Administration Guidelines

- Only given by or under the supervision of your child's doctor or another authorized health care professional.

- Give acetaminophen 45 minutes before vaccination and every 4 hours for 24 hours following vaccination to help prevent pain and fever.

- Usually given at 2, 4, 6, and 12 to 15 months of age, and again at 4 to 6 years of age as part of the DTP (diphtheria, tetanus, pertussis) vaccine; then as a booster between ages 11 and 12 and again every 5 to 10 years.

- The single tetanus vaccine is only administered to those 7 years of age and older.

- Usually given into a muscle

Side Effects

Tell your child's doctor about any side effects that are persistent or particularly bothersome.

More Common. Fever up to 102°F, irritability, loss of appetite, redness and/or tenderness at the site of injection, fatigue, hard lump at site of injection

Less Common. Tell the doctor if your child experiences fever higher than 102°F; difficulty breathing or swallowing; hives; itching; swelling of eyes, face, or inside of nose; reddening of skin (especially around ears); diarrhea; swelling, or warmth at the site of injection; skin rash; or vomiting.

Possible Drug Interactions

- Immunosuppressants may decrease the effectiveness of this vaccine.

Tell Your Child's Doctor If

- Your child has had an allergic reaction to this vaccine or any other vaccine.

- Your child has severe illness.

- Your child is allergic to preservatives, especially thimerosal.

- Your child has any serious illness involving lungs or bronchial tubes.

- Your daughter is or becomes pregnant.

Brand Names: Tetanus Toxoid Adsorbed (various manufacturers)

Generic Available: No

Use: Immunizes against tetanus

Time Required for Vaccine to Take Effect: 2 to 4 weeks after immunization

Dosage Form: Injection

How This Vaccine Works: Causes the body to produce its own protection (antibodies) against the disease.

Brand Name: Varivax

Generic Available: No

Use: Immunizes against chicken pox

Time Required for Vaccine to Take Effect: 4 to 6 weeks after immunization

Dosage Form: Injection

How This Vaccine Works: Causes the body to produce its own protection (antibodies) against the disease.

VARICELLA ZOSTER VACCINE

Administration Guidelines
• Only given by or under the supervision of your child's doctor or another authorized health care professional.

• Give acetaminophen 45 minutes before vaccination and every 4 hours for 24 hours following vaccination to help prevent pain and fever.

• Usually given at 12 to 18 months of age or at 13 years of age for children not vaccinated previously and who lack a reliable history of chicken pox.

• Children younger than 13 years of age should receive a single dose.

• Children older than 13 years of age should receive 2 doses 4 to 8 weeks apart.

Side Effects
Tell your child's doctor about any side effects that are persistent or particularly bothersome.

More Common. Fever up to 102°F, irritability, loss of appetite, redness and/or tenderness at the site of injection, fatigue

Less Common. Varicellalike rash. Tell the doctor if your child experiences fever higher than 102°F; difficulty breathing or swallowing; hives; itching; swelling of eyes, face, or inside of nose; reddening of skin (especially around ears); diarrhea; hard lump, swelling, or warmth at the site of injection; skin rash; or vomiting.

Tell Your Child's Doctor If
• Your child has had an allergic reaction to this vaccine or any other vaccine.

• Your child has a hypersensitivity to gelatin or a history of anaphylactoid reaction to neomycin.

• Your child has blood dyscrasias, leukemia, lymphoma, or malignant neoplasm.

• Your child has had a blood or plasma transfusion

Special Instructions
• Avoid salicylate (aspirin) use for 6 weeks after vaccination.

Canadian Brand Name Index

The following list contains the generic names of drugs included in *Children's Prescription Drugs* and the brand names under which they are sold in Canada. When the Canadian brand name and the American brand name is the same, it is listed in parentheses. Drugs for which no Canadian brand name could be found are excluded from this list.

acetaminophen	Atasol, Campain, (Panadol), (Tempra)	cefaclor	(Ceclor)
		cefadroxil	(Duricef)
acetazolamide	(Diamox)	cefixime	(Suprax)
acyclovir	(Zovirax)	cephalexin	Ceporex, (Keflex), Novo-lexin, Apo-Cephalex, Nu-Cephalex
albuterol	Novosalmol, (Ventolin)		
amantadine	(Symmetrel)		
amitriptyline	Amiline, Deprex, (Elavil), Levate, Meravil, Norotriptyn	chloral hydrate	Chloralex, Chloralvan, (Noctec), Novochlorhydrate
		chloramphenicol (systemic)	(AK-Chlor), (Chlormycetin), (Chloroptic)
amoxicillin	Amoxican, (Amoxil), Amoxi, Moxilean, Novamoxin, Penamox		
		chlorpheniramine	Chlorphen, Chlor-Tripolon
amoxicillin and clavulanic acid	Clavulin	chlorpromazine	Chlorprom, Chlorpromanyl, Largactil, Novochlorpromazine
ampicillin	(Amcill), Ampicin, Apo-Ampi, (Penbritin)		
aspirin	Acetophen, Asadrine C-200, Astrin, Coryphen	cimetidine	(Tagamet), Novocimetine, Peptol
astemizole	(Hismanal)	cisapride	Prepulsid
atenolol	(Tenormin)	clindamycin (systemic and topical)	Dalacin C, Dalacin T
attapulgite	(Kaopectate)		
azathioprine	(Imuran)	clonazepam	Rivotril
bacitracin	(Baciguent), Bacitin	clonidine	(Catapres), Dixarit
baclofen	(Lioresal)	clotrimazole (topical)	Canesten, Myclo
beclomethasone dipropionate	Beclodisk, (Beclovent)	codeine	Paveral
		cromolyn sodium (inhalation, nasal)	Fivent, (Intal), Nalcrom, Rynacrom
bisacodyl	Bisacolax, (Dulcolax)		
brompheniramine	(Dimetane)	cyclosporine	(Sandimmune)
budesonide	Pulmicort, (Rhinocort)	cyproheptadine	(Periactin), Vimicon
captopril	(Capoten)	dapsone	Avlosulfon
carbamazepine	Mazepine, (Tegretol)	desipramine	(Norpramine), Pertofrane
cascara sagrada	Fibyrax, (Glysennid)		

dexamethasone (systemic)	AK-Dex, (Decadron), Deronil, (Hexadrol)
dextroamphetamine	(Dexedrine)
dextromethorphan	Deca-Toux, (Delsym)
diazepam	Diazemuls, D-Tran, E-Pam, Meval, Neo-Calme, Novodipam
dicloxacillin	(Dynapen)
didanosine	(Videnx)
digoxin	(Lanoxin)
diltiazem	(Cardizem)
dimenhydrinate	(Dramamine), Gravol, Nauseatol
diphenhydramine	(Allerdryl), (Benadryl), (Benylin), Insomnal, Somnium
dipivefrin	Propine
docusate sodium	(Colace), (Docusate Sodium)
doxepin	(Sinequan), Triadapin
doxycycline	(Vibramycin)
droperidol	(Inapsine)
erythromycin	
Estolate:	(Ilosone), Novorythro
EES:	Apo-Erythro-ES, (EES)
Stearate:	Apo-Erythro-S, (Erythrocin), Novorythro
erythromycin and sulfisoxazole combination	(Pediazole)
ethambutol	Etibi, (Myambutol)
fluconazole	(Diflucan)
flunisolide (nasal)	Bronalide, Rhinalar
furosemide	Furoside, (Lasix), Neo-Renal, Novosemide, Uritol
griseofulvin	Fulvicin, Grisaltin, Grisovin-FP
guaifenesin	Balminil Expectorant, Broncho-Grippex
haloperidol	(Haldol), Novoperidol, Peridol
hydrochlorothiazide	Apo-Hydro, Diuchlor-H, Esidrex, Hydro-Aquil, (Diuril)
hydrocodone	Biohisdex DHC , Novahistex DH
hydrocortisone (systemic)	(Solu-cortef)
hydroxyzine	(Atarax), Multipax
ibuprofen	Amersol, (Motrin), Novoprofen
imipramine	Impril, Novopramine, (Tofranil)
indomethacin	(Indocid), Novomethacin
insulin	(Humulin), (Iletin), Initard, Insulatard
ipratropium bromide	(Atrovent)
isoniazid	Isotamine, Rimifon
isotretinoin	(Accutane)
ketoconazole	(Nizoral)
ketoprofen	(Orudis)
labetalol	(Trandate)
lactulose	Acilac, (Cephulac)
levothyroxine	Eltroxin, (Synthroid)
lindane	GBH, Kwellada
lithium	Carbolith, Duralith, (Lithane), Lithizine
loperamide	(Imodium)
loratadine	(Claritin)
lorazepam	(Ativan), Novolorazem
mebendazole	(Vermox)
medroxyprogesterone	(Depo-Provera), (Provera)
meperidine	(Demerol), Demer-Idine
mesalamine	Asacol, Salofalk
metaproterenol	(Alupent)
methenamine	(Mandelamine), Methandine
methylphenidate	Methidate, (Ritalin)
methylprednisolone (systemic)	(Depo-Medrol), (Medrol), (Sieropresol)

metoclopramide	Emex, Maxeran, (Reglan)
metolazone	(Zaroxolyn)
metoprolol	Betaloc, (Lopressor), Novometoprol
metronidazole	(Flagyl), Neo-Metric, Neo-Tric
Milk of Magnesia	(Phillips' Milk of Magnesia), Phillips' Magnesia Tablets
minocycline	(Minocin), Ultramycin
morphine	Epimorph, Morphitec, MOS, (Roxanol)
naproxen	(Anaprox), (Naprosyn), Naxen, Novonaprox
nedocromil sodium	(Tilacle)
neomycin (topical)	Myciguent
nifedipine	(Adalat)
nitrofurantoin	Furatine, (Macrodantin), Nephronex
nortriptyline	(Aventyl)
nystatin	(Mycostatin), Nadostine, (Nilstat)
omeprazole	Losec
ondansetron	(Zofran)
oxybutynin	(Ditropan)
oxycodone	Supeudol
oxymetazoline	Drixoral Nasal Spray, Nafrine
pancrelipase	Cotazym, (Pancrease)
pemoline	(Cylert)
penicillamine	(Cuprimine), (Depen)
penicillin VK	Apo-Pen-VK, (Ledercillin VK), Nadopen-V, Novopen-VK
permethrin	(Nix)
phenobarbital	Gardenal, Nova-Pheno
phenylephrine	AK-Dilafe, (Mydrifin)
phenylpropanolamine	Coldecon
phenytoin	Dantoin, (Dilantin)

prednisolone (systemic)	AK-Tate, Inflamase, (Pred-Forte)
prednisone (systemic)	Colisone, (Deltasone), Paracort
primidone	(Mysoline), Sertan
procainamide	(Procan SR), (Pronestyl)
prochlorperazine	Stemetil
promethazine	Histantil, (Phenergan)
propranolol	Detensol, (Inderal), Novopranol
propylthiouracil	Propyl-Thyracil
pseudoephedrine	Eltor, Pseudofrin, Robidrine, (Sudafed)
psyllium	(Citrucel), Normacol
pyrazinamide	Tebrazid
pyrethrin	R& II Spray, R&C Shampoo, Scabene
pyrimethamine	(Daraprim)
ranitidine	(Zantac)
rifampin	(Rifadin), (Rimactane)
simethicone	(Phazyme), Simecon
sodium bicarbonate	Normogastryl
sodium phosphate (phosphosoda)	Citro-carbonate, pHos-pHaid
sodium sulfacetamide (ophthalmic)	(AK-Sulf), (Bleph-10), Sulfex
sucralfate	Sulcrate
sulfadiazine silver	Flamazine
sulfamethoxazole and trimethoprim	Apo-Sulfatrim, (Bactrim), Protrin
sulfasalazine	Salazopyrin, (SAS)
terbutaline	(Bricanyl)
terfenadine	(Seldane)
tetracycline	(Achromycin), (Achromycin V), Apo-Tetra
theophylline	Asthmophylline, Elixophylline, (Respid), (Somophyllin)
thiabendazole	(Mintezol)

thiethylperazine	(Torecan)
thioridazine	(Mellaril), Thioril
thiothixene	(Navane)
thyroid hormone	(Thyroid)
tobramycin (ophthalmic)	(Tobrex)
tolmetin	(Tolectin)
trazodone	(Desyrel)
triamterene	(Dyrenium)
trifluoperazine	Clinazine, Novoflurazine, Pentazine
trimethobenzamide	(Tigan)
trimipramine	Surmontil
triprolidine	(Actidil)
valproic acid	(Depakene)
verapamil	(Isoptin)
warfarin	Athrombin-K, (Coumadin)
zidovudine (AZT)	Retrovir

INDEX